Biological and Hormonal Therapies of Cancer

Cancer Treatment and Research
Steven T. Rosen, M.D., *Series Editor*

Surwit EA, Alberts DS (eds): Endometrial Cancer. 1989. ISBN 0-7923-0286-9.
Champlin R (ed): Bone Marrow Transplantation. 1990. ISBN 0-7923-0612-0.
Goldenberg D (ed): Cancer Imaging with Radiolabeled Antibodies. 1990. ISBN 0-7923-0631-7.
Jacobs C (ed): Carcinomas of the Head and Neck. 1990. ISBN 0-7923-0668-6.
Lippman ME, Dickson R (eds): Regulatory Mechanisms in Breast Cancer: Advances in Cellular and Molecular Biology of Breast Cancer. 1990. ISBN 0-7923-0868-9.
Nathanson L (ed): Malignant Melanoma: Genetics, Growth Factors, Metastases, and Antigens. 1991. ISBN 0-7923-0895-6.
Sugarbaker PH (ed): Management of Gastric Cancer. 1991. ISBN 0-7923-1102-7.
Pinedo HM, Verweij J, Suit HD (eds): Soft Tissue Sarcomas: New Developments in the Multidisciplinary Approach to Treatment. 1991. ISBN 0-7923-1139-6.
Ozols RF (ed): Molecular and Clinical Advances in Anticancer Drug Resistance. 1991. ISBN 0-7923-1212-0.
Muggia FM (ed): New Drugs, Concepts and Results in Cancer Chemotherapy. 1991. ISBN 0-7923-1253-8.
Dickson RB, Lippman ME (eds): Genes, Oncogenes and Hormones: Advances in Cellular and Molecular Biology of Breast Cancer. 1992. ISBN 0-7923-1748-3.
Humphrey G, Bennett, Schraffordt Koops H, Molenaar WM, Postma A (eds): Osteosarcoma in Adolescents and Young Adults: New Developments and Controversies. 1993. ISBN 0-7923-1905-2.
Benz CC, Liu ET (eds): Oncogenes and Tumor Suppressor Genes in Human Malignancies. 1993. ISBN 0-7923-1960-5.
Freireich EJ, Kantarjian H (eds): Leukemia: Advances in Research and Treatment. 1993. ISBN 0-7923-1967-2.
Dana BW (ed): Malignant Lymphomas, Including Hodgkin's Disease: Diagnosis, Management, and Special Problems. 1993. ISBN 0-7923-2171-5.
Nathanson L (ed): Current Research and Clinical Management of Melanoma. 1993. ISBN 0-7923-2152-9.
Verweij J, Pinedo HM, Suit HD (eds): Multidisciplinary Treatment of Soft Tissue Sarcomas. 1993. ISBN 0-7923-2183-9.
Rosen ST, Kuzel TM (eds): Immunoconjugate Therapy of Hematologic Malignancies. 1993. ISBN 0-7923-2270-3.
Sugarbaker PH (ed): Hepatobiliary Cancer. 1994. ISBN 0-7923-2501-X.
Rothenberg ML (ed): Gynecologic Oncology: Controversies and New Developments. 1994. ISBN 0-7923-2634-2.
Dickson RB, Lippman ME (eds): Mammary Tumorigenesis and Malignant Progression. 1994. ISBN 0-7923-2647-4.
Hansen HH (ed): Lung Cancer. Advances in Basic and Clinical Research. 1994. ISBN 0-7923-2835-3.
Goldstein LJ, Ozols RF (eds): Anticancer Drug Resistance. Advances in Molecular and Clinical Research. 1994. ISBN 0-7923-2836-1.
Hong WK, Weber RS (eds): Head and Neck Cancer. Basic and Clinical Aspects. 1994. ISBN 0-7923-3015-3.
Thall PF (ed): Recent Advances in Clinical Trial Design and Analysis. 1995. ISBN 0-7923-3235-0.
Buckner CD (ed): Technical and Biological Components of Marrow Transplantation. 1995. ISBN 0-7923-3394-2.
Winter JN (ed): Blood Stem Cell Transplantation. 1997. ISBN 0-7923-4260-7.
Muggia FM (ed): Concepts, Mechanisms, and New Targets for Chemotherapy. 1995. ISBN 0-7923-3525-2.
Klastersky J (ed): Infectious Complications of Cancer. 1995. ISBN 0-7923-3598-8.
Kurzrock R, Talpaz M (eds): Cytokines: Interleukins and Their Receptors. 1995. ISBN 0-7923-3636-4.
Sugarbaker P (ed): Peritoneal Carcinomatosis: Drugs and Diseases. 1995. ISBN 0-7923-3726-3.
Sugarbaker P (ed): Peritoneal Carcinomatosis: Principles of Management. 1995. ISBN 0-7923-3727-1.
Dickson RB, Lippman ME (eds): Mammary Tumor Cell Cycle, Differentiation and Metastasis. 1995. ISBN 0-7923-3905-3.
Freireich EJ, Kantarjian H (eds): Molecular Genetics and Therapy of Leukemia. 1995. ISBN 0-7923-3912-6.
Cabanillas F, Rodriguez MA (eds): Advances in Lymphoma Research 1996. ISBN 0-7923-3929-0.
Miller AB (ed): Advances in Cancer Screening. 1996. ISBN 0-7923-4019-1.
Hait WN (ed): Drug Resistance. 1996. ISBN 0-7923-4022-1.
Pienta KJ (ed): Diagnosis and Treatment of Genitourinary Malignancies. 1996. 0-7923-4164-3.
Arnold AJ (ed): Endocrine Neoplasms. 1997. 0-7923-4354-9.
Pollock RE (ed): Surgical Oncology. 1997. 0-7923-9900-5.
Verweij J, Pinedo HM, Suit HD (eds): Soft Tissue Sarcomas: Present Achievements and Future Prospects. 1997. ISBN 0-7923-9913-7.

Biological and Hormonal Therapies of Cancer

edited by

Kenneth A. Foon, M.D.
Lucille Parker Markey Cancer Center
University of Kentucky
Lexington, Kentucky

Hyman B. Muss, M.D.
University of Vermont, College of Medicine
Vermont Cancer Center
Burlington, Vermont

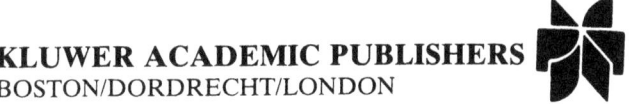

KLUWER ACADEMIC PUBLISHERS
BOSTON/DORDRECHT/LONDON

Distributors for North America:
Kluwer Academic Publishers
101 Philip Drive
Assinippi Park
Norwell, Massachusetts 02061 USA

Distributors for all other countries:
Kluwer Academic Publishers Group
Distribution Centre
Post Office Box 322
3300 AH Dordrecht, THE NETHERLANDS

Library of Congress Cataloging-in-Publication Data
Biological and hormonal therapies of cancer/edited by
Kenneth A.
  Foon, Hyman B. Muss.
    p. cm. — (Cancer treatment and research; v. 94)
  Includes bibliographical references and index.
  ISBN 0-7923-9997-8 (alk. paper)
    1. Cancer–Hormone therapy.   2. Cancer–Chemoprevention.
  3. Biological response modifiers.   I. Foon, Kenneth A.   II. Muss,
Hyman B.   III. Series.
    [DNLM: 1. Neoplasms–drug therapy.   2. Antineoplastic
Agents-therapeutic use.   W1 CA693 v. 94 1998/QZ 267 B6149 1998]
RC271.H55B54 1998
616.99'406 — dc21
DNLM/DLC
for Library of Congress   97-28807
                                                                            CIP

Copyright © 1998 by Kluwer Academic Publishers

All rights reserved. No part of this publication may be reproduced, stored in a retrieval system or transmitted in any form or by any means, mechanical, photocopying, recording, or otherwise, without the prior written permission of the publisher, Kluwer Academic Publishers, 101 Philip Drive, Assinippi Park, Norwell, Massachusetts 02061

Printed on acid-free paper.

PRINTED IN THE UNITED STATES OF AMERICA

Contents

Preface		xi
1.	Interferon therapy of hematologic malignancies KENNETH A. FOON	1
2.	Interferon Use in Solid Tumors WILLIAM J. JOHN and KENNETH A. FOON	23
3.	Cellular vaccine therapies for cancer MICHAEL J. MASTRANGELO, TAKAMI SATO, EDMUND C. LATTIME, HENRY C. MAGUIRE JR. and DAVID BERD	35
4.	Anti-idiotype antibody vaccine therapies of cancer MALAYA BHATTACHARYA-CHATTERJEE and KENNETH A. FOON	51
5.	Endocrine therapy of prostate cancer RICK L. BARE and FRANK M. TORTI	69
6.	Endocrine therapy of endometrial cancer SAMUEL S. LENTZ	89
7.	Phytochemicals for the prevention of breast and endometrial cancer J. MARK CLINE and CLAUDE L. HUGHES, JR.	107
8.	Hormonal strategies for the prevention of breast cancer MARK R. OLSEN and RICHARD R. LOVE	135

9. Ovarian ablation as adjuvant therapy for early-stage breast cancer 159
KATHLEEN I. PRITCHARD

10. The duration of adjuvant tamoxifen therapy 181
MALCOLM M. BILIMORIA and V. CRAIG JORDAN

11. Tamoxifen and the endometrium 195
RICHARD R. BARAKAT

12. Hormone replacement therapy and nonhormonal control of menopausal symptoms in breast cancer survivors 209
MELODY A. COBLEIGH

13. Endocrine therapy in metastatic breast cancer 231
GRETCHEN G. KIMMICK and HYMAN B. MUSS

14. The regulation of estrogen receptor expression and function in human breast cancer 255
ANNE T. FERGUSON, RENA G. LAPIDUS, and NANCY E. DAVIDSON

List of contributors

Richard R. Barakat, M.D.
c/o Academic Office
Gynecology Service
Department of Surgery
Memorial Sloan-Kettering Cancer Center
1275 York Avenue
New York, NY 10021

Rick L. Bare, M.D.
Department of Urology and The Comprehensive Cancer Center
The Bowman Gray School of Medicine
Wake Forest University
Winston-Salem, NC 27157-1094

David Berd, M.D.
Division of Neoplastic Diseases
Jefferson Medical College
Suite 1024, Curtis Building
1015 Walnut Street
Philadelphia, PA 19107

Malaya Bhattacharya-Chatterjee, Ph.D.
Department of Internal Medicine
Markey Cancer Center
800 Rose Street, Room 207 Combs Bldg
Lexington, KY 40536-0093

Malcolm M. Bilimoria
Department of Surgery and Robert H. Lurie Comprehensive Cancer Center
Northwestern University Medical School
303 E. Chicago Avenue
8258 Olson Pavilion
Chicago, IL 60611

J. Mark Cline, D.V.M., Ph.D.
Bowman Gray School of Medicine
Department of Comparative Medicine
Comprehensive Cancer Center of Wake Forest University
Medical Center Boulevard
Winston-Salem, NC 27157

Melody A. Cobleigh, M.D.
Rush Presbyterian — St. Luke's Medical Center
105 Michaux Road
Riverside, IL 60546-1827

Nancy E. Davidson
Johns-Hopkins Oncology Center
Johns-Hopkins Hospital
600 North Wolfe Street
Baltimore, MD 21287-0002

Anne T. Ferguson
Johns-Hopkins Oncology Center
Johns-Hopkins Hospital
600 North Wolfe Street
Baltimore, MD 21287-0002

Kenneth A. Foon, M.D.
Director, Lucille Parker Markey Cancer Center
Professor & Chief, Division of Hematology and Oncology
Department of Internal Medicine
University of Kentucky School of Medicine
800 Rose Street, Room CC140
Lexington, Kentucky 40536-0093

Claude L. Hughes, M.D., Ph.D.
Department of Obstetrics and Gynecology
Duke University Medical Center
Durham, NC 27710

William J. John, M.D.
Deputy Director,
Assistant Professor of Medicine
Lucille P. Markey Cancer Center
University of Kentucky
Lexington, Kentucky 40536

V. Craig Jordan, Ph.D., D.Sc.
Robert H. Lurie Comprehensive Cancer Center
Northwestern University Medical School
303 E. Chicago Avenue
8258 Olson Pavilion
Chicago, IL 60611

Gretchen G. Kimmick, M.D.
Comprehensive Cancer Center of Wake Forest University
The Bowman Gray School of Medicine
Medical Center Boulevard
Winston-Salem, NC 27157

Rena G. Lapidus
Johns Hopkins Oncology Center
Johns Hopkins Hospital
600 North Wolfe Street
Baltimore MD 21287-0002

Edmund C. Lattime, Ph.D.
Division of Neoplastic Diseases
Jefferson Medical College
Suite 1014, College Building
1025 Walnut Street
Philadelphia, PA 19107

Samuel S. Lentz, M.D.
Section on Gynecologic Oncology
Comprehensive Cancer Center of Wake Forest University
Medical Center Boulevard
Winston-Salem, NC 27157-1065

Richard R. Love, M.D.
Cancer Prevention Program
University of Wisconsin
7C Medical Sciences Center
1300 University Avenue
Madison, WI 53706

Henry C. Maguire, Jr., M.D.
Division of Neoplastic Diseases
Jefferson Medical College
Room 1008, College Building
1025 Walnut Street
Philadelphia, PA 19107

Michael J. Mastrangelo, M.D.
Division of Neoplastic Diseases
Jefferson Medical College
Suite 1024, College Building
1025 Walnut Street
Philadelphia, PA 19107

Hyman B. Muss, M.D.
Professor of Medicine
Comprehensive Cancer Center of Wake Forest University
The Bowman Gray School of Medicine
Medical Center Boulevard
Winston-Salem, NC 27157

Mark R. Olsen, M.D., Ph.D.
••
••
••

Kathleen I. Pritchard, M.D., FRCPC
Division of Medical Oncology/Haematology
Toronto-Sunnybrook Regional Cancer Centre
University of Toronto
2075 Bayview Avenue
Toronto, Ontario
M4N 3M5 Canada

Takami Sato, M.D.
Division of Neoplastic Diseases
Jefferson Medical College
Room 1011, College Building
1025 Walnut Street
Philadelphia, PA 19107

Frank M. Torti, M.D.
Bowman Gray School of Medicine
Comprehensive Cancer Center
Medical Center Boulevard
Winston-Salem, NC 27157

Preface

This volume, *Biological and Hormonal Therapies of Cancer*, which is part of the series *Cancer Treatment and Research*, presents selected new information concerning biologic and hormonal therapy of cancer. We have attempted to provide the reader with topics of major interest in a timely fashion.

There is renewed interest in biologic therapy of cancer. Two chapters review the role of interferon in the hematologic malignancies and in solid tumors. Vaccine therapies have come to the forefront of cancer therapy recently, and two chapters approach different strategies of vaccine therapies; one reviews the cellular vaccine therapies and another the anti-idiotype approach.

The hormonal therapy chapters focus on current uses of endocrine therapy in endometrial, breast, and prostate cancer. In addition, hormonal strategies for the prevention of breast cancer and endometrial cancer, including exciting information relating to phytochemicals, are presented. The effects of tamoxifen on endometrium is a topic of major interest and is discussed in detail. Finally, there is a chapter on estrogen receptor expression and regulation in human breast cancer. These chapters are all written by experts in the field and contain timely and relevant information of interest to laboratory and clinical scientists and practitioners alike.

Biologic and endocrine therapies represent major areas of cancer research interest. The advent of newer biologic therapies, including new antibody-targeted treatments, and the use of biologics as tumor modulators to enhance the effects of other treatment regimens is an exploding avenue of research. Moreover, there is renewed interest in hormonal therapy of cancer, especially with regard to prevention and adjuvant therapy. It is expected that such therapies will continue to proliferate and will eventually lead to further improvements in the treatment of cancer.

Biological and Hormonal Therapies of Cancer

1. Interferon therapy of hematologic malignancies

Kenneth A. Foon

1. Chronic myelogenous leukemia

Chronic myelogenous leukemia (CML) is a hematologic neoplasm characterized by the proliferation and accumulation of mature myeloid cells and their progenitors. It is a clonal disorder caused by somatic mutation in a pluripotent hematopoietic stem cell; consequently, there is involvement of myeloid and erythroid cells, monocytes/macrophages, megakaryocytes, and lymphocytes. Clonality has been conclusively demonstrated by polymorphic genetic systems such as glucose 6-phosphate dehydrogenase (G6PD) in heterozygous individuals with CML, X-chromosome DNA restriction fragment-length polymorphism of hypoxanthine glucuronyl ribosyl phosphoryl transferase, and the presence of the Philadelphia (Ph^1) chromosome and other clonal cytogenetic markers [1–5].

1.1. The Ph^1 chromosome

The Ph^1 chromosome is the result of breaks on chromosomes 9 and 22, t(9;22)(q34;q11), with a reciprocal translocation of the distal genetic material [6,7]. The *C-ABL* proto-oncogene is transposed from its normal location on chromosome 9 to chromosome 22 in proximity to the breakpoint cluster region (*BCR*) [8]. A new hybrid *BCR–ABL* oncogene is formed that produces an abnormal 8.5-kb RNA that encodes for a 210-kDa (p 210) fusion protein. This abnormal fusion protein has increased tyrosine kinase activity and altered intracellular distribution [9] and presumably is critical in the pathogenesis of CML. The expression of the *BCR–ABL* gene in a transgenic mouse model results in polyclonal myeloid or lymphoid acute leukemias [10,11].

1.2. Clinical features

CML is characterized by two distinct phases, namely, a chronic phase that lasts a median of three years and an acute phase that lasts from 6 to 12 months and is fatal. In approximately half the patients, there is an intervening accelerated phase associated with increased myelopoiesis and resistance or inability to tolerate therapy. In the chronic phase, increased myelopoiesis is restricted predominately to granulocytes, monocytes/macrophages, and platelets; increased erythrocyte production is rare. The affected cells usually retain the ability to mature normally without dividing, having normal or slightly increased lifespan, and respond appropriately to growth factors. In the acute phase, in contrast, the cells lose the ability to differentiate and mature and retain the ability to divide.

Transition from the chronic to the acute phase is usually gradual, but it may occur abruptly. Moreover, the distinction between chronic and acute phase is somewhat arbitrary, since patients in chronic phase may, by definition, have up to 20% immature myeloid cells in the blood and up to 30% in the bone marrow. Patients with higher numbers are often classified as being in the acute phase. However, there are often other differences between the chronic and acute phases. For example, during the chronic phase of CML, the granulocyte-associated enzyme leukocyte alkaline phosphatase (LAP) is usually absent or low, while the acute phase is characterized by a normal or elevated LAP. In some instances, an increase in LAP may be the first indication of transition to the acute phase. Furthermore, in the acute phase, in addition to the Ph^1 chromosome, there are typically additional chromosome abnormalities. Perhaps of greatest importance, once patients enter the acute phase, there is resistance to chronic phase therapies and a rapid downhill course.

The typical presenting symptoms in chronic-phase CML include fatigue, malaise, headache, and weight loss. Infections and bleeding are uncommon. Rare patients will present with leukostasis, typically when the total leukocyte count exceeds $100 \times 10^9/L$. Leukostasis may be associated with cerebral vascular accidents, infarctions, venous thrombosis, and pulmonary insufficiency. Physical examination may demonstrate splenomegaly; hepatomegaly is unusual at diagnosis. Lymphadenopathy is very infrequent. Many patients are diagnosed from routine leukocyte counts performed for other reasons. With disease progression, there are increasing problems with fevers, weight loss, infections, bone and joint pain, bleeding, and increasing hepatosplenomegaly. Extramedullary disease may herald transformation to the acute phase. Frequent sites of extramedullary disease include soft tissue, skin, central nervous system, lymph nodes, and bone.

The laboratory hallmark of chronic-phase CML is leukocytosis with mature and immature myeloid cells in the peripheral blood with less than 5% blasts. As described, the LAP score is absent or low. Typically, there is an elevated serum LDH, uric acid, vitamin B_{12}, and B_{12} binding capacity; the latter findings reflect the increased granulocytic pool. There may be eosinophilia, basophilia, and monocytosis. The bone marrow is hypercellular with myeloid and megakaryocytic hyperplasia and high myeloid erythroid ratios. The percentage of blasts is normal or minimally increased.

With acceleration, there is increasing anemia, thrombocytopenia, blasts, and cytogenetic evolution. Collagen fibrosis in the bone marrow may be associated with megakaryocytopenia, thrombocytopenia, and marrow failure, which is the terminal event in a minority of patients. Acute crisis is defined by the presence of 30% or more blasts in the blood or bone marrow. Sixty percent of cases are myeloid blast crisis with myeloperoxidase-positive blast cells. Twenty percent are lymphoid blast crisis that is myeloperoxidase-negative and terminal deoxynucleotidyl transferase (TdT) positive. Most cases of lymphoid blast crisis are pre-B cell and positive for the common acute lymphoblastic leukemia antigen (CD10). T-cell cases of lymphoid blast crisis have been reported [12,13]. The remaining cases represent either undifferentiated, megakaryocytic, or erythroid blast crisis.

1.3. Therapy

The drugs most commonly used to treat chronic-phase CML are busulfan and hydroxyurea. Busulfan is an alkylating agent, and the usual dose is 2–8 mg per day. Busulfan should be discontinued when the leukocyte count is under 20×10^9/L because of its protracted effect. Hydroxyurea is a ribonucleotidase inhibitor. It differs from busulfan in that it induces rapid disease control for a short duration. The initial dose is 0.5–2 g per day. The dose is reduced by half with each 50% reduction of the leukocyte count. If the leukocyte count is not reducing adequately, the dose can be increased up to 4 g per day. A leukocyte count of 20×10^9/L is a reasonable goal. There is no obvious survival advantage to either busulfan or hydroxyurea, and both will control the blood counts in the vast majority of patients. However, busulfan is associated with more serious side effects, which include severe myelosuppression; pulmonary, endocardial, and bone marrow fibrosis; and an Addison-like wasting syndrome. It is rare for patients treated with these drugs to experience disappearance of the Ph^1 chromosome. Other drugs rarely used for chronic-phase CML include chlorambucil, melphalan, 6-mercaptopurine, and cyclophosphamide. These offer no advantage except in situations where the side effects of busulfan or hydroxyurea are unacceptable or when these agents are no longer effective in disease control.

Intensive combination chemotherapy has also been used in CML [14]. The goal is elimination of the Ph^1 chromosome clone. Combination chemotherapy regimens have included cytarabine and an anthracycline, similar to AML treatment regimens. Typically, 30%–50% of patients have had suppression of the Ph^1 chromosome-positive clone, but there is no obvious survival advantage.

Leukapheresis has been used in emergencies to rapidly lower blood counts where leukostasis-related complications such as pulmonary failure or cerebral vascular accidents are likely. Leukapheresis may also have a role in pregnant women (particularly during the first trimester), for whom avoidance of potentially teratogenic drugs is important [15]. Its disadvantage is that it is expensive and cumbersome.

Splenectomy was used in CML because of the suggestion that acute-phase evolution might occur in the spleen. However, splenectomy is not effective and is reserved for symptomatic splenomegaly unresponsive to chemotherapy or for significant anemia or thrombocytopenia associated with hypersplenism. Splenic radiation is occasionally used to reduce the size of the spleen.

The goal of allogeneic bone marrow transplantation is to cure CML [16]. Transplantations are typically from monozygotic twins or HLA-identical siblings. Typical conditioning regimens include high-dose cyclophosphamide and total body radiation. Modifications such as busulfan and cyclophosphamide without radiation or the addition of high-dose cytarabine, an anthracycline, or etoposide produces similar results. Results of identical-twin transplantations (syngeneic) in the chronic phase include a seven-year disease-free survival in 55%, with a 30% relapse rate. HLA-identical sibling transplantations in chronic-phase CML have a five-year disease-free survival in the 40%–60% range, with a 5%–30% relapse rate [17]. The higher relapse rate in syngeneic transplantation is likely due to the absence of a graft-versus-leukemia effect. The outcome is considerably less favorable in accelerated and acute phase CML.

Acute myeloid-phase CML is usually resistant to chemotherapy. Nevertheless, induction of bone marrow aplasia to allow CML chronic-phase cells to repopulate the bone marrow is usually attempted with regimens similar to those used for acute myelogenous leukemia. Drugs such as an anthracycline and cytarabine are usually given in the myeloid acute phase. Remission rates are 20%–30% but are generally short-lived. High-dose cytarabine may yield higher remission rates but likely does not significantly benefit survival [18]. Therapy of the lymphoid acute phase is thought to be more successful, but at best a median survival of 9–12 months is reported. Remissions have been noted in up to 70% of patients treated with vincristine and prednisone with or without an anthracycline or cytarabine. Unfortunately, all patients eventually relapse. While a second remission is sometimes achieved, no patients are cured. The results of bone marrow transplantation in the accelerated and acute phases of CML are much less favorable than in the chronic phase [16,19]. Relapse rates as high as 80% are reported. Five-year disease-free survivals are reported in the 10%–20% range. Autotransplantation has been performed in accelerated or blast-phase CML; results are generally disappointing [19]. Approximately 50% of patients obtain a second chronic phase; it is typically short-lived, and less than 25% of patients survive for more than one year.

Interferons have a direct antiproliferative effect on the leukemia clone in CML. Therapy with partially purified human leukocyte interferon-alpha in CML patients in chronic phase have demonstrated a complete hematologic response in 70% of patients and a cytogenetic response in 40% [20]. Subsequent studies with recombinant interferon-alphas confirmed these early results with partially purified interferon-alpha [17,21–27]. Cytogenetic responses are generally divided into three groups: 1) complete disappearance of the Ph^1-positive cells, 2) a partial response, namely, greater than 65% disappearance of the Ph^1 clone, and 3) a minor response from 10%–65%. In most studies, the interferon-alpha dose has been 5×10^6 units/m^2/day or three times a week. However, one nonradomized phase II trial suggested that 2×10^6 units/m^2 was equally effective [28]. Typical side effects are the flulike symptoms typically associated with interferon-alpha, which are generally not dose limiting and are managed by bedtime doses and acetaminophen. These symptoms will usually disappear after 1–2 weeks of therapy. Later, side effects such as fatigue, weight loss, neurotoxicity, depression, insomnia, and rare immune-mediated complications may be seen. The immune-mediated complication [29–31] have included autoimmune anemia, thrombocytopenia, collagen vascular disorders, nephrotic syndrome, and hypothyroidism. Rare cases of cardiac arrhythmia and congestive heart failure have led to discontinuation of interferon-alpha. Porphyria cutaneous tarda, membranous glomerulonephritis, and vitiligo have also been reported [31].

Of critical importance is the long-term effect of the cytogenetic response. Cytogenetic responses have been durable in approximately 25% of patients [17]. This outcome is restricted primarily to those patients who have had a complete cytogenetic response, although one study reported that the benefits are not confined to cytogenetic responses but rather accrue to all patients who have received interferon-alpha [32]. Whether a cytogenetic response translates into prolonged remission duration and survival has been controversial. In one large-group, nonrandomized study, there was no significant correlation between cytogenetic response and remission duration or survival [24]. In another study, patients were randomized to interferon-alpha 5×10^6 units/m^2/day or hydroxyurea. A major cytogenetic response was found in 25% of patients receiving interferon-alpha but in none of the patients on hydroxyurea. Median survival was significantly better for patients receiving interferon-alpha [26]. In another large randomized trial, interferon-alpha was superior to busulfan and as effective as hydroxyurea [33]. Another randomized trial demonstrated superiority of interferon-alpha over busulfan [34]. In another study [27], patients were randomized to interferon-alpha or chemotherapy with either hydroxyurea or busulfan. Patients treated with interferon-alpha had more cytogenetic responses, delayed disease progression, and prolonged overall survival. These latter studies support the association between interferon-alpha and improved survival. A critical issue is whether the effects of interferon-alpha affect the total population or are restricted to those patients (i.e., 25%) that have had a complete cytogenetic response. If the survival benefit for all patients is not confirmed, then the recommendation may be to continue interferon only in patients who have developed a complete cytogenetic response.

Combination therapy of interferon-alpha and chemotherapy agents has also been studied. Interferon-alpha combined with hydroxyurea leads to rapid and excellent control of blood counts but is not associated with improved cytogenetic responses [27]. The combination of low-dose cytarabine and interferon-alpha also demonstrated excellent control of blood counts [34–36], and in a randomized study of patients with early chronic-phase CML, those treated with combined therapy had better cytogenetic responses and disease control [37].

The mechanisms of action of interferon-alpha in CML are not entirely known. In vitro, interferon-alpha suppresses normal and CML myeloid stem cell proliferation, probably by a direct growth-inhibitory effect. This finding does not explain the in vivo effects, which appear to be more selective. The direct effect of interferon-alpha is mediated through a specific cell receptor [38]. Receptor binding affinity and downregulation following therapy were studied in CML cells from responding and resistant patients and did not reveal a receptor binding defect [39]. In another study, it was demonstrated that the interferon inducible enzyme 2′,5′-oligoadenylate synthetase was increased in 7 of 9 responders and 0 of 3 resistant patients [40]. In another report, it was demonstrated that interferon-alpha induces a dose-dependent increase in the adhesion of long-term culture-initiating cells and committed colony-forming cells from CML bone marrow to normal stroma [41]. This adhesion was specifically inhibited by $\alpha 4$, $\alpha 5$, and β_1 integrin antibodies, suggesting that interferon-alpha induces normalization of progenitor–stroma interactions in CML. Immune flow cytometry showed that interferon-alpha did not change the level of $\alpha 4$, $\alpha 5$, and β_1 integrin expression, suggesting that interferon-alpha restores normal β_1 integrin function. Several genes have been demonstrated to be induced by interferon, but none of these genes has yet to be ascribed to the antiproliferative effect of interferon-alpha [42–44].

Interferon-gamma has been studied in patients with chronic-phase Ph^1-positive CML [45]. Patients were treated with $0.25–0.5 \, mg/m^2/day$ I.M. of interferon-gamma; 6 of 26 patients achieved a complete hematologic response, and four had partial responses. Five patients had cytogenetic improvement. Fever and flulike symptoms were the most common side effects. Some patients who had failed interferon-alpha responded to interferon-gamma and vice versa. Combination of interferon-alpha and interferon-gamma has not been encouraging [46,47]. Limited studies with interferon-beta in CML have had negative results [48].

1.4. Recommendations

Interferon-alpha is clearly effective in controlling blood counts and cytogenetic responses in patients in the chronic phase of CML. Nonetheless, it is still recommended that for younger patients who have an HLA-matched sibling donor and who are in early chronic phase, bone marrow transplantation is the treatment of choice. For chronic-phase CML patients who are not transplanted, an initial trial of an interferon-alpha regimen is considered reasonable and should be continued if there is a major cytogenetic response until this response is lost. It is also suggested that if the patient has a complete and durable cytogenetic response and does not have a related matched donor, autologous bone marrow storage should be considered. Patients in late chronic phase who are not transplant candidates should be transplanted with matched unrelated donors, mismatched related donors, or autologous marrow transplants, or considered for treatment with new agents or regimens.

2. Ph[1]-negative myeloproliferative diseases

Similar to CML, essential thrombocythemia, polycythemia vera, and agnogenic myeloid metaplasia are diseases of a pluripotent hematopoietic stem cell. Also similar to CML, many of these diseases progress to acute leukemia, even though to a considerably lesser degree than CML. These diseases suffer the complications of overproduction of red blood cells or platelets and may be complicated by thrombohemorrhagic complications [49–51].

It was first observed that interferon-alpha led to a dramatic decline in platelets in patients with longstanding Ph[1]-positive CML complicated by thrombocytosis [52]. It has been similarly observed that in patients with primary thrombocythemia, platelet counts dropped dramatically within 2–3 weeks of initiating interferon-alpha therapy. In order to continue to control platelet counts, therapy is continued in a maintenance fashion. In some patients, platelets responded even in the face of rising white blood cell counts. Overall, responses have been in the range of 90% [53–60].

Polycythemia vera is characterized by increased red cell mass and thrombohemorrhagic complications. Standard therapy has been phlebotomy to reduce the red cell mass; however, phlebotomy is associated with an approximately 40% incidence of thrombohemorrhagic complications [61]. Chlorambucil and radioactive phosphorus have also been used to control disease, but both are leukemogenic [62]. Hydroxyurea may also be used but may also be leukemogenic [63]. Many patients with polycythemia vera will experience night sweats and pruritis and will develop iron deficiency secondary to multiple phlebotomies. Patients also have progressive splenomegaly and myelofibrosis. For all these reasons, newer treatment agents are necessary. Eleven consecutive patients with prior phlebotomy therapy were treated with recombinant interferon-alpha 2b 3×10^6/units/m^2 three times weekly [64]. In addition to elevated hemoglobin, the majority of these patients had thrombocytosis and modest leukocytosis. Over a course of 6–12 months, most of the patients had improvement in all parameters, including decline in spleen size. None of the patients had a thrombohemorrhagic event while on interferon-alpha. These results suggest that interferon-alpha may be an important new treatment for polycythemia vera.

Preliminary data exist that suggest responses in some patients with agnogenic myeloid metaplasia [65,66]. In one patient, there was improvement in bone marrow histology, partial resorption of myelofibrosis, and cytogenetic improvement [66].

3. Hairy cell leukemia

Hairy cell leukemia (HCL), or leukemic reticuloendotheliosis, was first described by Borouncle and coworkers in 1958 [67]. This is a malignant B-cell lymphoproliferative disease that typically presents with pancytopenia, prominent splenomegaly, and circulating mononuclear cells with irregular cytoplasmic projections in the blood, bone marrow, spleen, and other organs. Remarkable progress in the diagnosis, biology, immunology, and therapy of this disease have occurred over the past 15 years.

3.1. Clinical and laboratory features

Typical presenting clinical features include weakness and fatigue secondary to anemia, bleeding secondary to thrombocytopenia, and recurrent infections secondary to neutropenia [68–71]. Some patients will have abdominal complaints related to splenomegaly. A few persons will have weight loss, fever, and night sweats. Splenomegaly is the most common physical finding at diagnosis and is found in 80%–90% of patients; massive enlargement is common. Approximately 10% of patients have lymphadenopathy, and 20% have hepatomegaly with abnormal liver function tests. The serum protein electrophoresis is abnormal in 25% of patients, but a monoclonal pattern is rare, although a small quantity of monoclonal protein is commonly detected by immunofixation [72]. Most patients present with mild to moderate normochromic, normocytic anemia secondary to replacement of the bone marrow by leukemia cells and to hypersplenism. Leukopenia is common; an absolute neutropenia (under 2×10^9/L) is found in 75% of patients, and monocytopenia is also characteristic. In approximately 20% of patients, platelet numbers are less than 100×10^9/L at presentation. Qualitative platelet abnormalities are also common [73]. Approximately 10% of patients will present with leukocytosis with more than a 10×10^9/L cell count of predominantly hairy cells in the peripheral blood. As described, patients are usually leukopenic, with a small percentage of circulating hairy cells.

One third of patients develop infections during the course of their disease; over half of these involve gram-negative organisms [70]. Atypical microbacterium is common, and open lung biopsy may be required. Disseminated fungal diseases may occur, whereas *Pneumococcus carinii* pneumonia is rare. Other complications of HCL include an autoimmune syndrome characterized most often by vasculitis, arthritis, and bone lesions. Systemic vasculitis is usually documented by biopsy of skin lesion. Long-bone involvement, usually of the femur, can result in lytic lesions and associated pain and pathologic fractures.

A rare variant [74] of HCL has been described, with morphologic features intermediate between those of HCL and prolymphocytic leukemia. The clinical course is chronic, with splenomegaly and high leukocyte counts (typically $> 50 \times 10^9$/L) but without significant neutropenia or monocytopenia. The cells differ from those of classic HCL in that they do not express the CD25 antigen and do not respond to therapies as dramatically as HCL (see below).

The typical HCL cell is irregular with a serrated border. The cytoplasm is sky blue without granules. The nuclear membrane is distinct and the chromatin spongy. Occasionally, a single nucleolus is present. Electron micrographs show pseudopods and long cytoplasmic villi resembling hairs on the cell surface [71]. The cytoplasm contains abundant oval or round mitochondria with well-developed Golgi apparatus, free ribosomes, and rough endoplasmic reticulum. The bone marrow cannot be aspirated in more than 50% of cases because of leukemic infiltration and/or fibrosis. Core biopsies are usually diagnostic, showing diffuse involvement with hairy cells and increased reticulum.

HCL is a clonal proliferation of malignant B cells [75]. There is typically intense staining of surface membrane immunoglobulin with a single light chain that confirms the clonality of the disease. B-cell-associated antigens, including CD19, CD20, CD22, and sometimes CD23 and CD24, are also present [76–78]. CD21, an antigen that is lost in the later stages of B-cell differentiation, is absent. The PCA-1 antigen, typically found on plasma cells, is present on hairy cells, suggesting that hairy cells may be preplasma cells [79,80]. Studies of immunoglobulin genes indicate clonal rearrangement of heavy chain immunoglobulin genes and at least one light chain immunoglobulin gene [81,82]. CD25 [82] and CD103 [83] are present in virtually every case of HCL. HCL cells contain the tartrate-resistant isoenzyme 5 of acid phosphatase (TRAP) [84]. The PAS and alpha-nathyl acetate esterase tests may be weakly positive, whereas naphthol-ASD-chloracetate esterase and peroxidase reactions are negative.

3.2. Therapy

Approximately 10% of patients with HCL will never require treatment. They are usually elderly with modest cytopenias [70]. The remainder ultimately require therapy.

Prior to the introduction of interferon-alpha therapy, splenectomy was the standard of care. Indications were typically cytopenias with hemoglobin less than 10 g/dL and/or neutrophils less than 1×10^9/L and/or platelets less than 100×10^9/L. Other less common indications for therapy were symptomatic splenomegaly and recurrent infections. Bone involvement and vasculitis were indications for therapy, but vasculitis was more likely to respond to steroids and bone involvement to radiation therapy. In the great majority of patients, cytopenias improve following splenectomy. While spleen size does not consistently correlate with hematologic improvement following splenectomy, the degree of marrow involvement with leukemia is predictive of response [70]. Median duration of response to splenectomy is approximately 18 months. Prior to the introduction of interferon-alpha therapy, there were no satisfactory systemic approaches to the treatment of HCL. Androgens, leukapheresis, combination chemotherapy, and single-agent therapy such as chlorambucil had all been tried but none of them with consistently positive results. The median survival of patients with HCL prior to interferon-alpha was approximately eight years.

The first report of responses to interferon-alpha was in 1984 with the use of purified human leukocyte interferon [85]. All seven patients treated had a significant improvement in their peripheral blood counts and reduction of HCL infiltration of the bone marrow. The toxicity to this low dose of interferon was minor. Additional studies using lymphoblastoid interferon-alpha [86,87], recombinant interferon-alpha 2a [88], and recombinant interferon-alpha 2b [89] demonstrated that approximately 75% of patients had either a complete or a partial response to interferon-alpha that lasted from 12 to 24 months. It is generally believed that interferon does not induce true complete remissions, and virtually all patients will eventually relapse following interferon-alpha therapy. Most of these patients will respond to a second course of interferon-alpha.

The mechanism of action of interferon-alpha in HCL is unknown. The two most extensive areas of investigation have been the direct antiproliferative effects on hairy cells and the effects on patient immune systems. The direct effect is believed to be mediated through binding to specific cell surface receptors. The number of interferon-alpha binding receptors on hairy cells is approximately 800 to 1000 per cell, which is approximately double the number detected on chronic lymphocytic leukemia cells (CLL) [90,91], a disease that is unresponsive to interferon-alpha. This difference in receptors, however, could also be explained by the significantly greater cell surface area of hairy cells compared with CLL cells [92]. In addition, the number of receptors on HCL cells is not necessarily correlated with response [92]. It also has been reported that, with binding to the receptor, there is a downregulation of the receptor that correlates with increased activity of $2',5'$-oligoadenylate synthetase [93–95]. It has also be noted that interferon-alpha induces RNA synthesis in HCL cells [91]. This outcome correlates with the synthesis of a number of specific cellular proteins. These proteins can be inhibited with actinomycin-D, indicating that new mRNA synthesis was required for the protein production [96,97]. Interferon-alpha also inhibits the proliferative response of HCL cells to B-cell growth factor [98,99] and appears to have an inhibitory effect on DNA synthesis [98]. The above studies support the notion that the antiproliferative effects of interferon-alpha play a role in its therapeutic efficacy in HCL.

Patients with HCL have a severe deficiency of natural killer (NK) cell activity that recovers following treatment with interferon-alpha [88,100]. This NK recovery is typically delayed 6–8 months. Interestingly, HCL cells have been shown to be resistant to NK cell lysis, and therefore the recovery of NK cells may play no role in the clinical effect [101,102]. Increased HLA-DR antigen expression has been demonstrated to occur in vitro following interferon-alpha exposure to HCL cells, and nonresponders have shown a reduction in HLA-DR antigen expression in vitro [103–105]. Class II HLA antigen expression of tumor cells is important in the generation of immune effector cell responses and may potentiate T-cell-mediated cytotoxic events that could contribute to the antitumor effect of interferon-alpha in HCL.

In summary, both antiproliferative and immunomodulatory effects have been demonstrated to occur in HCL patients treated with interferon-alpha. Their significance in the therapeutic role of interferon-alpha is not known but is suggested.

There are two interferon-alpha preparations for the treatment of HCL that have been approved by the United States Food and Drug Administration (FDA). Interferon-alpha 2a is recommended at a dose of 3 million units per day I.M. or subcutaneously for approximately six months followed by an additional 6–8 months of 3 million units given three times per week. Interferon-alpha 2b is recommended to be given as 2 million units/m^2 three times per week for a period of 12–18 months.

The pattern of response to interferon is quite predictable, with platelets recovering within approximately two months, hemoglobin within 3–4 months, and granulocytes in 4–5 months. With the rise in granulocytes, the incidence of infections correspondingly decreases. The circulating hairy cells clear from the peripheral blood within a few months of therapy, and the bone marrow improves over 6–9 months [104–106]. As mentioned above, it is rare that the bone marrow is completely cleared of hairy cells. In some patients, there may be improvement in the reticulin fibrosis involvement of the marrow.

Interferon-alpha is rarely given for more than two years. Interestingly, following the discontinuation of interferon-alpha, patients may even have a further improvement in their peripheral blood counts. However, over time, there is gradual bone marrow progression of HCL following the discontinuation of interferon-alpha. Ultimately, all patients will relapse within a matter of months to years following discontinuation of interferon-alpha. Once a hematologic relapse has occurred, patients will generally respond to a second course of interferon-alpha.

Toxicity to interferon-alpha includes flulike symptoms with fever, malaise, and headaches that may resolve after the first few courses of therapy. Rashes and mild injection-site erythema are common. Mild nausea, vomiting, and diarrhea may be seen in a relatively small proportion of patients. Asymptomatic elevation of hepatic transaminases are frequently reported. Mild neurological complaints have been reported along with memory loss and depression. A very small percentage of patients have more severe central nervous system complications accompanied with confusion and lethargy. Decreased libido has been seen in some men treated with interferon-alpha. The most significant problem with prolonged therapy with interferon-alpha is chronic fatigue.

There have been reports of antibody formation to interferon, and in a small number of these patients, these antibodies were neutralizing [107]. This incidence appears to be greater in patients treated with interferon-alpha 2a compared to interferon-alpha 2b.

Pentostation or 2-deoxycoformycin, an adenosine deaminase inhibitor, is also approved by the FDA for the treatment of HCL. Treatment with $4\,mg/m^2$ every two weeks produces complete responses in approximately 50% of patients and partial responses in 25% [108,109]. Pentostatin leads to more rapid and more complete responses than interferon-alpha. Toxicities include rash, diarrhea, nausea, and vomiting; these are generally mild. Data suggest that treatment with pentostatin causes a profound decrease in all lymphocyte subsets that is associated with a marked decrease in proliferative responses to mitogens and alloantigens and an increased incidence of herpes infections [110]. The treatment period has generally ranged from 3 to 6 months, and the responses appear to be quite durable. Patients treated with prior interferon-alpha respond to pentostatin [111].

Cladribine, or 2-chlorodeoxyadenosine, differs from pentostatin in that it is not an adenosine deaminase inhibitor but rather an adenosine deaminase-resistant purine substrate analogue. At a dose of 0.1 mg/kg/day by continuous intravenous infusion for seven days, 80% of patients with HCL have complete responses, with the majority of the remaining 20% partial responders [109,112]. Thus far, even the partial responses have been durable following a single seven-day course of therapy. Responses are independent of previous splenectomy or interferon-alpha therapy. Toxicity has been limited to transient fevers and neutropenia. A very small number of patients have required second treatments, and most respond. There is a profound effect on T cells following treatment with cladribine, with a decrease in total T cells that typically recovers within 12 months. Surprisingly, major infections have not been reported. Cladribine has been approved by the FDA for the treatment of HCL.

3.3. Recommendations

Interferon-alpha represented the first highly effective systemic therapy for HCL. The responses have been excellent, with modest toxicity. Pentostatin has had more complete responses as well as more durable responses than interferon-alpha, but significant toxicity is reported in some patients. Responses to a single seven-day course of cladribine are excellent and durable with minimal toxicity. It would appear at this time that cladribine, rather than splenectomy, should be considered to be the first-line therapy for HCL patients.

4. Multiple myeloma

Multiple myeloma is caused by neoplastic plasma cells that synthesize abnormal amounts of immunoglobulin or immunoglobulin fragments. The clinical manifestations typically include monoclonal immunoglobulin production, decreased immunoglobulin secretion by normal plasma cells leading to hypogammaglobulinemia, impaired hematopoiesis, osteolytic bone lesions, and renal dysfunction. Tumor formation in the form of plasmacytomas may also be seen.

4.1. Clinical and laboratory features

Patients may present with symptoms of pain, most frequently from vertebral compression fractures, sites of osteopenia, or lytic bone lesions. These are likely due to excessive osteoclastic-activating-factor activity stimulated by IL-1-beta, TNF-beta, and/or IL-6 [113–115]. Pain can also be caused by cord compression from plasmacytomas. Amyloid may cause pain by infiltrating nerve sheaths or organs. Abnormalities in cellular and immune function may lead to serious infections [116,117]. Because of the inability to opsonize by specific antibody, *Streptococcus pneumoniae* is quite common. Renal abnormalities resulting from light chains causing interstitial nephritis with light chain casts is quite common [118]. The second most common cause of nephropathy is hypercalcemia with hypercalciuria. Hypercalcemia may also lead to calcium deposits in the renal tubules, producing interstitial nephritis [119]. Amyloidosis associated with light chain proteinuria typically presents as a nephrotic syndrome and can lead to renal failure [120]. Neurologic abnormalities are generally caused by regional tumor growth that presses the spinal cord or cranial nerves. Polyneuropathies may be associated with amyloid deposition. Plasma cell leukemia is rare but may be seen in end-stage disease. Disease involving the meninges or intracerebral masses are rare [121]. Hyperviscosity occurs in less than 10% of patients with myeloma [122,123]. The symptoms due to circulatory problems lead to cerebral, pulmonary, renal, and other organ dysfunction. Bleeding is reported in 15% of patients with IgG myeloma and in over 30% of patients with IgA myeloma [124,125].

Most patients with myelomas secrete a monoclonal immunoglobulin that is detected by immunoelectrophoresis or immunofixation. Approximately 60% have monoclonal IgG, 20% have IgA, and 20% have only light chains. Myelomas producing a monoclonal IgD, IgE, and IgM or more than one immunoglobulin class are rare. Decreased levels of normal immunoglobulin classes are common. Often there is very low to no expression of heavy and light chain on the cell surface, but it can be detected intracellularly. B-cell markers such as CD19 and CD20 may be detected, while CD38 is virtually always detected. CD10 and CD11b may be present on the cell surface, and sometimes adhesions molecules such as CD56 and CD54 are present. Cytogenetic abnormalities may be seen, but there is no classic single abnormality.

4.2. Therapy

Standard therapy for myeloma still remains oral melphalan and prednisone, which was introduced over 25 years ago [126,127]. This therapy controls symptoms and reduces tumor mass by at least 50% in over one half of patients. A variety of combination regimens have also been used, including nitrosoureas, doxorubicin, vinca alkaloids, and cyclophosphamide in addition to melphalan and prednisone [128,129]. Most studies have not demonstrated that these regimens improve survival, although there is evidence that they lead to a more rapid tumor response. Some patients respond to high doses of glucocorticoids [130]. Autologous and allogeneic bone marrow transplantation are considered in selected patients.

Interferon-alpha has been used as both part of the induction therapy and as a maintenance therapy. Overall, results are controversial. In one study, patients were randomized to receive melphalan and prednisone versus melphalan and prednisone and interferon-alpha at 5 mU three times weekly. There was no evidence of improved response rate or survival in the interferon-alpha arm [131]. In another, similarly randomized trial, there was no difference in response or survival in patients with IgG myeloma, although the survival in 72 patients with IgA or Bence Jones myeloma who were randomized to receive interferon-alpha was significantly longer [132]. In a third, similarly randomized trial, there was no difference between the two groups [133]. In another study, those patients who responded to melphalan and prednisone were randomized to receive maintenance interferon-alpha at $2 mU/m^2$ subcutaneously three times per week or no maintenance therapy [134]. In this trial, interferon-alpha maintenance therapy improved the progression and overall survival of patients who responded to melphalan and prednisone. The authors noted that the toxicity was substantial and needed to be weighed against potential benefits in response duration and survival. Other trials using a similar design have controversial results [135]. In summary, interferon-alpha does not appear to have a role during the initial phase of therapy, and its role as a maintenance therapy is controversial and continues to be under investigation.

5. Lymphoma

Lymphomas of low-grade histology include diffuse small lymphocytic lymphoma, follicular small cleaved lymphoma, and follicular mixed-cell lymphoma and represent approximately 25% of patients with lymphoma. Most studies with interferon-alpha therapy have been of patients with low-grade lymphomas. Interferon-alpha has activity in low-grade lymphomas [136]. In some studies of low-grade lymphoma, an advantage has been reported for combination chemotherapy with interferon-alpha, but these results remain controversial [137,138]. A number of trials have been opened to evaluate the role of interferon-alpha maintenance therapy following successful chemotherapy in patients with low-grade lymphoma [139–141]. Preliminary results appear promising; however, confirmatory trials are required before this therapy can be recommended. Activity in patients with cutaneous T-cell lymphoma, adult T-cell lymphoma, and lymphoblastic lymphoma have also been reported [142–146].

References

1. Fialkow PJ, Jacobson RJ, Papayannopoulou T. 1977. Chronic myelocytic leukemia. Clonal origin in a stem cell common to the granulocyte, erythrocyte, platelet and monocyte/macrophage. Am J Med 63:125–130.
2. Champlin RE, Golde DW. 1985. Chronic myelogenous leukemia: recent advances. Blood 65:1039–1047.
3. Fauser AA, Kanz L, Bross KJ, Löhr GW. 1985. T cells and probably B cells arise from the malignant clone in chronic myelogenous leukemia. J Clin Invest 75:1080–1082.
4. Nitta M, Kato Y, Strife A, Wachter M, Fried J, Perez A, Jhanwar S, Duigou-Osterndorf R, Chaganti RSK, Clarkson B. 1985. Incidence of involvement of the B and T lymphocyte lineages in chronic myelogenous leukemia. Blood 66:1053–1061.
5. Jones D, Lübbert M, Kawasaki ES, Henke M, Bross KJ, Mertelsmann R, Herrmann F. 1992. Clonal analysis of bcr-abl rearrangement in T lymphocytes from patients with chronic myelogenous leukemia. Blood 79:1017–1023.
6. Nowell PC, Hungerford DA. 1960. A minute chromosome in human chronic granulocytic leukemia. Science 132:1497–1501.
7. Rowley JD. 1973. A new consistent chromosomal abnormality in chronic myelogenous leukemia identified by quinacrine fluorescence and Giemsa staining. Nature 243:290–293.
8. Kurzrock R, Gutterman JU, Talpaz M. 1988. The molecular genetics of Philadelphia chromosome-positive leukemias. N Engl J Med 319:990–998.
9. Van Etten RA, Jackson P, Baltimore D. 1989. The mouse type IV c-abl gene product is a nuclear protein and activation of transforming ability is associated with cytoplasmic localization. Cell 58:669–678.
10. Heisterkamp N, Jenster G, ten Hoeve J, Zovich D, Pattengale PK, Groffen J. 1990. Acute leukaemia in bcr/abl transgenic mice. Nature 344:251–253.
11. Daley GQ, Van Etten RA, Baltimore D. 1990. Induction of chronic myelogenous leukemia in mice by the p210 bcr-abl gene of the Philadelphia chromosome. Science 247:824–830.
12. Herrmann F, Komischke B, Kolecki P, Ludwig WD, Sieber G, Teichmann H, Rühl H. 1984. Ph¹ positive blast crisis of chronic myeloid leukaemia exhibiting features characteristic of early T blasts. Scand J Haematol 32:411–416.
13. Griffin JD, Tantravahi R, Canellos GP, Wisch JS, Reinherz EL, Sherwood G, Beveridge RP, Daley JF, Lane H, Schlossman SF. 1983. T-cell surface antigens in a patient with blast crisis of chronic myeloid leukemia. Blood 61:640–644.
14. Clarkson B. 1985. Chronic myelogenous leukemia: Is aggressive treatment indicated? J Clin Oncol 3:135–139.
15. Fitzgerald D, Rowe JM, Heal J. 1986. Leukapheresis for control of chronic myelogenous leukemia during pregnancy. Am J Hematol 22:213–218.
16. Goldman JM, Grosveld G, Baltimore D, Gale RP. 1990. Chronic myelogenous leukemia — the unfolding saga. Leukemia 4:163–167.
17. Kantarjian HM, Deisseroth A, Kurzrock R, Estrov Z, Talpaz M. 1993. Chronic myelogenous leukemia: a concise update. Blood 82:691–703.
18. Herzig RH, Phillips GL, Lazarus HM, et al. 1985. High-dose cytarabine for the treatment of blastic phase chronic myelogenous leukemia. Cancer Treat Rep 69:881–883.
19. Delage R, Ritz J, Anderson KC. 1990. The evolving role of bone marrow transplantation in the treatment of chronic myelogenous leukemia. Hematol Oncol Clin North Am 4:369–388.
20. Talpaz M, Kantarjian HM, McCredie KB, et al. 1987. Clinical investigation of human alpha interferon in chronic myelogenous leukemia. Blood 69:1280–1288.

21. Talpaz M, Kantarjian HM, McCredie K, et al. 1986. Hematologic remission and cytogenetic improvement induced by recombinant human interferon alpha A in chronic myelogenous leukemia. N Engl J Med 314:1065–1069.
22. Alimena G, Morra E, Lazzarino M, et al. 1988. Interferon alpha-2b as therapy for Ph[1]-positive chronic myelogenous leukemia. A study of 82 patients treated with intermittent or daily administration. Blood 72:642–647.
23. Niederle N, Kolki O, Osieka KR, et al. 1987. Interferon alpha-2b in the treatment of chronic myelogenous leukemia. Semin Oncol 16:29–35.
24. Ozer H, George SL, Schiffer CA, et al. 1993. Prolonged subcutaneous administration of recombinant α2b interferon in patients with previously untreated Philadelphia chromosome-positive chronic-phase chronic myelogenous leukemia: effect on remission duration and survival: Cancer and Leukemia Group B Study 8583. Blood 82:2975–2984.
25. Freund M, Von Wussow P, Diedrich H, et al. 1989. Recombinant human interferon (IHN) alpha-2b in chronic myelogenous leukemia — dose dependency of response and frequency of neutralizing anti-interferon antibodies. Br J Haematol 72:350–356.
26. Kluin-Nelemans JC, Louwagie A, Delannoy A, et al. 1992. CML treated by interferon alpha-2b vs hydroxyurea alone — preliminary report of a large multicenter randomized trial (abstract). Blood 80 (Suppl 1):358a.
27. Tura S, Baccarani M, Zuffa E, et al. 1994. Interferon alfa-2a as compared with conventional chemotherapy for the treatment of chronic myeloid leukemia. N Engl J Med 330:820–825.
28. Schofield JR, Robinson WA, Murphy JR, Rovira DK. 1994. Low doses of interferon-α are as effective as higher doses in inducing remissions and prolonging survival in chronic myeloid leukemia. Ann Intern Med 121:736–744.
29. Ronnblom LE, Alm FV, Oberg KE. 1991. Autoimmunity after alpha-interferon therapy for malignant carcinoid tumors. Ann Intern Med 115:178–183.
30. Conlon KC, Urba WJ, Smith JW, Steis RG, Longo DL, Clark JW. 1990. Exacerbation of symptoms of autoimmune disease in patients receiving alpha-interferon therapy. Cancer 65:2237–2242.
31. Sacchi S, Kantarjian H, O'Brien S, Cohen PR, Pierce S, Talpaz M. 1995. Immune-mediated and unusual complications during interferon alfa therapy in chronic myelogenous leukemia. J Clin Oncol 13:2401–2407.
32. Allan NC, Richards SM, Shepherd PCA. 1995. UK Medical Research Council randomised, multicentre trial of interferon-αn1 for chronic myeloid leukaemia: improved survival irrespective of cytogenetic response. Lancet 345:1392–1396.
33. Hehlmann R, Heimpel H, Hasford J, Kolb HJ, et al. 1994. Randomized comparison of interferon-α with busulfan and hydroxyurea in chronic myelogenous leukemia. Blood 84:4064–4077.
34. Ohnishi K, Ohno R, Tomonaga M, Kamada N, et al. 1995. A randomized trial comparing interferon-α with busulfan for newly diagnosed chronic myelogenous leukemia in chronic phase. Blood 86:906–916.
35. Cannistra S, Tantravahi R, Robertson MJ, Griffin J, Canellos GP. 1990. Low-dose cytosine arabinoside induces cytogenetic remissions in patients with stable phase chronic myeloid leukemia (abstract). Blood 76 (Suppl 1):259a.
36. Kantarjian HM, Keating MJ, Estey EH, et al. 1992. Treatment of advanced stages of Philadelphia chromosome-positive chronic myelogenous leukemia with interferon-α and low-dose cytarabine. J Clin Oncol 10:772–778.
37. Guilhot F, Tanzer J, Bauters F, et al. 1991. A multicenter randomized study of alpha 2b interferon and hydroxyurea with or without cytosine-arabinoside in previously untreated patients with Ph+ CML. Leuk Lymphoma 11 (Suppl 1):181–183.
38. Lengyel P. 1982. Biochemistry of interferons and their actions. Annu Rev Biochem 51:251–282.
39. Maxwell B, Talpaz M, Gutterman JU. 1985. Down-regulation of peripheral blood cell interferon receptors in chronic myelogeneous leukemia patients undergoing human interferon (HuIFN) therapy. Int J Cancer 36:23–28.

40. Rosenblum M, Maxwell B, Talpaz M, et al. 1986. *In vivo* sensitivity and resistance of chronic myelogenous leukemia cells to alpha interferon: correlation with receptor binding and induction of 2'5' oligoadenylate synthetase. Cancer Res 46:4848–4852.
41. Bhatia R, Wayner EA, McGlave PB, Verfaillie CM. 1994. Interferon-α restores normal adhesion of chronic myelogenous leukemia hematopoietic progenitors to bone marrow stroma by correcting impaired β1 integrin receptor function. J Clin Invest 94:384–391.
42. McMahon M, Stark GR, Kerr IM. 1986. Interferon-induced gene expression in wild-type and interferon-resistant human lymphoblastoid (Daudi) cells. J Virol 57:362–366.
43. Dron M, Modjtahedi N, Brison O, et al. 1986. Interferon modulation of c-myc expression in cloned daudi cells: relationship to the phenotype of interferon resistance. Mol Cell Biol 6:1374–1378.
44. Friedman RL, Stark GR. 1985. α-Interferon-induced transcription of HLA and metallothionein genes containing homologous upstream sequences. Nature 314:637–639.
45. Kurzrock R, Talpaz M, Kantarjian H, et al. 1987. Therapy of chronic myelogenous leukemia with recombinant interferon-gamma. Blood 70:943–947.
46. Wandl UB, Kloke O, Nagel-Hiemke M, et al. 1992. Combination therapy with interferon alpha-2b plus low-dose interferon-gamma in pretreated patients with Ph-positive chronic myelogeneous leukemia. Br J Haematol 81:516–519.
47. Talpaz M, Kurzrock R, Kantarjian H, Rothberg J, Saks S, Evans L, Gutterman JU. 1991. A phase II study alternating alpha-2a-interferon and gamma-interferon therapy in patients with chronic myelogenous leukemia. Cancer 68:2125–2130.
48. Ratain MJ, Larson RA, Hooberman A, Pape L, Wallenberg J, Marcus S. 1988. Phase II study of recombinant beta interferon in chronic myelogenous leukemia (abstract). Blood 72 (Suppl 1):797a.
49. Kessler CM, Klein HG, Havlik RJ. 1982. Uncontrolled thrombocytosis in chronic myeloproliferative disorders. Br J Haematol 50:157–167.
50. Hehlmann R, Jahn M, Baumann B, et al. 1988. Essential thrombocythemia: clinical characteristics and course of 61 patients. Cancer 61:2487–2496.
51. Wu KK. 1978. Platelet hyperaggregability in patients with thrombocythemia. Ann Intern Med 88:7–11.
52. Talpaz M, Mavligit G, Keating M, et al. 1983. Human leukocyte interferon to control thrombocytosis in chronic myelogenous leukemia. Am J Med 99:789–792.
53. Talpaz M, Kurzrock R, Kantarjian H, et al. 1989. Recombinant interferon-alpha therapy of Philadelphia chromosome-negative myeloproliferative disorders with thrombocytosis. Am J Med 86:554–558.
54. Giles FJ, Gray AG, Brozovic M, et al. 1989. Alpha-interferon therapy for essential thrombocythaemia. Lancet 1:634–637.
55. Velu T, Delwiche F, Gangji D, et al. 1985. Therapeutic effect of human recombinant interferon-alpha-2c in essential thrombocythaemia. Oncology 42:10–14.
56. Gisslinger H, Linkesch W, Fritz E, et al. 1989. Long-term interferon therapy for thrombocytosis in myeloproliferative diseases. Lancet 1:634–637.
57. May D, Wandl UB, Niederle N. 1989. Treatment of essential thrombocythaemia with interferon alpha-2b. Lancet 1:96.
58. Bellucci S, Harousseau JL, Brice P, et al. 1988. Treatment of essential thrombocythaemia by alpha2a interferon. Lancet 2:960–961.
59. Kasparu H, Reisner R, Bernhart M, et al. 1987. Recombinant alpha-2b interferon in the treatment of essential thrombocythaemia. Blut 55:284–287.
60. Middlehoff G, Boll I. 1992. A long-term clinical trial of interferon alpha-therapy in essential thrombocythemia. Ann Hematol 64:207–209.
61. Berk PD, Goldberg JD, Donovan PB, Fruchtman SM, Berlin NI, Wasserman LR. 1986. Therapeutic recommendations in polycythemia vera based on Polycythemia Vera Study Group protocols. Semin Hematol 23:132–143.
62. Donovan PB, Kaplan ME, Goldberg JD, et al. 1984. Treatment of polycythemia vera with hydroxyurea. Am J Hematol 17:329–334.

63. Silver RT. 1993. Interferon-alpha-2b: A new treatment for polycythemia vera. Ann Intern Med 119:1091–1092.
64. Jimenez SA, Freundlich B, Rosenbloom J. 1984. Selective inhibition of human diploid fibroblast collagen synthesis by interferons. J Clin Invest 74:1112–1116.
65. Wickramasinghe SN, Peart S, Gill DS. 1987. Alpha-interferon in primary idiopathic myelofibrosis. Lancet 2:1524–1525.
66. Radin AI, Buckley P, Duffy TP. 1991. Interferon therapy for agnogenic myeloid metaplasia complicated by immune hemolytic anemia. Hematol Pathol 5:83–88.
67. Bouroncle BA, Wiseman BK, Doan CA. 1958. Leukemic reticuloendotheliosis. Blood 13:609–611.
68. Golomb HM, Catovsky D, Golde DW. 1978. Hairy cell leukemia: a clinical review based on 71 cases. Ann Intern Med 89:677–683.
69. Golomb HM, Catovsky D, Golde DW. 1983. Hairy cell leukemia: a five-year update on seventy-one patients. Ann Intern Med 99:485–486.
70. Golomb HM. 1983. Hairy cell leukemia: lessons learned in twenty-five years. J Clin Oncol 1:652–656.
71. Catovsky D, Pettit JE, Galton DAG, Splers SD, Harrison CV. 1974. Leukaemic reticuloendotheliosis ('hairy' cell leukaemia): a distinct clinicopathological entity. Br J Haematol 26:9–27.
72. Fitzpatrick J, O'Donnell A, DiLoro A, Bhargava A. 1986. Serum M-proteins in hairy cell leukemia, chronic lymphocytic leukemia and free ligh chain myeloma causing high resolution electropheresis/immunofixation (abstract). Blood 69:208A.
73. Rosove MH, Naeim F, Harwig S, Zighelboim J. 1980. Severe platelet dysfunction in hairy cell leukemia with improvement after splenectomy. Blood 55:903–906.
74. Cawley JC, Burns GF, Hayhoe RGH. 1980. A chronic lymphoproliferative disorder with distinctive features: a distinct variant of hairy cell leukemia. Leuk Res 4:547–559.
75. Catovsky D, Pettit JE, Galetto J, Okos A, Galton DAG. 1974. The B-lymphocyte nature of the hairy cell of leukemic reticuloendotheliosis. Br J Haematol 26:29–37.
76. Jansen J, LeBien TW, Kersey JH. 1982. The phenotype of the neoplastic cells of hairy cell leukemia studies with monoclonal antibodies. Blood 59:609–614.
77. Worman CP, Brooks DA, Hogg N, Zola H, Beverley PCL, Cawley JD. 1983. The nature of hairy cells: a study with a panel of monoclonal antibodies. Scand J Haematol 30:223–226.
78. Divine M, Farcet JP, Gourdin MF, et al. 1984. Phenotype study of fresh and cultured hairy cells with the use of immunologic markers and electron microscopy. Blood 64:547–552.
79. Anderson KC, Park EK, Bates MP, et al. 1983. Antigens on human plasma cells identified by monoclonal antibodies. J Immunol 130:1132–1138.
80. Anderson KA, Boyd AW, Fisher DC, et al. 1985. Hairy cell leukemia: a tumor of pre-plasma cells. Blood 65:620–629.
81. Cleary ML, Woods GS, Warnke R, Chao J, Sklar J. 1984. Immunoglobulin gene rearrangements in hairy cell leukemia. Blood 64:99–104.
82. Korsmeyer SJ, Greene WC, Cossman J, et al. 1983. Rearrangement and expression of immunoglobulin genes and expression of Tac antigen in hairy leukemia. Proc Natl Acad Sci USA 80:4522–4526.
83. Visser L, Shaw A, Slupsky J, Vos H, Poppema S. 1989. Monoclonal antibodies reactive with hairy cell leukemia. Blood 74:320–325.
84. Li CY, Yam LT, Lam KW. 1970. Studies of acid phosphatase isoenzymes in human leukocytes: demonstration of isoenzyme cell specificity. J Histochem Cytochem 18:901–910.
85. Quesada JR, Reuben J, Manning JT, et al. 1984. Alpha interferon for induction of remission in hairy cell leukemia. N Engl J Med 310:15–18.
86. Worman CP, Catovsky D, Cawley JC, et al. 1987. The U.K. experience with human lymphoblastoid interferon in HCL: a report of the first 50 cases. Leukemia 1:320–322.
87. Kamasio EE, Bernasconi C, Castoldi GL, et al. 1987. Human lymphoblastoid interferon for hairy cell leukemia: results from the Italian cooperative group. Leukemia 1:331–333.
88. Foon KA, Maluish AE, Abrams PG, et al. 1986. Recombinant leukocyte A interferon

therapy for advanced hairy cell leukemia: therapeutic and immunologic results. Am J Med 80:351–356.
89. Golomb HM, Jacobs A, Fefer A, et al. 1986. Alpha-2 interferon therapy of hairy cell leukemia: a multicenter study of 64 patients. J Clin Oncol 4:900–905.
90. Dadmarz R, Evans T, Secher D, et al. 1987. Hairy cells possess more interferon receptors than other lymphoid cell types. Leukemia 1:357–361.
91. Schwarzmeier JD, Schwabe M, Wagner L, et al. 1987. Effect of alpha-2-interferon on hairy cells and cell lines: a role for type I interferon receptors and RNA synthesis. Leukemia 1:361–365.
92. Faltynek CR, Princler GL, Rossio JL, et al. 1986. Relationship of the clinical response and binding of recombinant interferon alpha in patients with lymphoproliferative diseases. Blood 67:1077–1082.
93. Billard C, Sigaux F, Castaigne S, et al. 1986. Treatment of hairy cell leukemia with recombinant alpha interferon: II. *In vivo* down-regulation of alpha interferon receptors on tumor cells. Blood 67:821–826.
94. Billard C, Ferbus D, Sigaux F, et al. 1988. Action of interferon-alpha on hairy cell leukemia: expression of specific receptors and $(2'-5')$ oligo (A) synthetase in tumor cells from sensitive and resistant patients. Leukemia Res 12:11–18.
95. Nielsen B, Hokland M, Justesen J, et al. 1989. Immunological recovery and dose evaluation in IFN-alpha treatment of hairy cell leukemia: analysis of leukocyte differentiation antigens, NK and $2',5'$-oligoadenylate synthetase activity. Eur J Haematol 42:50–59.
96. Samuels BL, Golomb HM, Brownstein BH. 1986. *In vitro* induction of proteins by alpha-interferon in hairy cell leukemia. Cancer Res 46:4151–4155.
97. Samuels BL, Golomb HM, Brownstein BH. 1987. *In vivo* induction of proteins during therapy of hairy cell leukemia with alpha-interferon. Blood 69:1570–1573.
98. Paganelli KA, Evans SS, Han T, et al. 1986. B cell growth factor-induced proliferation of hairy cell lymphocytes and inhibition by type I interferon *in vitro*. Blood 67:937–942.
99. Mongini P, Seremetis S, Blessinger C, et al. 1988. Diversity in inhibitory effects of IFN-gamma and IFN-alpha A on the induced DNA synthesis of a hairy cell leukemia B lymphocyte clone reflects the nature of the activating ligand. Blood 72:1553–1559.
100. Ruco LP, Procopio A, Maccallini V, et al. 1983. Severe deficiency of natural killer activity in the peripheral blood of patients with hairy cell leukemia. Blood 61:1132–1137.
101. Griffiths SD, Cawley JC. 1987. The beneficial effects of alpha-interferon in hairy cell leukemia are not attributable to NK cell-mediated cytoxicity. Leukemia 1:372–376.
102. Starling GC, Nimmo JC, Hart DNJ. 1988. Hairy cell leukemia cells are relatively NK-resistant targets. Pathology 20:361–365.
103. Baldini L, Cortelezzi A, Polli N, et al. 1986. Human recombinant interferon alpha-2c enhances the expression of class II HLC antigens on hairy cells. Blood 67:458–464.
104. Naeim F, Jacobs AD. 1985. Bone marrow changes in patients with hairy cell leukemia treated by recombinant alpha-2-interferon. Human Pathol 16:1200–1205.
105. Bardawil RG, Ratain MJ, Golomb HM, et al. 1987. Changes in peripheral blood and bone marrow specimens during and after alpha-2b-interferon therapy for hairy cell leukemia. Leukemia 1:340–343.
106. Flandrin G, Sigaux F, Castaigne S, et al. 1986. Treatment of hairy cell leukemia with recombinant alpha interferon: I Quantitative study of bone marrow changes during the first months of treatment. Blood 67:817–820.
107. Steis RG, Smith JW II, Urba JW, et al. 1988. Resistance to recombinant interferon alfa-2a in hairy cell leukemia associated with neutralizing anti-interferon antibodies. N Engl J Med 318:1409–1413.
108. Spiers SDC, Moore D, Cassileth PA, et al. 1987. Hairy cell leukemia: complete remission with pentostatin (2'deoxycoformycin). N Engl J Med 316:825–830.
109. Saven A, Piro LD. 1992. Treatment of hairy cell leukemia. Blood 79:1111–1120.
110. Urba WJ, Baselor MW, Kopp WC, et al. 1989. Deoxycoformycin-induced immunosuppression in patients with hairy cell leukemia. Blood 73:38–46.

111. Foon KA, Nakano GM, Koller CA, Longo DL, Steis RG. 1986. Response to 2'-deoxycoformycin after failure of interferon-α in nonsplenectomized patients with hairy cell leukemia. Blood 68:297–300.
112. Piro LD, Carrera CJ, Carson DA, Butler E. 1990. Lasting remissions in hairy cell leukemia induced by a single infusion of 2-chlorodeoxyadenosine. N Engl J Med 322:1117–1121.
113. Cozzolino F, Torcia M, Adinucci D, et al. 1989. Production of interleukin-1 by bone marrow myeloma cells. Blood 74:380–387.
114. Garrett IR, Durie BGM, Nedwin GE, et al. 1989. Production of lymphotoxin, a bone resorbing cytokine, by cultured human myeloma cells. N Engl J Med 317:526–530.
115. Bataille R, Klein B. 1991. The bone resorbing activity of interleukin-6. J Bone Miner Res 9:1143–1146.
116. Jacobson DR, Zolla-Pazner S. 1986. Immunosuppression and infection in multiple myeloma. Semin Oncol 2:282–290.
117. Broder S, Humphrey R, Durm M, et al. 1975. Impaired synthesis of (non-paraprotein) immunoglobulins by circulating lymphocytes from patients with multiple myeloma. N Engl J Med 293:887–892.
118. Solomon A, Weiss DT, Kattine AA. 1991. Nephrotoxic potential of Bence Jones proteins. N Engl J Med 324:1845–1851.
119. Alexanian R, Barlogie B, Dixon D. 1990. Renal failure in multiple myeloma: pathogenesis and prognostic implications. Arch Intern Med 150:1693–1695.
120. Kyle RA, Greipp PR. 1983. Amyloidosis (AL): clinical and laboratory features in 229 cases. Mayo Clinic Proc 58:665–683.
121. Spiers ASD, Halpern R, Ross SC, et al. 1980. Meningeal myelomatosis. Arch Intern Med 140:256–259.
122. Pruzanski W, Watt JG. 1972. Serum viscosity and hyperviscosity syndrome in IgG multiple myeloma. Ann Intern Med 77:853–860.
123. Chandy KG, Stockley RG, Leonard RCF, et al. 1981. Relationships between serum viscosity and intravascular IgA polymer concentration in IgA myeloma. Clin Exp Immunol 46:653–661.
124. Perkins HA, MacKenzie MR, Fudenberg HH. 1970. Haemostatic defects in dysproteinaemias. Blood 35:695–707.
125. Lackner H. 1973. Haemostatic abnormalities associated with dysproteinaemias. Serum Haematol 10:125–133.
126. Bergsagel DE, Sprague CC, Austin C, Griffith KM. 1962. Evaluation of new chemotherapeutic agents in the treatment of multiple myeloma IV: L-Phenylalanine mustard. Cancer Chemother Res 21:87–93.
127. Alexanian R, Haut A, Khan AU, et al. 1969. Treatment of multiple myeloma: combination chemotherapy with different melphalan dose regimens. JAMA 208:1680–1685.
128. Boccadoro M, Marmont F, Tribalto M, et al. 1991. Multiple myeloma: VMCP/VBAP alternating combination chemotherapy is not superior to melphalan and prednisone even in high-risk patients. J Clin Oncol 9:444–448.
129. Gregory WM, Richards MA, Malpas JS. 1992. Combination chemotherapy versus melphalan and prednisolone in the treatment of multiple myeloma: an overview of published trials. J Clin Oncol 10:334–342.
130. Salmon SE, Shadduck RK, Schilling A. 1967. Intermittent high dose prednisone therapy for multiple myeloma. Cancer Chemother Rep 51:179–187.
131. Cooper MR, Dear K, McIntyre OR, et al. 1993. A randomized clinical trial comparing melphalan/prednisone with or without interferon alfa-2b in newly diagnosed patients with multiple myeloma: a cancer and leukemia group B study. J Clin Oncol 11:155–160.
132. Österborg A, Björkholm M, Björeman M, et al. 1993. Natural interferon-α in combination with melphalan/prednisone versus melphalan/prednisone in the treatment of multiple myeloma stages II and III: a randomized study from the myeloma group of central Sweden. Blood 81:1428–1434.
133. Hjorth M, Westin J, Dahl IMS, et al. 1996. Interferon-α2b added to melphalan–prednisone for initial and maintenance therapy in multiple myeloma. Ann Intern Med 124:212–222.

134. Browman GP, Bergsagel D, Sicheri D, et al. 1995. Randomized trial of interferon maintenance in multiple myeloma: a study of the National Cancer Institute of Canada Clinical Trials Group. J Clin Oncol 13:2354–2360.
135. Westin J, Rödjer S, Turesson I, et al. 1995. Interferon alfa-2b versus no maintenance therapy during the plateau phase in multiple myeloma: a randomized study. Br J Haematol 89:561–568.
136. Foon KA, Sherwin SA, Abrams PG, et al. 1984. Treatment of advanced non-Hodgkin's lymphoma with recombinant leucocyte A interferon. N Engl J Med 311:1148–1152.
137. McLaughlin P. 1993. The role of interferon in the therapy of low grade lymphoma. Leuk Lymphoma 10:17–20.
138. Ozer H, Anderson JR, Peterson BA, et al. 1994. Combination trial of subcutaneous recombinant $\alpha_2\beta$ interferon and oral cyclophosphamide in follicular low-grade non-Hodgkin's lymphoma. Med Pediatr Oncol 22:228–235.
139. Anderson JW, Smalley RV. 1993. Interferon alfa plus chemotherapy for non-Hodgkin's lymphoma: five-year follow-up. N Engl J Med 329:1821–1822.
140. McLaughlin P, Cabanillas F, Hagemeister FB, et al. 1993. CHOP-bleo plus interferon for stage IV low-grade lymphoma. Ann Oncol 4:205–211.
141. Hagenbeek A, Carde P, Somers R, et al. 1992. Maintenance of remission with human recombinant alpha-2 interferon (Roferon-A) in patients with stages III and IV low-grade malignant non-Hodgkin's lymphoma: results from a prospective, randomized phase III clinical trial in 331 patients. Blood 80:288A.
142. Bunn PA, Foon KA, Inde DC, et al. 1984. Recombinant leukocyte A interferon: an active agent in advanced cutaneous T-cell lymphomas. Ann Intern Med 101:484–487.
143. Bunn PA Jr, Hoffman SJ, Norris D, et al. 1994. Systemic therapy of cutaneous T-cell lymphomas (mycosis fungoides and the Sézary syndrome). Ann Intern Med 121:592–602.
144. Ross C, Tingsgaard P, Jorgensen H, Vejlsgaard GL. 1993. Interferon treatment of cutaneous T-cell lymphoma. Eur J Haematol 51:63–72.
145. Gill PS, Ilarkington W, Kaplan MH, et al. 1995. Treatment of adult T-cell leukemia-lymphoma with a combination of interferon alfa and zidovudine. N Engl J Med 332:1744–1748.
146. Lauer SJ, Ochs J, Pollock BH, Buchanan GR. 1994. Recombinant alpha-2B interferon treatment for childhood T-lymphoblastic disease in relapse. Cancer 74:197–202.

2. Interferon use in solid tumors

William J. John and Kenneth A. Foon

1. Introduction

Interferon-alpha as a single agent has been shown to have little activity in solid tumors. No responses were reported in gastrointestinal tumors and non-small cell lung cancer [1–4]. Interferon-alpha also failed to prolong disease-free and overall survival as maintenance therapy in patients with small cell lung cancer [5]. In vitro studies have suggested significant cytotoxic interactions between interferon-alpha and chemotherapeutic agents such as fluorouracil [6]. Recent clinical research has focused on combinations of interferon-alpha with chemotherapeutic agents. The review in this chapter will focus on interferon-alpha in combination with cytotoxic chemotherapy in the treatment of gastrointestinal malignancies and lung cancer.

2. Colorectal cancer

Thirty patients, 17 previously untreated, were given a combination of fluorouracil and interferon-alpha in the first report of combined fluorouracil and interferon-alpha in the treatment of advanced colorectal cancer [7]. Encouraging results, including 13 responses in 17 previously untreated patients, were reported. However, none of these responses was a complete response. The dosing schedule was fluorouracil $750\,mg/m^2$ daily for five days. After one week of rest, the patients were given the same dose of fluorouracil weekly. Interferon was administered at 9 million units subcutaneously three times each week starting on the first day. None of the previously treated patients responded to chemotherapy. Median survival of the previously untreated group was 16 months, and toxicity was quite manageable, with one toxic death. After this initial report, there were five subsequent phase II studies using the same dose and treatment schedule [8–12]. These studies are summarized in table 1. Responses varied from 24% to 64%, and median survival ranged from 10 to 18 months. Treatment-related toxicities are summarized in table 2. Significant differences in these experiences included a 34% neurologic toxicity characterized by unstable gait, delirium, dizziness, memory loss, and subsequent

Table 1. Fluorouracil and interferon in advanced colorectal cancer

Patient number	Response rate	Survival	Reference
38	26%	13 months	8
45	35%	16 months	9
59	31%	10 months	10
35	24%	NR	11
38	42%	18 months	12

Table 2. Fluorouracil and interferon-alpha: toxicity

Mucositis
Diarrhea
Leukopenia
Thrombocytopenia
Neurotoxicity
Fever
Chills
Myalgias
Fatigue

Table 3. Fluorouracil and interferon-alpha: alternative schedules

Regimen	Response	Duration
5-FU 750 mg/m^2 × 5d, INF 9 mu d1,3,5 repeat q 14d	31%	7.5 mo
5-FU 250 mg/m^2 Cl × 6 wks, IFN 3 mu tiw	33%	5 mo

dementia [8]. This degree of neurologic toxicity was not noted in any of the other trials despite the identical treatment schedule. The etiology of the neurologic toxicity as seen in this one study was not delineated.

It is important to remember that the dose and schedule of fluorouracil and interferon-alpha were empirically derived, and many studies were subsequently undertaken that changed the dose and schedule in order to improve results. Table 3 summarized the results of 39 previously untreated patients who were treated with 750 mg/m^2 per day of fluorouracil as a continuous infusion for five days with 9 million units of interferon-alpha on day 1, 3, and 5 [13]. This program was repeated at 14-day intervals. One complete and 11 partial responses were reported, with a median duration of response at 7.5 months. Toxicities were relatively unchanged from those reported with the first treatment schedule. Thirty patients received 250 mg/m^2 per day of fluorouracil as a continuous low-dose infusion with interferon-alpha at 3 million units three times per week for six-week intervals [14]. The toxicity of this regimen was more significant than the original schedule, with all patients treated for more than two months requiring dose reductions due to toxicity.

Table 4. Fluorouracil and interferon-alpha: salvage in colorectal cancer

Number of patients	Response	Duration
12	36%	2 mo
13	0%	NA
9	11%	4 mo

Ten patients achieved a partial response, but the duration of the response was short and no clinical improvement of survival was realized.

Based on the limited results summarized in table 4, it is clear that systemic interferon-alpha and fluorouracil has no role in the salvage therapy of patients with colorectal cancer. Responses were minimal, side effects were significant, and no benefit and survival was realized. Forty-eight patients were treated with hepatic-artery interferon-alpha at $5\,Mu/m^2/day$ over six hours and fluorouracil at $1500\,mg/m^2/day$ over 18 hours, after failure of system fluorouracil and leucovorin [16]. Cycles were repeated every 28–35 days. There were 3 (6.6%) complete and 12 (26.6%) partial responses in 45 evaluable patients. Duration of response was seven months, and survival was 15 months. Toxicity was acceptable, with grade III and IV toxicity as follows: 40% mucositis, 42% neutropenia, and 12% thrombocytopenia. The investigators felt that the efficacy was promising and that treatment was well tolerated.

More recent investigations in colorectal cancer have introduced leucovorin to 5-FU and interferon as dual modulation for advanced disease. Dual modulation has the advantage of incorporating different mechanisms of action for the treatment of advanced colorectal cancer. The initial protocol treatment schedule was interferon-alpha $5\,mu/m^2$ on days 1–7, fluorouracil $370\,mg/m^2$ on days 2–6, and leucovorin $500\,mg/m^2$ on days 2–6 [17]. The initial program emphasized the higher doses of interferon to achieve to complete modulation of fluorouracil. This treatment was based on in vitro testing that showed that at least 5 million units/m^2 was necessary for pharmacological modulation [18].

Table 5 summarizes the results of double modulation [17,19–26]. Results vary from 10% to 54%. Toxicity, mainly stomatitis and diarrhea, was moderate but was considered manageable. Median time to treatment failure ranged from 8 to 16 months. Investigators have published results of phase II studies utilizing both bolus and infusion fluorouracil, leucovorin, and interferon [23]. The response rate was comparable to trials without interferon. However, toxicity was significantly worse. The recently completed NSABP trial utilized 5-FU, leucovorin, and interferon for the treatment of stage II and III colon cancer after definitive resection; results are shown in figure 1. Results of this trial are still preliminary at this time.

Fifteen patients were treated with a similar schedule after failing 5-FU and

Table 5. Fluorouracil, leucovorin, and interferon-alpha in colorectal cancer

Number of patients	Response	Duration
46	54%	7.8 mo
43	10%	NR
45	25%	11 mo
15	20%	NR
45	51%	NR

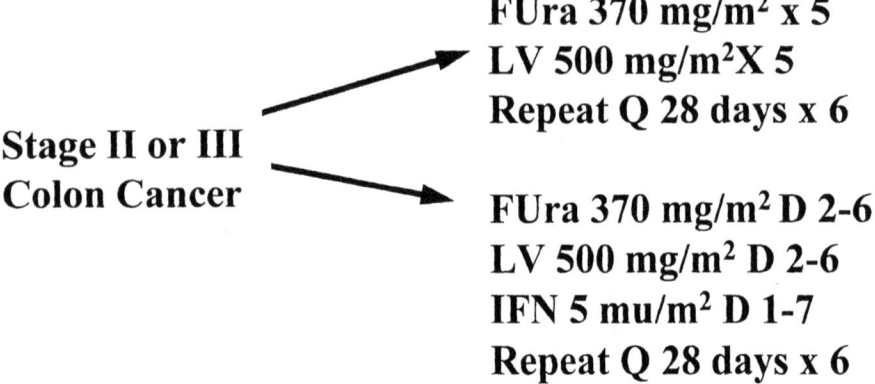

Figure 1. Fluorouracil, leucovorin, and interferon-alpha in the treatment of colon cancer: the NSABP trial.

leucovorin [27]. No responses were recorded, and significant toxicities developed. As with all other interventions including interferon and fluorouracil, this schedule was unsuccessful in salvage therapy for colorectal cancer.

In an effort to more clearly define the role of interferon in the treatment of previously untreated advanced colorectal cancer, two large phase III trials have been reported [28,29]. The treatment schemas are detailed in figures 2 and 3. In the first study, 245 patients were treated with fluorouracil with or without interferon-alpha. Response rates, time to treatment failure, and survival were not significantly different in the two treatment groups. Both groups had a response rate of less than 35%. In the second large trial, 496 patients were randomized to receive either 5-FU and interferon or 5-FU and leucovorin. Responses in both studies were less than 20%, and no significant differences between the two arms were seen either in the time to treatment failure or in overall survival, the former being seven months and the latter 11 months. These results do not compare favorably with other survival seen in patients with advanced colorectal cancer treated with various forms of biochemical modulation of fluorouracil.

Investigators have retrospectively reviewed the cost of various treatments

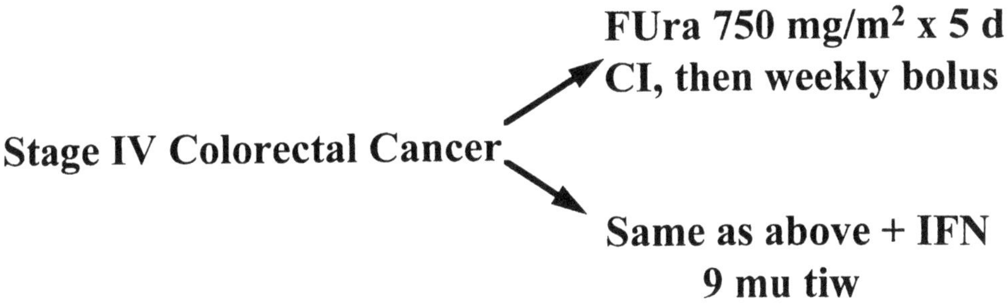

Stage IV Colorectal Cancer
→ FUra 750 mg/m² x 5 d CI, then weekly bolus
→ Same as above + IFN 9 mu tiw

Figure 2. Fluorouracil and interferon-alpha, phase III [28].

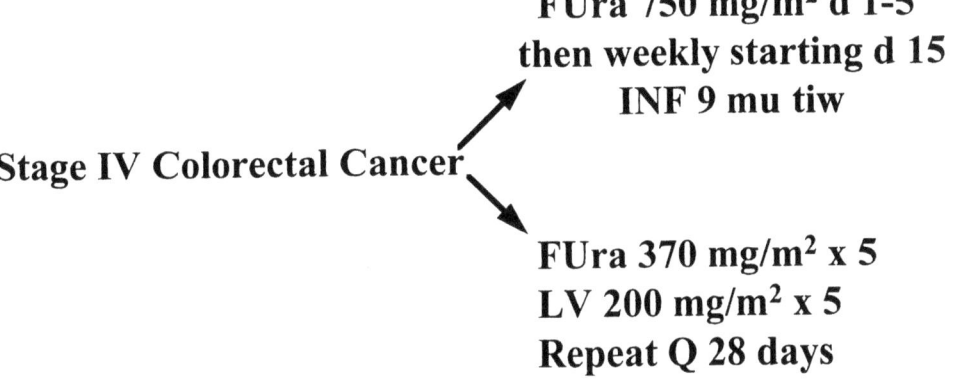

Stage IV Colorectal Cancer
→ FUra 750 mg/m² d 1-5 then weekly starting d 15 INF 9 mu tiw
→ FUra 370 mg/m² x 5 LV 200 mg/m² x 5 Repeat Q 28 days

Figure 3. Fluorouracil and interferon-alpha, phase III [29].

Table 6. Fluorouracil in advanced colorectal cancer: cost

Method	Cost without drug charges	Cost with drug charges
Protracted infusion	$1344	$1408
FUra and LV	$1064	$1124
FUra and IFN	$490	$1930

of colorectal cancer, including, specifically, fluorouracil and interferon-alpha, fluorouracil and either high-dose leucovorin or low-dose leucovorin, and protracted venous infusion of fluorouracil [30]. Results are shown in table 6. When charges other than drug costs were calculated, treatment with fluorouracil and interferon proved to be a very cost-effective therapy. However, when the cost of the drugs were included, fluorouracil and interferon was the most costly treatment.

Current data would suggest that interferon-alpha has no role in the treatment of stage IV colorectal cancer. Based on the available data, interferon-alpha cannot be routinely recommended in the management of advanced colorectal cancer.

3. Esophageal cancer

Interferon-alpha has no single-agent activity in the treatment of either squamous cell or adenocarcinoma of the esophagus. Two phase II studies report the treatment of 61 patients with fluorouracil and interferon-alpha [31–33]. Forty patients were treated with the same schedule reported by Wadler in his treatment of colorectal cancer. Of those patients, 27% responded to therapy, and toxicity was similar to that seen in colorectal cancer. Duration of response was 6–7 months. Eight adenocarcinomas and 13 squamous carcinomas were treated with an identical regimen. Ten of those patients had local regional disease, and 11 had metastatic disease. The response rate was 25%. Cisplatin probably has the best single-agent response in patients with esophageal cancer. Twenty-one patients were treated with cisplatin, fluorouracil, and interferon-alpha [29]. The response rate in 15 evaluable patients was 50%. Long-term survival data were not recorded in this trial. With these limited data, no long-range conclusions can be made regarding the use of interferon-alpha in the treatment of esophageal cancer. It is unclear that interferon-alpha will have a lasting role in the treatment of esophageal cancer.

4. Gastric cancer

Table 7 gives the overall experience of interferon-alpha in the treatment of gastric cancer [34–36]. The dosage and schedule were similar except that the interferon dose was reduced to 5 million units three times a week. Four of 13 patients were noted to have objective responses with similar toxicity. In the second study, 44 patients were treated, with a response rate of 25% and a median survival of 29 weeks. The third phase II study utilized six courses of weekly fluorouracil with double modulation utilizing leucovorin and interferon-alpha. Seventeen of 44 patient responded, with six complete responders. The duration of response and survival have not been reported. As with esophageal tumors, the data are insufficient to draw a conclusion regarding the role of interferon in the treatment of gastric cancer.

Table 7. Fluorouracil and interferon: gastric cancer

Number of patients	Response
14	31%
44	25%
41	41%[a]

[a] Received leucovorin.

Table 8. Fluorouracil, leucovorin, and interferon: pancreas cancer

Number of patients	Response
13	23%
32	12%
24	8%

5. Pancreas cancer

Interferon-alpha has no single-agent activity in pancreas cancer. In one report, fluorouracil was utilized with interferon-alpha in 49 previously untreated patients with locally advanced unresectable disease or metastatic disease [37]. The response rate was 4%. Nineteen patients suffered grade III or IV toxicity with diarrhea, inanition, neutropenia, and stomatitis. The conclusion of this study was that this regimen had no activity in pancreas cancer and that the toxicity was significant. Table 8 summarizes the phase II experience of fluorouracil, interferon-alpha, and leucovorin in pancreas cancer [38–40]. Sixty-nine patients were treated in three trials, with a response rate ranging anywhere from 8% to 23%. No complete responders were seen. Survival was not affected. Toxicity was significant, with up to 50% of patients having fever, leukopenia, diarrhea, stomatitis, and decreased performance status. In one study of 13 patients treated with protracted venous infusion 5-FU and interferon, one responder was noted with a duration of response of three months. The overall survival was eight months. Toxicity was significant. Interferon does not appear to have any role in the treatment of pancreas cancer.

6. Hepatoma

Treatment of hepatoma was initiated in 71 patients with interferon-alpha 50 million units/m^2 as supportive care [41]. Patients receiving interferon achieved a survival that was twice as long as supportive care — 14 versus 7 weeks. Thirty-one percent achieved an objective tumor response. Thirty-four percent required dose reductions due to toxicity. Interferon was felt to be a potentially reasonable alternative to other cytotoxic chemotherapy. Fluorouracil and interferon have been used in treating hepatoma, along with doxorubicin and interferon [42]. Eighteen patients were treated with fluorouracil, with three objective responders and modest toxicity. Thirty-one patients were treated with doxorubicin and interferon, with one objective responder and no effect on survival [43].

The disparity between phase II studies with combinations and the promising potential single-agent activity of interferon-alpha is difficult to explain. Further studies are necessary to define the role of interferon-alpha in the treatment of hepatoma.

7. Non-small cell lung cancer

Treatment of stage IV non-small cell lung cancer with interferon-alpha alone has been unsuccessful. Responses are exceedingly rare, and there has been no impact on survival. Phase II experience with cisplatin and interferon-alpha has been more encouraging [44]. Sixty patients were treated with interferon-alpha 3–5 million units weekly and cisplatin $100\,mg/m^2$ every 21 to 28 days. Eighteen patients received a partial response, and toxicity was manageable, although it was felt that the nausea and vomiting was more severe.

One hundred eighty-two patients were treated with chemotherapy with or without interferon, as outlined in figure 4 [45]. Ninety-two patients received chemotherapy alone, while 90 received chemotherapy plus interferon. The primary endpoint of this study was survival, and patients receiving chemotherapy alone lived significantly longer than those that received interferon (6 versus 5.5 months), despite significantly more responses in the interferon group (8% versus 19%). The addition of interferon also increased the incidence of leukopenia, thrombocytopenia, nausea, vomiting, mucositis, inanition, and anorexia. No toxic deaths were observed. It was felt by the investigators that interferon potentially was effective chemotherapy but that this effect was not associated with improved survival and was associated with increased toxicity. There has also been a limited 25-patient experience with continuous infusion cisplatin given at $20\,mg/m^2/day$ for five days with interferon on day 1, 3, and 5. These cycles were repeated every 28 days. With this dose and schedule, the response rate was less than 20%, and survival was unchanged. Toxicity was significant and included nausea, vomiting, and renal dysfunction.

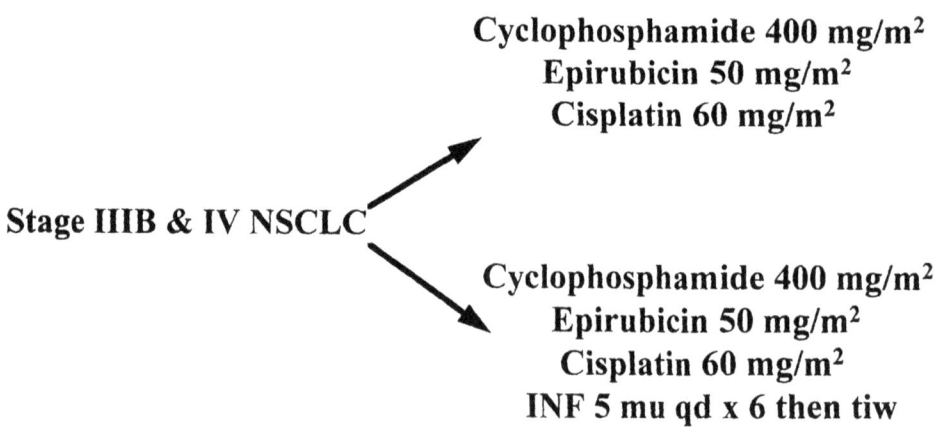

Figure 4. Chemotherapy and interferon-alpha in non-small cell lung cancer, phase III.

8. Conclusions

There is no treatment benefit for solid tumors with interferon-alpha. Except for colorectal cancer, all the data consist of phase I or phase II experience. The consensus of available information suggests no role for the use of interferon-alpha in the treatment of patients with colorectal cancer. There may be some additive effect in patients given 5-FU and leucovorin, however, the added toxicity is significant. The initial optimism fueled by phase II studies has not been confirmed in phase III trials.

References

1. Neefe JR, Silgals R, Ayoob M, Schein PS. 1984. Minimal activity of recombinant clone a interferon in metastatic colon cancer. J Biol Respir Mod 3(4):366–370.
2. Figlin RA. 1987. Biotherapy with interferon in solid tumors. Oncol Nurs Forum (Suppl 6): 23–26.
3. Gilewski TA, Golomb HM. 1989. Interferon in the treatment of malignant disease. In Zenser TV, CoE RM, eds. Cancer and Aging: Progress in Research and Treatment. New York: Springer, 1989.
4. Foon KA. 1989. Biological response modifiers: the new immunotherapy. Cancer Res 49:1621–1639.
5. Kelly K, Crowley JJ, Bunn PA, et al. 1995. Role of recombinant interferon alfa-2a maintenance in patients with limited-stage small-cell lung cancer responding to concurrent chemoradiation: a Southwest Oncology Group study. J Clin Oncol 13:2924–2930.
6. Wadler S, Wersto R, Weinberg V, et al. 1990. Interaction of fluorouracil and interferon in human colon cancer cell lines: cytotoxic and cytokinetic effects. Cancer Res 50:5735–5739.
7. Wadler S, Schwartz EL, Goldman M, et al. 1989. Fluorouracil and recombinant-alfa-2a-interferon: an active regimen against advanced colorectal carcinoma. J Clin Oncol 7:1769–1775.
8. Kemeny N, Younes A. 1992. Alfa-2a interferon and 5-fluorouracil for advanced colorectal carcinoma: the Memorial Sloan–Kettering experience. Sem Oncol 19 (2, Suppl 3):171–175.
9. Pazdur R, Moore DF Jr, Bready B. 1992. Modulation of fluorouracil with recombinant alfa interferon: M.D. Anderson clinical trial. Sem Oncol 19 (2, Suppl 3):176–179.
10. Weh HJ, Platz D, Braumann D, et al. 1992. Phase II trial of 5-fluorouracil and recombinant interferon alfa-2b in metastatic colorectal carcinoma. Eur J Cancer 28A:1820–1823.
11. Diaz Rubio E, Jimeno J, Camps C, et al. 1992. Treatment of advanced colorectal cancer with recombinant interferon alpha and fluorouracil: activity in liver metastasis. Cancer Invest 10:259–264.
12. Wadler S, Lembersky B, Atkins M, et al. 1991. Phase II trial of fluorouracil and recombinant interferon alfa-2a in patients with colorectal carcinoma: an Eastern Cooperative Oncology Group study. J Clin Oncol 9:1806–1810.
13. Pazdur R, Ajani JA, Patt YZ, et al. 1993. Phase II evaluation of recombinant alpha-2a-interferon and continuous infusion fluorouracil in previously untreated metastatic colorectal adenocarcinoma. Cancer 71:1214–1218.
14. John WJ, Neefe JR, Macdonald JS, et al. 1993. 5-fluorouracil and interferon-alpha-2a in advanced colorectal cancer: Results of two treatment schedules. Cancer 72:3191–3195.
15. Pavlick AC, DelGaudio D, Harper H, Rosenbluth R, Pecora AL. 1992. Salvaged therapy with continuous infusion 5-fluorouracil and alpha interferon in patients with colorectal cancer. Proc Am Soc Clin Oncol 11:A565.

16. Patt YZ, Hoque A, Lozano R, et al. 1997. Phase II trial of hepatic arterial infusion of fluorouracil and recombinant human interferon alfa-2b for liver metastases of colorectal cancer refractory to systemic fluorouracil and leucovorin. J Clin Oncol 15:1432–1438.
17. Grem JL, McAtee N, Murphy RF, et al. 1991. A pilot study of interferon alfa-2a in combinantion with fluorouracil plus high-dose leucovorin in metastatic gastrointestinal carcinoma. J Clin Oncol 9:1811–1820.
18. Yee LK, Allegra CJ, Steinberg SM, et al. 1992. Decreased catabolism of 5-fluorouracil in peripheral blood monocytes during therapy with 5-fluorouracil, leucovorin and interferon alpha-2a. J Natl Cancer Inst 84:1820–1825.
19. Grem JL, Hoth D, Hamilton MJ, et al. 1987. An overview of the current status and future direction of clinical trials of 5-fluorouracil and folinic acid. Cancer Treat Rep 71:1249–1264.
20. Taylor CW, Modiano MR, Woodson ME, et al. 1992. A phase I trial of fluorouracil, leucovorin, and recombinant interferon alpha-2B in patients with advanced malignancy. Semin Oncol 19 (2, Suppl 3):185–190.
21. Grem JL, Jordan E, Robson ME, et al. 1993. Phase II study of fluorouracil, leucovorin and interferon-alfa-2a in metastatic colorectal carcinoma. J Clin Oncol 11:1737–1745.
22. Schmoll JH, Kohne-Wompner CH, Hiddeman W, et al. 1992. Interferon alpha-2b, 5-fluorouracil and folinic acid combination therapy in advanced colorectal cancer: preliminary results of a phase I/II trial. Semin Oncol 19 (2, Suppl 3):191–196.
23. Tournigand C, Louvat C, de Gramont A, et al. 1997. Bimonthly high-dose leucovorin and 5-fluorouracil 48-hour infusion with interferon-alpha-2a in patients with advanced colorectal cancer. Cancer 79:1094–1099.
24. Punt CJ, Burhouts JT, Croles JJ, et al. 1993. Continuous infusion of high-dose 5-fluorouracil in combination with leucovorin and recombinant interferon-Alpha-2b in patients with advanced colorectal cancer. A multicenter phase II study. Cancer 72:2107–2111.
25. Sobrero A, Nobile MT, Guglielmi A, et al. 1992. Phase II study of 5-fluorouracil plus leucovorin and interferon alpha-2b in advance colorectal cancer. Eur J Cancer 28A:850–852.
26. Cascinu S, Fedeli A, Fedeli SL, et al. 1992. Double biochemical modulation of 5-fluorouracil leucovorin and cyclic low dose interferon alpha-2b in advanced colorectal cancer patients. Ann Oncol 3:489–491.
27. Bernhard H, Klein O, Meyer zum Buschenfeld KH, et al. 1992. Treatment of refractory colorectal carcinomas with fluorouracil, folinic acid, and interferon alfa-2a. Semin Oncol 19 (2, Suppl 3):204–207.
28. Corfu-A Study Group. Phase III randomized study of two fluorouracil combinations with either interferon alfa-2a or leucovorin for advanced colorectal cancer. J Clin Oncol 13:921–928.
29. Hill M, Norman A, Cunningham D, et al. 1995. Fluorouracil with or without interferon alfa-2b on tumor response, survival and quality of life in advanced colorectal cancer. J Clin Oncol 13:2317–2323.
30. Lokich J, Anderson N, Bern M, et al. 1991. Comparison cost of three chemotherapy regimens for advanced colon cancer: 5-fluorouracil (5FU)+leucovorin (LCV), 5-FU + interferon (IFN), and protracted-infusion 5FU (PIF). Proc Am Soc Clin Oncol 10:A436.
31. Kelsen D, Lovett D, Wong J, et al. 1992. Interferon alfa-2a and fluorouracil in the treatment of patients with advanced esophageal cancer. J Clin Oncol 10:269–274.
32. Wadler S, Fell S, Haynes H, et al. 1993. Treatment of carcinoma of the esophagus with 5-fluorouracil and recominant alfa-2a-interferon. Cancer 71:1726–1730.
33. Sirott MN, Kelsen D, Johnson B, et al. 1992. Alpha-interferon (IFN) 5-fluorouracil (FU) and cisplatin (CDDP): an active regimen in advanced adenocarcinoma (adenoca) and squamous cancer (SCC) of the esophagus (meeting abstract). Proc Am Soc Clin Oncol 11:A501.
34. Lee KH, Lee JS, Suh C, et al. 1992. Combination of fluorouracil and recombinant interferon alpha-2b in advanced gastric cancer. A phase I trial. Am J Clin Oncol 15:141–145.
35. Pazdur R, Ajani JA, Winn R, et al. 1992. A phase II trial of 5-fluorouracil and recombinant alpha-2a-interferon in previously untreated metastatic gastric carcinoma. Cancer 69:878–882.
36. Jager-Arand E, Bernhard H, Klein O, et al. 1993. Combination 5-fluorouracil (FU), folinic

acid (FA), and alpha-interferon 2B (IFN) in advanced gastric cancer (meeting abstract). Proc Am Soc Clin Oncol 12:A559.
37. Pazdur R, Ajani JA, Abbruzzese JI, et al. 1992. Phase II evaluation of fluorouracil and recombinant alpha-2a-interferon in previously untreated patients with pancreatic adenocarcinoma. Cancer 70:2073–2076.
38. Knuth A, Bernhard H, Klein O, et al. 1992. Combination fluorouracil, folinic acid, and interferon-alfa-2a: an active regimen in advanced pancreatic carcinoma. Semin Oncol 19 (2, Suppl 3):211–214.
39. Scheithauer W, Pfeffel F, Kornek G, et al. 1992. A phase II trial of 5-fluorouracil, leucovorin and recombinant alfa-2b interferon in advanced adenocarcinoma of the pancreas. Cancer 70:1864–1866.
40. Cascinu S, Fedeli A, Fedeli SL, et al. 1993. 5-fluorouracil, leucovorin and interferon alpha-2b in advanced pancreatic cancer: a pilot study. Ann Oncol 4:83–84.
41. Lai CL, Lau JY, Wu PC, et al. 1993. Recombinant interferon-alpha in inoperable hepatocellular carcinoma: a randomized controlled trial. Hepatology 17:389–394.
42. Patt YZ, Noonan C, Pazdur R, et al. 1991. Phase II trial of 5-FU and R interferon-alpha (RIFN) in hepatocullular carcinoma (HCC) (meeting abstract). Proc Am Soc Clin Oncol 10:A442.
43. Kardinal CG, Moertel CG, Wieand HS, et al. 1993. Combined doxorubicin and alpha-interferon therapy of advanced hepatocellular carcinoma. Cancer 71:2187–2190.
44. Olsen BK, Ernst P, Nissen MH, et al. 1987. Recombinant interferon-alpha therapy of small cell and squamous cell carcinoma of the lung: a phase II study. Eur J Cancer Clin Oncol 23:987–989.
45. Ardizzoni A, Salvati F, Rosso R, et al. 1993. Combination of chemotherapy and recombinant alpha-interferon in advanced non-small cell lung cancer: multicenter randomized FONICAP trial report. Cancer 72:2929–2935.

3. Cellular vaccine therapies for cancer

Michael J. Mastrangelo, Takami Sato, Edmund C. Lattime,
Henry C. Maguire, Jr., and David Berd

1. Introduction

The presence of functionally specific tumor-associated antigens was first convincingly demonstrated by Prehn and Main [1]. These investigators immunized syngeneic mice with a chemically induced sarcoma using a technique whereby the transplanted tumor was allowed to grow but was excised before it killed the host. These now surgically cured mice were able to reject a subsequent transplant of the same tumor yet accepted a skin graft from a mouse of the same strain as that in which the tumor had arisen. This experiment provided a scientific foundation for the pursuit of active specific immunization as a cancer treatment (i.e., antigens existed on tumor cells that could be targeted to effect tumor rejection) as well as a caution (i.e., tumors can grow progressively in the presence of concomitant immunity) that until recently seems to have gone unnoticed. Investigators have narrowly focused on improving the immunogenicity of their vaccines and are only now coming to recognize the emerging evidence that human tumors can and do grow in the presence of an immune response.

Tumor cells not only were the sole source of antigens available to early investigators but also were a logical first choice, since they display not one or a few epitopes but all the rejection-related antigens expressed by the tumor and do so in the context of the appropriate major histocompatibility complex (MHC) molecules. Since tumor cells (especially autologous tumor cells) are of limited availability and are cumbersome to use, investigators are exploring more 'practical' alternatives. However, tumor cells, particularly autologous tumor cells, remain the benchmark against which the performance of all other vaccines must be compared. Cutaneous melanoma has served as a focus for clinical trials of active specific immunization because of the well-documented spontaneous regression of primary and also, rarely, of metastatic tumors and because of the accessibility of tumor tissue. Renal cell cancer has attracted interest for similar reasons. A few studies have been carried out in patients with adenocarcinoma of the large bowel and in patients with non-small cell lung cancer. This chapter reviews the development of tumor cell-based vaccines, describes their promise, defines their limitations, and attempts to identify reasonable avenues for further development. Only those trials reporting a clinical outcome are considered.

2. Trials in patients with clinically evident residual disease

The usual goal of vaccine strategies is disease prevention. However, the early trials of active specific immunization with tumor cell-based vaccines were conducted in a therapy setting.

2.1. Melanoma

The results of active specific immunization with whole tumor cell vaccines in patients with clinically evident residual melanoma are presented in table 1. Only 1 of 64 patients [2–5] immunized intradermally or subcutaneously with autologous tumor cells alone experienced objective tumor regression. The use of the intralymphatic route for administration seemingly enhanced the objective response rate (18%), but this report by Ahn et al. [6] has not been confirmed.

The addition of microbial adjuvants such as bacille Calmette–Guerin (BCG) to whole melanoma cell vaccines appeared to have improved the response, rate with six complete and nine partial remissions among 79 patients (19%) [7–9]. However, in our experience [8], even the complete remissions were disappointingly brief, lasting just 3–4 months.

Berd and coinvestigators [10] exploited the immunopotentiating effects of cyclophosphamide to enhance the cutaneous delayed-type hypersensitivity (DTH) response to autologous melanoma cells. Nineteen melanoma patients were treated either with vaccine (autologous tumor + BCG) alone or with

Table 1. Active specific immunization with whole tumor cell vaccines in patients with clinical evidence of residual melanoma

Investigators	Vaccine	Response rate
Ikonopisov et al. [2]	Rad AU TC, SC	0/13
Krementz et al. [3]	Rad AU TC, ID	1 CR/19
Currie et al. [4]	Rad AU TC, SC	0/22
McCarthy et al. [5]	Rad AU TC, SC	0/10
Ahn et al. [6]	Rad AL TC, Ily	7 PR/38
Gerner & Moore [7]	Au or AL TC, ID + microbial antigens, IL	1 CR, 1 PR/21
Laucius et al. [8]	Rad AU TC + BCG, ID	2 CR, 2 PR/18
Morton et al. [9]	Rad AL TC + BCG, ID	3 CR, 6 PR/40
Berd et al. [11]	Rad AU TC + BCG, ID post-cy	4 CR, 1 PR/40

Abbreviations: Rad, x-irradiated; AU, autologous; AL, allogeneic; TC, tumor cells; SC, subcutaneous; ID, intradermal; IL, intralesional; ILY, intralymphatic; CR, complete response; PR, partial response; BCG, bacille Calmette-Guerin; Cy, Cyclophosphamide.

vaccine injected three days after the intravenous administration of cyclophosphamide ($300\,mg/m^2$). Of the patients who completed two vaccine treatments, 7 of 8 cyclophosphamide pre-treated patients but only 2 of 7 control patients had DTH reactions to autologous tumor greater than 5 mm ($p = 0.034$).

Active specific immunization with cyclophosphamide-induced immunopotentiation has undergone limited evaluation in humans. Berd et al. [11] noted four complete responses and one partial response among 40 evaluable patients (table 1). This response rate is no better than the previously reported results of this group [8] with autologous tumor cells plus BCG without cyclophosphamide: two complete and two partial responses in 18 evaluable patients. However, the remission duration was prolonged: 10 months (range 7–120) for the cyclophosphamide-treated group versus three months (range 2–4) for the group treated without cyclophosphamide.

Working with whole tumor cells is cumbersome. Mitchell and his coworkers have explored a therapeutic vaccine composed of mechanically disrupted melanoma cells from two cell lines combined with the adjuvant DETOX (a mixture of *M. phlei* cell wall skeletons, monophosphoryl lipid A, and squalane). The several trials conducted with this material in patients with clinically evident residual disease have been reviewed by Mitchell [12]. In his personal experience over nine years, five complete and 15 partial responses were observed in 106 patients (19%). The median duration of response was 21 months. In a multicenter trial, there were five complete and seven partial responses among 139 patients (8%). Median survival was 23 months. Likewise, in the phase III comparison with chemotherapy, only one partial and two complete responses were noted in 70 patients (4.4%). In aggregate, there were 12 complete and 35 partial responses in 315 patients (11%).

Tumor cells, particularly autologous tumor cells, are weakly immunogenic. The various efforts to enrich the tumor cell surface with foreign proteins are grouped here under the rubric of *antigen supplementation*, and the clinical trials [5,15–19] are summarized in table 2. The goal of antigen supplementa-

Table 2. Active specific immunization with antigen-supplemented tumor cell-based vaccines in patients with clinically evident residual melanoma

Investigator	Vaccine	Outcome
Livingston et al. [15]	AU and/or AL VSV lysate	0/9 resp
Wallack et al. [16]	AU vaccinia oncolysate	3/9 lack of prog
Murray et al. [17]	AU(11) or AL(2) NDV oncolysate	6/13 MR
Czajkowski et al. [18]	AU TC — rabbit globulin + IFA, ID and IM	0/2 resp
McCarthy et al. [5]	Rad AU TC-goat globulin, ID	1 CR, 1 PR/50
Berd et al. [19]	Rad DNP-AU TC + BCG, ID post-cy	5 PR/46

Abbreviations: AU, autologous; AL, allogeneic; TC, tumor cell; Rad, x-irradiated; VSV, vesicular stomatitis virus; NDV, Newcastle disease virus; MR, mixed response; resp, response; prog, progression; CR, complete responses; PR, partial response; DNP, dinitrophenyl; BCG, bacille Calmette–Guerin; CY, cyclophosphamide; IFA, incomplete Freund's adjuvant; ID, intradermal; IM, intramuscular; DTH, delayed-type hypersensitivity.

tion is to generate T-lymphocyte help to augment the antitumor immune response by eliciting the release of critical cytokines at the vaccination site [13]. This approach has been shown to enhance tumor rejection in experimental systems [14].

Viral xenogenization is the approach to antigen supplementation that has been most extensively studied. The results of trials in patients with melanoma are summarized in table 2. Although 9 of 31 melanoma-bearing patients were reported to have improved, the magnitude of tumor regression (mixed or stable disease) was modest.

Czajkowski et al. [18] conjugated rabbit globulin to autologous tumor cells that were mixed with incomplete Freund's adjuvant prior to immunization. Neither of the two melanoma patients responded. The frequency of response (2 of 50) achieved by McCarthy et al. [5] (table 2) in melanoma patients using goat globulin as a conjugate suggested a marginal improvement over the results that they had achieved with tumor cells alone (0 of 10) (table 1).

The tumor cell surface also can be antigen supplemented by use of a hapten, a molecule that is itself not immunogenic but that combines with a native protein to yield a new immunogen. The hypothesis is that the T-lymphocyte response to a strongly immunogenic, hapten-modified tumor antigen will be followed by development of immunity to unmodified tumor antigen.

Berd et al. [19] added dinitrophenyl (DNP) as a hapten to their autologous tumor cell vaccine (+ BCG); the vaccine was administered three days following low-dose cyclophosphamide. Patients were first sensitized to dinitrofluorobenzene. Once again, objective remissions were noted, but they were no more frequent than those seen without DNP conjugation [11]. However, a major difference from the prior trial was the development of clinically evident inflammatory responses in nodal, subcutaneous, and intradermal metastases in 20 of 46 patients. Inflamed metastatic lesions varied in size from 0.5 cm to 10–12 cm, and the number of inflamed lesions on a single patient ranged from one to more than one hundred. Flow-cytometric analysis of dissociated inflamed tumor nodules revealed that, on average, 40% ± 2.7% (mean ± SE) of the viable cells were T cells. This is a marked increase over the 10.2% ± 2.2% of T cells found in subcutaneous metastases of untreated patients. Paradoxically, only a small percentage of those metastases that were heavily infiltrated with CD8+ lymphocytes regressed. This finding suggested the presence of tumor cell defense mechanisms. Using the reverse transcription polymerase chain reaction and primers specific for cytokines, Lattime et al. [20] demonstrated, in both melanoma metastases and melanoma cell lines, the presence of mRNA for IL-10, which is known to suppress cell-mediated immunity.

2.2. Renal cell carcinoma

Trials of active specific immunization with whole tumor cell vaccines in patients with clinically evident residual renal cell cancer are summarized in table

Table 3. Active specific immunization with whole tumor cell vaccines in patients with clinical evidence of residual renal cell cancer

Investigators	Treatment	Outcome
McCune et al. [21]	Rad AU TC + C. parvum	4 MR/14
Rauschmeier [22]	Rad AU or AL TC + Candida antigen	2 CR, 2 PR/16
Adler et al. [23]	(A) Primostat alone or with	A, 1 PR/8
	(B) Rad AU TC + BCG, ID/ILY	B, 1 PR/12
Sahasrabudhe et al. [24]	Rad AU TC + C. Parvum post-cy	1 CR, 4 PR/20

Abbreviations: Primostat, 17-alpha hydroxy-19 norprogesterone caproate; Rad, radiation; AU, autologous; AL, allogeneic; TC, tumor cells; ID, intradermal; ILY, intralymphatic; CR, complete response; PR, partial response; MR, mixed response; BCG, bacille Calmette–Guerin; Cy, cyclophosphamide.

3. A few bonafide tumor regressions were observed in all four studies [21–24]. However, these trials are heterogeneous regarding the source of tumor cells, the adjuvant employed, pretreatment with cyclophosphamide, route of admnistration, and concurrent therapy. These differences preclude meaningful comparisons or meta-analysis. Definitive assessment requires further study.

Objective tumor regressions have been documented to occur coincident with active specific immunization with a variety of tumor cell-based vaccines in patients with melanoma and renal cell cancer. Even though remissions were infrequent and an immunologic basis was not documented, we consider these observations to constitute *proof of principle* that tumor growth can be modulated by active specific immunization.

3. Adjuvant trials in patients surgically free of disease but at high risk for recurrence

The occurrence of at least a few well-documented cases of objective regression of measurable melanoma and renal cell cancer metastases following active specific immunization with whole tumor cells is encouraging, since this is the clinical circumstance — that is, large tumor burden — in which this approach is least likely to be effective. A more reasonable therapeutic challenge is the eradication of micrometastases after surgical excision of clinically evident disease.

3.1. Melanoma

Active specific immunization with whole tumor cell vaccines has also been employed after surgical removal of all clinically evident melanoma. Elias et al. [25] used a complex schema to immunize melanoma patients at very high risk of recurrence following surgical excision of extensive regional lymph node metastases (2–14 nodes positive and often matted). Patients were first sensitized with BCG. Three weeks later, monthly (×3) intradermal vaccinations were begun with three sets of vaccines (mitomycin-C-treated tumor cells, each from a different donor to minimize development of anti-HLA immunity) and purified protein derivative of tuberculin. Five of nine patients were alive at five years and free of disease. This outcome is difficult to place in perspective in the absence of suitable controls or confirmatory trials.

The results of controlled trials [27–33] are presented in table 4. The favorable outcome noted by Hedley et al. [26] with chemoimmunotherapy in patients with metastatic melanoma was not reproduced when the same treatment was used in an adjuvant setting and compared with a randomized control [29]. Indeed, these investigators and McIllmurray et al. [27] both halted accrual early (few patients, brief follow-up) because it appeared that patients in the

Table 4. Randomized trials of adjunctive active specific immunotherapy with whole cell vaccines in melanoma patients who were surgically free of disease but at high risk for recurrence

Investigators: Mc Illmurray et al. [27,28]			
Treatment	WE + RLND RAD AU TC + BCG	WE + RLND	
Total patients	8	7	
Recurrences (24 mos)	6	5	
Deaths (24 mos)	5	3	
Investigators: Hedley et al. [29]			
Treatment	WE + RLND DTIC + VCR + BCG RAD AL TC	WE + RLND DTIC + VCR + BCG	
Total patients	16	12	
Median DFS (mos)	5	8	
Investigators: Morton et al. [30,31]			
Treatment	WE + RLND BCG + AL TC	WE + RLND	
Total patients	49	46	
Recurrences	23 (47%)	27 (59%)	
Deaths	22 (45%)	24 (52%)	
Investigators: Aranha et al. [32]			
Treatment	WE + RLND VCN-AU TC + BCG	WE + RLND	
Total patients	14	17	
Median DFS (mos)	15	15	
Median survival (mos)	22	30	
Investigators: Terry et al. [33]			
Treatment	WE + RLND BCG + VCN-AL TC	WE + RLND + MeCCNU	WE + RLND alone
Total patients	45	46	43
Median DFS (mos)	30	22	12
% DF @ 4 yrs	40	40	27

Abbreviations: WE, wide excision; RLND, regional lymph node dissection; Rad, x-irradiation; AL, allogeneic; AU, autologous; TC, tumor cell; BCG, bacille Calmette–Guerin; DTIC, dimethyl triazeno imidazole carboxamide; VCR, vincristine; MeCCNU, methyl CCNU or semustine; VCN, *Vibrio cholerae neuraminidase* treated; DF(S), disease free (survival).

Table 5. Adjunctive active specific immunization with antigen-supplemented tumor cell-based vaccines in melanoma patients who were surgically free of disease but at high risk for recurrence

Investigators	Treatment	Patients	Outcome
Cassell et al. [34]	AL NDV oncolysate	NED post RLND	DFS @ 36 mos RXed, 28/32 HC, 3/48
Hersey et al. [35]	AL vaccinia oncolysate	486 pts NED post RLND	5-yr. sur: RXed, 52% RC, 52%
Wallack et al. [36]	AL vaccinia oncolysate	217 pts NED post RLND	DFS @ 5 yrs: RXed, 32% RC, 36%
Berd et al. [37]	Rad DNP-AU TC + BCG + CY, ID	NED post RLND	53/92 relapses at 48 mos; 4-yr DFS 42%

Abbreviations: AU, autologous; AL, allogeneic; TC, tumor cell; Rad, x-irradiated; NDV, Newcastle disease virus; NED, no evidence of disease; RLND, regional lymph node dissection; DFS, disease-free survival; RXed, treated; HC, historical control; RC, randomized control; DNP, dinitrophenyl; BCG, bacille Calmette–Guerin; CY, cyclophosphamide; ID, intradermal.

immunotherapy arms were failing more frequently than patients in the respective control arms. With additional follow-up, this proved not to be so [28]. The most interesting of this series of trials is that of Terry et al. [33]. Here, patients in the chemotherapy-alone arm fared better than patients treated with surgery alone ($p = 0.048$). It is likely that this observation was not pursued, because methyl CCNU (semustine) was subsequently shown to be significantly carcinogenic. Inexplicably, a similar outcome in the BCG + tumor cells arm was not statistically significant.

Trials of antigen-supplemented tumor cells used as adjunctive therapy [34–37] are summarized in table 5. Although viral oncolysates did demonstrate some antitumor activity in patients with clinically evident residual disease, this modest level of antitumor activity could not be confirmed in randomized prospective trials of postsurgical adjuvant immunization [35,36].

The DNP-conjugated autologous whole melanoma cell vaccine is being used as an adjuvant in patients undergoing resection of clinically positive regional lymph nodes [37]. Of 92 evaluable patients, 39 were disease free at 48 months. This outcome is clinically and statistically significant when compared with the 22% disease-free survival achieved on an earlier trial with unconjugated vaccine [11]. Similarly, total survival at four years was improved compared with that of patients treated with surgery alone (60% and 27%, respectively). Seemingly, haptenization is more effective in overcoming tumor cell defenses when the tumor burden is minimal.

3.2. Other cancers

The results of clinical trials of adjunctive active specific immunization with whole cell vaccines in patients with renal cell, colorectal, and non-small cell lung cancers are summarized in table 6 [38–45]. In 1987, Galligioni et al. [38] initiated a prospective randomized clinical trial of adjuvant active specific

Table 6. Adjunctive active specific immunization with whole cell vaccines in patients with renal cell, colorectal and non-small cell lung cancers

Investigators	Tumor	Treatment	Outcome
Galligioni et al. [38] (R)	Renal	Rad AU TC, ID W BCG X 2, W/O BCG X 1 vs. observation	25/60 treated and 20/60 control pts relapsed at 61 mos MFU (p = NS)
Hoover et al. [39,40] (R)	Colorectal	(A) Surgery alone (39 pts) versus (B) Surgery + BCG + AU TC, ID (41 pts)	10-yr DFS— colon: (A) 43% (B) 75% p = 0.03 rectum: (A) 37% (B) 35%
Harris et al. [41,42] (R)	Colorectal	(A) Surgery alone versus (B) Surgery + BCG + AU TC, ID	Deaths— Dukes B: 12/123 (A) 18/123 (B) Dukes C: 22/52 (A) 18/51 (B)
Jessup et al. [43]	Colorectal	Rad AU TC (3×10^6 or 1×10^7) + BCG, ID	DTH to AU TC: 10/11 + 30 mos DFS— Dukes B2: 6/6 vs. 7/29 HC Dukes C: 3/5 vs. 6/12 HC
Schulof et al. [44]	NSCLC	Rad AU TC + BCG, ID	Pos DTH (AU TC): 7/13 relapses Neg DTH (AU TC): 3/5 relapses p = NS
Perlin et al. [45] (R)	NSCLC	(A) Surgery alone or with (B) AL TC + BCG, ID/SC	3-yr DFS— (A) 42% (B) 70% p = 0.06

Abbreviations: Rad, x-irradiation; AU, autologous; AL, allogeneic; TC, tumor cells; BCG, bacille Calmette–Guerin; W, with; W/O, without; ID, intradermal; SC, subcutaneous; NSCLC, non-small cell lung cancer; R, randomized; MFU, median follow-up; DFS, disease-free survival; DTH, delayed-type hypersensitivity; HC, historical control, +, positive.

immunization with enzymatically prepared autologous tumor cells in 120 patients following radical surgery for renal cell cancer. The treated patients received one intradermal vaccination per week ($\times 2$) of 10^7 viable, irradiated, autologous tumor cells and 10^7 viable BCG organisms. BCG was omitted from the third weekly injection, and a 21-day course of isoniazed was started. One month after completing active specific immunotherapy, 38 of 54 immunized and evaluable patients showed a significant DTH response to autologous tumor but not to autologous normal renal cells (43.2 mm^2 vs. 6.9 mm^2 mean area of induration, $p < 0.01$). Despite this rather remarkable result, disease-free survival and overall survival were not improved in immunized patients, even when analyzed by the magnitude of the DTH response. Indeed, the results of the DTH responses are surprising. Since both tumor and control tissues were prepared by enzymatic digestion, as was the tumor for vaccine, one would have expected a marked DTH to the contaminating enzyme in the control cells. An enzyme-alone control was not used.

Several investigators have attempted adjuvant active specific immunization with whole tumor cell vaccines in patients surgically free of colorectal cancer but at high risk for recurrence (table 6). The most mature of these is the randomized trial of Hoover et al. [39,40] comparing surgery with or without adjuvant BCG + autologous tumor cell vaccine. These investigators reported a clinically and statistically significant increase in 10-year disease-free survival for patients with colon cancer. No benefit was seen in patients with rectal cancer. The explanation proffered, that the pelvic radiation administered to the rectal cancer patients was immunosuppressive, was quite plausible. However, of the 20 immunized patients tested preimmunization and postimmunization for DTH with autologous tumor cells (versus normal mucosal cells), 16 (80%) became positive, with somewhat similar distribution between those with colon and rectal primary cancers (86% and 67%, respectively).

The Eastern Cooperative Oncology Group (ECOG) conducted a multi-institution, randomized trial to further assess this treatment. This trial [41] included only patients with colon cancer (Dukes B2, B3, C). The demonstration of a therapeutic benefit for adjunctive 5FU + levamisole in patients with Dukes C colon cancer subsequent to the initiation of this trial halted the accrual of this group at 115. At the time of interim analysis, 266 Dukes stage B2/3 and 103 Dukes stage C patients were considered evaluable. There are no significant differences between treatments with respect to overall survival or time to relapse. Substantial difficulties were found with vaccine preparation in this multi-institutional trial: 'When an analysis is performed just on the subset of patients who had adequate vaccine preparation and significant 3rd vaccination induration, there is evidence of a trend towards better survival in (Dukes) C patients treated with vaccine. A similar trend was seen in a small group of C patients who had initially been treated with vaccination followed by 5FU' [42].

In a small separate study, Jessup et al. [43] vaccinated 11 patients (nine rectal cancer, three colon cancer) with autologous tumor cells plus BCG. Almost all patients were successfully immunized (positive DTH) to autologous tumor cells (mean of the averages of two perpendicular diameters in mm ± SEM: high dose, 8.5 ± 1.4; low dose, 9.6 ± 1.9), and survival was improved by comparison with a historical control for those patients with Dukes B2 lesions, 4 of 6 of whom had rectal cancer. The authors do not indicate whether or not the rectal cancer patients received perioperative pelvic radiation. Additional trials of active immunization in rectal cancer patients are made difficult by the current standard of care, which mandates radiation and chemotherapy, both of which are generally immunosuppressive.

The prospective randomized study by Perlin et al. [45] of postsurgical adjunctive immunization with BCG plus allogeneic tumor cells in patients with non-small cell lung cancer is of interest in that a strong trend ($p = 0.06$) was seen towards improved disease-free survival in the immunotherapy group. A follow-up report on this now mature trial would be welcomed.

4. Future directions

4.1. Genetically engineered cancer vaccines

Adjuvants (e.g., BCG) and foreign proteins (e.g., viral xenogenization) are incorporated into cancer vaccines because of their ability to generate appropriate cytokine-based help to aid the development of an anti-tumor immune response. Cytokines provide costimulatory signals important for T-lymphocyte activation. Enrichment of the cytokine milieu by local injection at the site of immunization can promote the acquisition of cellular immunity to a variety of antigens [46]. Reasoning that higher and perhaps more effective cytokine levels could be sustained at the immunization site by local production rather than by local injection, tumor cells or fibroblasts genetically engineered to produce the molecule(s) of interest were included in vaccine preparations. Tepper et al. [47] were the first to introduce a cytokine gene in a tumor cell as an anti-tumor strategy. In a seminal study, Golumbek et al. [48] were able to show in a murine system that immunization with IL-4 transfected RENCA (renal carcinoma) cells resulted in elimination of a preexisting wild-type tumor, which was, however, the result of a small inoculum and only a few days growth.

Rosenberg et al. [49,50] were the first to use tumor cells engineered to secrete cytokines to immunize patients. Autologous melanoma cells were established in culture, transduced with either the IL-2 or TNF (tumor necrosis factor) genes, and then used to immunize the donors. Several weeks later, the lymph nodes draining the immunization site were removed. The cytotoxic lymphocytes were expanded in culture and then reintroduced into the patient. The therapeutic efficacy of these lymphocytes remains to be defined. Jaffee et al. [51] conducted a phase I trial in 17 patients with renal cancer to compare autologous irradiated tumor cells with autologous irradiated GM-CSF-secreting tumor cells for safety and the induction of tumor immunity. The GM-CSF-secreting vaccine produced DTH responses that were fourfold greater than those achieved with the control vaccine. One partial tumor response was observed. Since tumor cells are often difficult to transduce, Lotze et al. [52] resorted to readily available fibroblasts for genetic modification and reintroduced these cells admixed with the unmodified tumor cells. Outcome results have not yet been reported. A further simplification would be the local injection of the cyotkine(s) at the vaccination site. Leong et al. [53] treated 20 melanoma patients with irradiated autologous tumor cells admixed with BCG preceded by cyclophosphamide. GM-CSF was injected concurrently at the vaccination site as well as daily for four days thereafter. Four patients (20%) had substantial tumor regression. This result seems not unlike those results reported by others using similar regimens without GM-CSF (table 1). A direct comparison in humans with transduced tumor cells has not been published.

4.2. In vivo in situ gene transfer

The use of ex vivo gene transfer techniques in the clinic is severely limited by the requirement that autologous tumor or fibroblasts be available, removed, grown in vitro, transfixed with the gene(s) of interest, etc. We and others are attempting to effect gene transfer in situ in vivo. Mastrangelo et al. [54] injected metastatic melanoma deposits with wild-type vaccinia (about twice weekly) for as long as 90 days and demonstrated viral gene function throughout this period. We have constructed a vaccinia recombinant virus that carries and expresses the gene for human GM-CSF, a cytokine that enhances antigen processing for presentation to cytotoxic T lymphocytes. A phase I clinical trial of intralesional injection of melanoma metastases with this recombinant virus has been initiated.

Stopeck et al. [55] explored a novel approach to improving tumor cell immunogenicity via the introduction of the MHC alloantigen HLA-B7. Melanoma metastases were injected with a DNA plasmid containing the HLA-B7 and beta 2-microglobulin genes in a cationic lipid vector. There were one complete (lymph node metastases) and two partial (lung metastases) remissions in 11 patients. Seven patients experienced reductions from 30% to 87% in the size of injected tumors.

These studies show that in situ gene transfer is feasible and less cumbersome than ex vivo transfer to autologous cells. It remains to be determined whether this approach will yield clinically useful systemic effects.

4.3. Tumor defense mechanisms

Bona fide remissions have been observed with various cell-based vaccines in all of the several tumor types studied. These remissions are infrequent, consistently ranging between 10% and 20%. The DNP-conjugated vaccine of Berd et al. [19] induced a dramatic inflammatory response in melanoma metastases in 40%–50% of the patients treated. Despite this outcome, the objective response rate was just 9.2%. The presence of viable tumor cells growing in a sea of lymphocytes that are demonstrably cytotoxic in vivo [19] leads inescapably to the conclusion that, in situ, tumor cells can effectively defend against immunologic attack. As originally demonstrated by Prehn and Main [1], tumors can and do grow in the presence of an antitumor immune response.

In an effort to define the mechanism(s) by which tumor cells evade immune destruction in vivo, investigators are studying cytokine production. Melanoma is again the focus of attention. Melanoma-derived cytokines have been reviewed by Bohm and Luger [56]. IL-10 is a candidate suppressor of cellular immunity, inhibiting antigen presentation and accessory cell function by macrophages and dendritic cells. Addition of IL-10 to cultures of monocytes or alveolar macrophages results in dose-dependent suppression of their cytotoxicity for tumor cells [57]. As cited above, Lattime et al. [20] found IL-10 mRNA in pretreatment and posttreatment specimens of metastatic melanoma. Sato et al. [58] found that IL-10 protein was produced by 26 of 30 single-cell suspensions of melanoma metastases. Melanoma cell-enriched (95% pure) fractions produced eight times more IL-10 protein than did the lymphocyte-enriched (95% pure) fractions. The functional significance of this observation remains to be demonstrated. The observation by Chen et al. [59] that anti-IL-10 monoclonal antibody did not completely restore immunologic reactivity in vitro suggests that additional factors may be involved.

The transforming growth factor (TGF) beta isoforms are potent regulators of the immune responses, cell proliferation, differentiation, and extracellular matrix synthesis and deposition. Melanoma cell lines produce and secrete TGF betas into the culture media [60], making these molecules good suspects for mediating in situ immunosuppression. There are likely multiple other regulatory molecules involved. It will be many years before this area is adequately understood.

5. Concluding remarks

Working with a murine tumor model, Prehn and Main [1] convincingly demonstrated that a naive animal can be successfully immunized to reject a strongly immunogenic tumor but cautioned that these same tumors, when preexisting, can and do grow in the presence of an antitumor immune response. It is encouraging, therefore, that active specific immunization with tumor cell-based vaccines, when formulated with adjuvants, did induce objective tumor regression in 10%–20% of patients bearing melanoma or renal cell cancer. There remains considerable room for improvement to reach our goal of an effective, safe, broadly applicable, and user friendly vaccine. We have the tools to allow identification of antigens of potential importance in immunologically mediated tumor regression. Genetic engineering affords an unprecedented opportunity to develop user friendly vaccines. Although more user friendly, these chemically defined, genetically engineered vaccines are not likely to be more effective than the benchmark cell-based vaccines. In attempting to understand why objective tumor regression is frustratingly infrequent, the work of Berd et al. [19] with the DNP-conjugated autologous melanoma vaccine is insightful. In approximately 50% of patients, tumor deposits become inflamed, often dramatically so. This finding provides de facto evidence that an antitumor response was generated. Enthusiam for this remarkable achievement is tempered by the disappointing observation that only 10% of treated patients experienced objective tumor regression. The tumor cells were not defenseless. Significant improvement in effectiveness must await a better understanding of tumor defense mechanisms and the formulation of methods of circumvention. In the interim, lives can be saved by the systemic implementation of currently available tumor cell-based vaccine strategies.

Acknowledgments

This work was supported by grants from the American Cancer Society (#EDT-98), the National Institutes of Health (R21-CA69253), and the Nat Pincus Fund.

References

1. Prehn RT, Main JM. 1957. Immunity to methylcholanthrene induced sarcomas. J Natl Cancer Inst 18:769–778.
2. Ikonopisov RL, Lewis MG, Hunter-Craig ID, et al. 1970. Autoimmunization with irradiated tumor cells in human malignant melanoma. Br Med J 2:752–754.
3. Krementz ET, Samuels MS, Wallace JH. 1971. Clinical experience in the immunotherapy of cancer. Surg Gynecol Obstet 133:209–217.
4. Currie GA, Lejeune F, Hamilton-Fairley G. 1971. Immunization with irradiated tumor cells and specific lymphocyte cytotoxicity in malignant melanoma. Br Med J 2:305–310.
5. McCarthy WH, Cotton G, Carlton A, et al. 1973. Immunotherapy of malignant melanoma. A clinical trial. Cancer 32:97–103.
6. Ahn SS, Irie RF, Weisenburger TH, et al. 1982. Humoral immune response to intralymphatic immunotherapy for disseminated melanoma: correlation with clinical response. Surgery 92:362–367.
7. Gerner FR, Moore GE. 1976. Feasibility study of immunotherapy in patients with solid tumors. Cancer 38:131–143.
8. Laucius JF, Bodurtha AJ, Mastrangelo MJ, et al. 1977. A phase II study of autologous irradiated tumor cells plus BCG in patients with metastatic malignant melanoma. Cancer 40:2091–2093.
9. Morton DL, Foshag LJ, Hoon DSB, et al. 1992. Prolongation of survival in metastatic melanoma after active specific immunotherapy with a new polyvalent melanoma vaccine. Ann Surg 216:463–482.
10. Berd D, Maguire HC Jr, Mastrangelo MJ. 1986. Induction of cell mediate immunity to autologous melanoma cells and regression of metastases after treatment with a melanoma cell vaccine preceded by cyclophosphamide. Cancer Res 46:2572–2577.
11. Berd D, Maguire HC Jr, McCue P, Mastrangelo MJ. 1990. Treatment of metastatic melanoma with an autologous tumor cell vaccine: clinical and immunological results in 64 patients. J Clin Oncol 8:1858–1867.

12. Mitchell MS. 1995. Active specific immunotherapy of melanoma. Br Med Bull 51:631–646.
13. Mitchison NA. 1970. Immunologic approach to cancer. Transplant Proc 11:92–103.
14. Galili ND, Naor B, Asjo B, Klein G. 1976. Induction of immune responsiveness in a genetically low-responsive tumor–host combination by chemical modification of the immunogen. Eur J Immunol 6:473–476.
15. Livington PO, Albino AP, Chung JJ, et al. 1985. Serological responses of melanoma patients to vaccines prepared from VSV lysates of autologous and allogeneic cultured melanoma cells. Cancer 55:713–720.
16. Wallack MK, Steplewski Z, Koprowski H, et al. 1977. A new approach in specific active immunotherapy. Cancer 39:560–564.
17. Murray DR, Cassel W, Torbin A, et al. 1977. Viral oncolysates in the management of malignant melanoma. Cancer 40:680–686.
18. Czajkowski NP, Rosenblatt M, Wolf PL, Vazquez J. 1967. A new method of active immunization to autologous human tumor tissue. Lancet 2:905–909.
19. Berd D, Maguire HC Jr, Mastrangelo MJ. 1993. Treatment of human melanoma with hapten-modified autologous vaccine. Ann NY Acad Sci 690:147–152.
20. Lattime EC, Mastrangelo MJ, Berd D. 1995. Expression of cytokine mRNA in human melanoma cells. Cancer Immunol Immunother 41:151–156.
21. McCune CS, Schapira DV, Henshaw EC. 1981. Specific immunotherapy of advanced renal carcinoma: evidence for the polyclonality of metastases. Cancer 47:1984–1987.
22. Rauschmeier HA. 1988. Immunotherapy of metastatic renal cancer. Semin Surg Oncol 4:169–173.
23. Adler A, Gillon G, Lurie H, et al. 1987. Active specific immunotherapy of renal cell carcinoma patients: a prospective randomized study of hormono-immuno- versus hormonotherapy. Preliminary report of immunological and clinical aspects. J Biol Respir Mod 6:610–624.
24. Sahasrabudhe DM, deKernion JB, Pontes JE, et al. 1986. Specific immunotherapy with suppressor function inhibition for metastatic renal cell carcinoma. J Biol Respir Med 5:581–594.
25. Elias EG, Tomazic VJ, Buda BS. 1992. Adjuvant immunotherapy in melanoma: a new approach. J Surg Oncol 50:144–148.
26. Hedley DW, McElwain TJ, Currie GA. 1977. Tumor regression and survival of patients with disseminated malignant melanoma treated with chemotherapy and specific active immunotherapy. Eur J Cancer 13:1169–1173.
27. Mc Illmurray MB, Embleton MJ, Reeves WB, et al. 1977. Controlled trial of active immunotherapy in management of stage IIB malignant melanoma. Br Med J 1:540–542.
28. Mc Illmurray MB, Reeves WG, Langman MJS, et al. 1978. Active immunotherapy in malignant melanoma (letter). Br Med J 1:579.
29. Hedley DW, McElwain TJ, Currie GA. 1978. Specific active immunotherapy does not prolong survival in surgically treated patients with stage IIB malignant melanoma and may promote early recurrence. Br J Cancer 37:491–496.
30. Morton DL, Holmes EC, Eilber FR, et al. 1982. Adjuvant immunotherapy: results of a randomized trial in patients with lymph node metastases. In Terry WD, Rosenberg SA, eds. Immunotherapy of Human Cancer. New York: Elsevier North Holland, pp 245–249.
31. Morton DL. 1986. Adjuvant immunotherapy of malignant melanoma: status of clinical trials at UCLA. Int J Immunother 2:31–36.
32. Aranha GV, McKhann CF, Grage TB, et al. 1979. Adjuvant immunotherapy of malignant melanoma. Cancer 43:1297–1303.
33. Terry WE, Hodes RJ, Rosenberg SA, et al. 1982. Treatment of stage I and II malignant melanoma with adjuvant immunotherapy or chemotherapy: preliminary analysis of a prospective randomized trial. In Terry WD, Rosenberg SA, eds. Immunotherapy of Human Cancer. New York: Elsevier North Holland, pp 252–257.
34. Cassel WA, Murray DR, Phillips HS. 1983. A phase II study of the post surgical management of stage II melanoma with a Newcastle disease virus oncolysate. Cancer 52:856–860.

35. Hersey P, Coates A, McCarthy WH. 1993. Active immuotherapy following surgical removal of high risk melanoma. Present status and future prospects (abstract). Proc Soc Biol Ther 8:24.
36. Wallack MK, Sivanandham M, Balch CM, et al. 1995. A phase III randomized, double-blind, multi-institutional trial of vaccinia melanoma oncolysate-active specific immunotherapy for patients with stage II melanoma. Cancer 75:34–42.
37. Berd D, Maguire HC, Nathan FE, Schuchter LM, Bloome E, Mastrangelo MJ. 1996. Autologous DNP-modified vaccine as post surgical adjuvant treatment of stages III and IV melanoma (abstract). Proc Am Soc Clin Oncol 15:554.
38. Galligioni E, Quaia M, Merlo A, et al. 1996. Adjuvant immunotherapy treatment of renal carcinoma patients with autologous tumor cells and bacillus Calmette–Guerin. Cancer 77:2560–2566.
39. Hoover HC Jr, Surdyke MG, Dangel RB, et al. 1985. Prospectively randomized trial of adjuvant active specific immunotherapy for human colorectal cancer. Cancer 55:1236–1243.
40. Hoover HC Jr, Brandhorst JS, Peters LC, et al. 1993. Adjuvant active specific immunotherapy for human colorectal cancer: 6.5 year median follow up of a phase III prospectively randomized trial. J Clin Oncol 11:390–399.
41. Harris J, Ryan L, Adams G, et al. 1993. Results of the ECOG trial of autologous colon cancer vaccine (abstract). J Immunother 14:358.
42. Harris J, Ryan L, Adams G, et al. 1994. Survival and relapse in adjuvant autologous tumor vaccine therapy for Dukes B and C colon cancer (abstract). Proc Am Soc Clin Oncol 13:294.
43. Jessup JM, McBride CM, Ames FC, et al. 1986. Active specific immuotherapy of Dukes B2 and C colorectal carcinoma: comparison of two doses of the vaccine. Cancer Immunol Immunother 3:233–239.
44. Schulof RS, Mai D, Nelson MA, et al. 1988. Active specific immunotherapy with an autologous tumor cell vaccine in patients with resected non-small cell lung cancer. Mol Biother 1:30–36.
45. Perlin E, Oldham RK, Weese JL, et al. 1980. Carcinoma of the lung: immunotherapy with intradermal BCG and allogeneic tumor cells. Int J Radiat Oncol Biol Phys 6:1033–1039.
46. Maguire HC Jr, Guidotti MB, Weiner WP. 1989. Local murine recombinant interferon heightens the acquisition of allergic contact dermatitis in the mouse. Int Arch Allergy 88:345–347.
47. Tepper RI, Pattengale PK, Leder P. 1989. Murine interleukin-4 displays potent anti-tumor activity in vivo. Cell 57:503–512.
48. Golumbek PT, Lazenby AJ, Levitsky HI, et al. 1991. Treatment of established renal cancer by tumor cells engineered to secrete interleukin-4. Science 254:713–716.
49. Rosenberg SA. 1992. The immunotherapy and gene therapy of cancer. J Clin Oncol 10:180–199.
50. Rosenberg SA, Anderson WF, Blaese RM, et al. 1992. Immunization of cancer patients using autologous cancer cells modified by the insertion of the gene for interleukin-2. Hum Gene Ther 3:75–90.
51. Jaffee EM, Marshall F, Weber C, et al. 1996. Bioactivity of a human GM-CSF tumor vaccine for the treatment of metastatic renal cell carcinoma (abstract). Proc Am Soc Clin Oncol 15:237.
52. Lotze MT, Rubin JT. 1994. Gene therapy of cancer: a pilot study of IL-4 gene modified fibroblasts with autologous tumor to elicit an immune response. Hum Gene Ther 5:41–55.
53. Leong SPL, Enders-Zohr P, Zhou YM, et al. 1996. Active specific immunotherapy with GM-CSF as an adjuvant to autologous melanoma vaccine in metastatic melanoma (abstract). Proc Am Soc Clin Oncol 15:437.
54. Mastrangelo MJ, Maguire HC Jr, McCue P, et al. 1995. A pilot study demonstrating the feasibility of using intratumoral vaccinia injections as a vector for gene transfer. Vaccine Res 4:58–69.
55. Stopeck AT, Hersh EM, Akopriaye T, et al. 1995. Phase I study of immunotherapy of malignant melanoma by direct gene transfer of an allogeneic histocompatibility antigen HLA-B7 (abstract). Proc Am Soc Clin Oncol 14:227.

56. Bohm M, Luger TA. 1996. Melanoma-derived cytokines. In Maio M, ed. Immunology of Human Melanoma. Amsterdam: IOS Press, pp 55–69.
57. Nabioullin R, Sone S, Mizuno K, et al. 1994. Interleukin-10 is a potent inhibitor of tumor cytotoxicity by human monocytes and alveolar macrophages. J Leuk Biol 55:437–440.
58. Sato T, McCue P, Masuoka K, et al. 1996. Interleukin-10 production by human melanoma. Clin Cancer Res 2:1383–1390
59. Chen Q, Daniel V, Maher DW, Hersey P. 1994. Production of IL-10 by melanoma cells: examination of its role in immunosuppression mediated by melanoma. Int J Cancer 56:755–760.
60. VanBelle P, Rodeck U, Nuamah I, et al. 1996. Melanoma-associated expression of transforming growth factor-beta isoforms. Am J Pathol 148:1887–1894.

4. Anti-idiotype antibody vaccine therapies of cancer

Malaya Bhattacharya-Chatterjee and Kenneth A. Foon

1. Introduction

Immunotherapy of cancer is divided into two overlapping categories: active and passive. The goal of active immunotherapy is the stimulation of host antitumor immunity, either cellular or humoral. This can be accomplished in a direct or specific fashion by using tumor vaccines to generate an immune response to tumor-associated antigens (TAAs). Nonspecific antitumor immunity can be propagated by compounds such as bacillus Calmette–Guerin (BCG). Passive immunotherapy relies on the administration of biologically active agents with innate antitumor properties, such as antibodies reactive with growth factor receptors. In most instances, host immunity is an important cofactor in active immunotherapy. In addition, some agents, such as antibodies, can exert anti-immune circuits that are set into motion by these therapies and account for the imperfect but nonetheless useful division into active and passive types.

Immunotherapy is very effective in certain animal model systems, and it has been used to treat human cancers for several decades [1]. The active immunotherapy of cancer patients with tumor-derived material has been studied by numerous investigators, with positive clinical responses reported. A number of problems exist with using tumor material for immunization, and TAAs are often found to be poorly immunogenic. A common explanation for the absence of antitumor immunity is that the immune system has been tolerized by the tumor antigen. If this is true, steps could be taken to break the existing antitumor tolerance. An effective method of breaking tolerance is to present the critical epitope in a different molecular environment to the tolerized host [2]. While this can be done easily with haptens and other small, well-defined antigens, it is impossible with most tumor antigens because they are chemically ill defined and difficult to purify — especially carbohydrate antigens, vaccines for which cannot be produced by recombinant techniques.

The immune network hypothesis offers a unique approach to transform epitope structures into idiotypic Id determinants expressed on the surface of antibodies. Immunoglobulin (Ig) molecules possess variable regions specific for antigen recognition. The variable region is encoded by V_H, D, and J_H genes for the heavy chains and V_L and J_L chains for the light chain [3]. The variable region contains determinants known as idiotypes (Ids), which are themselves immunogenic. Antibodies can be made to many structures in the variable region that are associated with the light chain, heavy chain, or a combination of both chains [4,5]. Early studies indicated that an Id was unique to a small set of antibody molecules [4,5]. However, the Id determinants may show a continuum of specificity from more or less private to semipublic [6,7]. For example, if different antibodies are coded by the same V_H gene segment, a shared or semipublic Id may be found. The Id is often defined by the antibody made against it, which is known as *anti-Id antibody*.

Jan Lindemann in 1973 [8] and Niels Jerne in 1974 [9] proposed theories that describe the immune system as a network of interacting antibodies and lymphocytes. According to this original network hypothesis, the Id–anti-Id interactions regulate the immune response of a host to a given antigen. Both Ids and anti-Ids have been used to manipulate cellular and humoral immunity.

The network hypothesis predicts that within the immune network the universe of external antigens is mimicked by Id expressed by antibodies and T-cell receptors. According to the network concept, immunization with a given antigen will generate the production of antibodies against this antigen, termed *Ab1*. This Ab1 can generate a series of anti-Id antibodies against Ab1, termed *Ab2*. Some of these Ab2 molecules can effectively mimic the three-dimensional structures of external antigens. These particular anti-Ids, called *Ab2β*, which fit into the paratopes of Ab1, can induce specific immune responses similar to responses induced by nominal antigen. Anti-Id antibodies of the β type express the internal image of the antigen recognized by the Ab1 antibody and can be used as surrogate antigens. Immunization with Ab2β can lead to the generation of anti-anti-Id antibodies (Ab3) that recognize the corresponding original antigen identified by the Ab1. Because of this Ab1-like reactivity, the Ab3 is also called *Ab1'* to indicate that it might differ in its other idiotypes from Ab1. This cyclic nature of complementary binding sites and idiotopes is the basis for the approach to Id vaccines. In figure 1, the relationships of antigen, idiotype (Ab1), anti-idiotype (Ab2), and anti-anti-idiotype (Ab3) are shown schematically.

The utilization of the Id network in tumor immunotherapy opens new perspectives and may enrich the therapeutic armamemtarium. There are two basic approaches that utilize the Id network for tumor immunotherapy. The first takes advantage of the existence of internal antigen images in the Id repertoire. This approach has already been used successfully by several investigators and has the advantage of not being genetically restricted. Internal-image Ids mimic the three-dimensional shapes of antigens and thus are effective across the species barrier. At the same time, antigens can be presented in a different molecular environment.

The other method of using the Id network rests on the existence of so-called *regulatory Ids* [10–12], which may also be linked to the regulatory network of

Immunize Mice with Human Tumor Cell to Generate Ab1

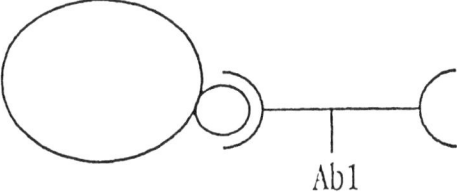

Ab1

Immunize Syngeneic Mice with Ab1 to Generate Anti-Idiotype (Ab2)

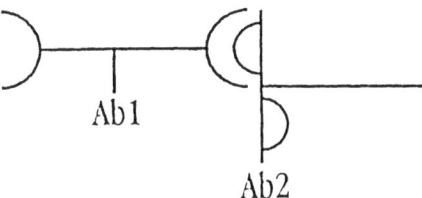

Ab1

Ab2

Immunize Patients with Ab2 Anti-Idiotype (with Adjuvant to Generate Ab3)

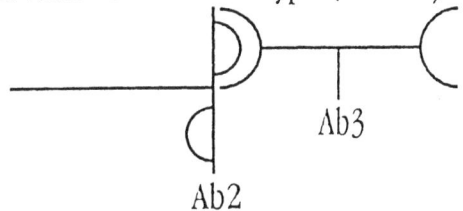

Ab3

Ab2

Figure 1. Relationships of antigen, Ab1, Ab2, and Ab3.

anticancer responses. This concept, initially proposed by Paul and Bona [13], suggests that a special class of idiotopes exist with unique regulatory functions before antigenic stimulation. Discovering the role of regulatory Ids in antitumor responses would be important and could be the first step in using these regulatory Ids to control tumor growth by immunologic means. A discussion of the potential mechanism of regulatory Id-based immunoregulation is beyond the scope of this chapter.

The administration of Ab2 as surrogate tumor-associated antigens represents another potential application of the Id vaccine concept. Id-based vaccines do not contain nominal antigen or antigen fragments; therefore, Id vaccines are more economical to produce and less prone to give rise to autoimmune reactions.

Because Id vaccines are proteins, they can be coupled to potent immunogenic carriers to become T-cell-dependent antigens that can receive full T help. Eventually, it might be possible to produce fully synthetic Id vaccines, for example, to design peptides that contain the relevant idiotypic structures necessary to induce the desired vaccination effect.

T-cell-dependent protein vaccines can become a decisive factor in situations where the responding immune system is immature or suppressed. From experimental studies in animals, we know that the response to T-cell-dependent antigens matures earlier than the T-cell-independent response to carbohydrate antigen and that often a genetically or acquired abnormal immune system responds better to T-cell-dependent than to T-cell-independent antigens.

Finally, data exist showing that an acquired tolerance to one antigen can be broken by using a different molecular form of the same antigenic moiety. This finding could become an important consideration in a broader context such as immunotherapy in cancer patients, who can often be immunodeficient against their own tumor-associated antigens.

In this chapter, we will briefly summarize the data on the use of internal image anti-Id antibodies in experimental tumor systems and then discuss the efforts towards the generation of anti-Id vaccines and subsequent clinical trials for human tumors.

2. Animal tumor model

Active immunization with tumor-specific Id vaccines has been shown to inhibit tumor growth in animals. In some, mechanisms responsible for inducing antitumor immunity have been studied in detail. An anti-Id antibody was used to induce immunity to SV-40 transformed cells. Mice vaccinated with this anti-Id demonstrated prolonged survival after tumor transfer [14].

The role of Id interactions in regulating the immune response of mice to chemically induced, syngeneic sarcomas has been studied [15]. Significant antitumor activity was seen following treatment with anti-Id monoclonal antibodies (mAbs) of mice with established sarcomas (MCA-490 and MCA-1511). One report on mouse leukemia model L1210 in DBA/2 mice has provided basic information on B- and T-cell-induced responses using the anti-Id approach [16–20]. A number of anti-Id mAbs against an mAb to the L1210 tumor were generated. These anti-Id mAbs induced tumor-specific delayed-type hypersensitivity, tumor growth inhibition, and T cells that were killer or helper cells. However, only 1 of 7 anti-Ids were able to induce protective immunity in mice against tumor challenge [19]. While there was no indication from immunochemical and biological testing of these anti-Id vaccines as to which might induce protection, there were correlations of the corresponding, cross-reactive idiotope levels in sera in protected animals as opposed to nonprotected animals [20]. In addition, certain idiotope recognizing T helper cells were found in tumor-immune mice. These data support the notion that antigens and internal-image anti-Ids induce changes in the network that regulates the tumor immunity.

Next, the investigators explored the use of soluble anti-Id mAbs as immunostimulators in tumor-bearing mice. Although this treatment did not induce cures, it significantly increased survival time. Interestingly, this anti-Id effect was dose dependent, whereby large and small doses had no effect. Finally, in a recent study, a 100% cure of established tumors was achieved in DBA/2 mice by combining anti-Id vaccines with cyclophosphamide, whereas a 50% cure rate was obtained with anti-Id therapy alone [18]. Similar findings have been obtained when dramatic survival benefit resulted from administering cyclophosphamide (100 mg/kg) in combination with anti-Id vaccines to mice that had 10-day-old, 1- to 2-cm diameter, subcutaneous B-cell lymphomas (38C13) [21]. These results provide guidelines for developing clinical protocols for cancer patients by using combination therapy of anti-Id and chemotherapy.

Vaccination of tumor-bearing mice with cytokine gene-inserted tumor cells [22] has been reported as a modality for cancer therapy. However, only limited success (about a 40% to 50% cure rate) has been obtained in most cases. Considering the amount of work and risk involved in introducing the gene through retroviral vectors into isolated tumor cells, the anti-Id approach might turn out to be safer, more effective, and less labor intensive. The greatest challenge in immunotherapy by means of anti-Id antibodies is to identify the right network antigen for a tumor-associated antigen system.

3. Anti-idiotype antibodies and human cancer

Limited experience in human trials using anti-Id to stimulate immunity against tumors has shown promising results. Polyclonal Ab2 antibodies that functionally mimic the antigens defined by the anticolorectal carcinoma antibodies 17-1A and GA733 have been generated [23]. Thirty patients with advanced colorectal carcinoma were immunized with alum-precipitated goat Ab2. The doses ranged from 0.5 to 4 mg per injection. All patients developed Ab3 that bound to cultured tumor cells. Furthermore, the Ab3 competed with Ab1 for binding to colorectal tumor cells. Ab3 antibodies were eluted from colorectal cancer cells and shown to bind to purified tumor antigen. Furthermore, clinical improvement was observed in 13 of the 30 patients [24]. No immediate or delayed hypersensitivity reaction or other adverse side effects were observed.

In a follow-up trial, a different goat polyclonal Ab2 was administered to 12 patients who had previously been diagnosed with colorectal carcinoma but whose tumors were excised prior to Ab2 therapy [25]. The Ab3 specifically inhibited binding of the Ab1 to tumor cells and therefore may bind to the same antigen as the Ab1. Two of the six patients who developed tumor-specific Ab3 also had antigen-specific T cells that proliferated in culture to stimulation with the GA733 antigen, but not with irrelevant control antigen. Seven of the 12 patients showed tumor remissions that lasted between 1.1 and 4.1 years after treatment.

In another study, an anti-Id mAb that mimics a high-molecular-weight human melanoma antigen elicited antitumor antibody responses in melanoma patients [26]. Repeated injections of murine anti-Id mAb were not associated with side effects. Reductions in the size of metastatic lesions were observed in 7 of the 37 immunized patients. Another 25 patients with stage IV melanoma were immunized with the mouse anti-Id mAb MK2-23, which bears the internal image of the determinant defined by antihuman high-molecular-weight melanoma antigen (HMW-MAA) mAb 763.74. Fourteen patients developed antibodies that were shown by serologic and immunochemical assays to recognize the same or a spatially close determinant as the anti-HMW-MAA mAb 763.74 and to express the idiotope defined by mAb MK2-23 in their antigen-combining sites. Side effects that are likely to be caused by BCG present in the immunogen consisted of erythema, induration, and ulceration at injection sites [27]. Patients occasionally complained of flulike symptoms, arthralgias, and myalgias. Three patients who developed anti-HMW-MAA antibodies achieved partial responses, consisting of decreases in metastatic lesion size that lasted 52 weeks in one patient and 93 weeks in two others. Survival of the 14 patients who developed anti-HMW-MAA antibodies was significantly longer than that of the nine patients without detectable humoral anti-HMW-MAA immunity development [27].

A human monoclonal Ab2 (105AD7) that interacts with the binding site of 791T/36, a mouse monoclonal antibody against gp72 antigen, was administered to six patients with advanced colorectal cancer in a phase I clinical study [28]. Cryopreserved blood mononuclear cells were tested for in vitro proliferative responses by [^{3}H] thymidine incorporation; plasma samples were tested by enzyme-linked immunosorbent assay for anti-anti-Id and antitumor antibodies and for interleukin 2. Proliferative responses to gp72-positive tumor cells were seen in 4 of 5 patients tested; parallel in vitro responses to 105AD7 anti-Id antibody were seen in most of these patients. Interleukin 2 was detected in the plasma of 4 of 6 patients after 105AD7 immunization, with peak levels up to 7 units/mL. No toxicity related to anti-Id immunization and no antitumor or anti-anti-Id antibodies were seen.

Another clinical trial involves vaccination with Ids derived from B-cell lymphomas. In this case, purified immunoglobulin derived from patients' tumors were used as the immunogen to generate an active immunity [29]. Nine patients who had minimal residual disease or a complete remission after chemotherapy received a series of subcutaneous injections of the Ig derived from his or her tumor cells (Ig Id), which had been conjugated to a protein carrier (KLH). The vaccine was administered in an adjuvant formlation (SAF-1). In 7 of the 9 patients, the immunization induced sustained Id-specific immunologic responses of the humoral type (two patients), the cell-mediated type (four patients), or both (one patient). The use of an adjuvant was essential for these immune responses. The induced antibodies bound specifically to autologous Ig–Id, inhibited the binding of murine mAb anti-Ids, and bound autologous tumor cells. The vaccine also induced cellular immunity against the tumor Id, as demonstrated by the ability of the Id to stimulate peripheral blood lymphocytes in culture obtained from the vaccinated patients. The tumors of both the patients with measurable disease regressed completely. Toxicity associated with the vaccine was minimal and consisted of mild reactions at the site of intramuscular injection. These results demonstrate that autologous Ig Id can be formulated into an immunogenic, tumor-specific antigen in humans with B-cell lymphoma and provide the background for large-scale trials of active specific immunotherapy of this disease.

Recently, we have generated monoclonal Id cascades for four different human tumor-associated antigens. The first cascade originated from a T-cell leukemia/lymphoma [30,31] and the second one from carcinoembryonic antigen (CEA) [32]. The third one originated from human milk fat globule (HMFG) membrane antigen overexpressed by breast and ovarian cancer cells and the fourth one from the ganglioside GD2 expressed by melanoma, sarcoma, small cell carcinoma of the lung, and neuroectodermal tumors. In all these cascades, we have produced TAA-mimicking monoclonal anti-Id [33–35] and monoclonal anti-anti-Ids (Ab3) that bind to that original TAA.

4. Anti-idiotype vaccine therapy of human T-cell lymphoma

We have generated an Ab2β anti-Id mAb [30,31] to a murine mAb, designated SN2 (Ab1), that identifies a highly restricted T-cell antigen designated gp37 that is found on 70% of T-cell acute lymphoblastic leukemia and approximately 30% of T-cell lymphoma but not on normal or activated T lymphocytes. The SN2 mAb does not have a cluster designation, and the function of the epitope is unknown. We have been unable to identify this antigen on any normal adult human tissues. The IgG1 anti-Id mAb generated to the SN2 mAb was shown to be an internal image by generating anti-anti-Id (Ab3) responses that recognized gp37 in three animal models, namely, mouse, rabbit [30,31], and nonhuman primates. This anti-Id mAb was used to treat T-cell lymphoma patients in a phase 1b clinical trial [36].

4.1. Selection of patients

All the patients had T-cell lymphoma primarily confined to the skin. Three of the four patients had clinically and histologically classic mycosis fungoides, while patient 2 had a diffuse large cell lymphoma. Patients were selected on the basis of SN2 (Ab1) antibody binding to their tumor. Baseline studies included complete physical examination, chest radiography, computer axial tomography examination of the abdomen, and routine blood counts and chemistries. Two of the patients (3 and 4) were anergic to intradermal skin testing with mumps, candida, and trichophytin antigens. All the patients had been off prior therapy for at least four weeks, and staging was repeated at the conclusion of therapy. Informed consent was obtained under a protocol approved by the Institutional Review Board.

4.2. Treatment schedule

The patients were treated with 1 mg of aluminum hydroxide-precipitated anti-Id antibody intracutaneous every other week for eight weeks and then every four weeks if they demonstrated a clinical or immunologic response. All the patients received four total injections except for patient 2, who received a total of 17 injections.

4.3. Disease assessment

The patient's cutaneous lesions were carefully mapped at the start of treatment and at each visit. Lesion size was specified by measurements of the major and minor axes of the infiltrates and volume by the product of these axes times the average thickness. The same observer performed the measurements.

4.4. Humoral responses to anti-idiotype

The development of humoral immunity induced by immunization with aluminum hydroxide precipitated Ab2, 4DC6, was assessed by testing sera obtained from patients before therapy and after each treatment with the vaccine. Hyperimmune sera (following the fourth injection of 4DC6) from 3 of 4 patients showed significant levels of total human antimouse antibody responses, including anti-iso/allo/and anti-anti-Id antibodies against immunizing Ab2, 4DC6, as determined by ELISA assay. Next, the sera from these immunized patients were treated with excess normal murine Ig (50 μg/mL) to block human antibodies against isotypic and allotypic determinants and tested against $F(ab')_2$ 4DC6 anti-Id antibody in an ELISA. Absorbed sera from 3 of the 4 patients demonstrated strong reactivity with the $F(ab')_2$ 4DC6, while there was no reactivity with $F(ab')_2$ fragment of an unrelated isotype and allotyped matched Ab2 desingated 3H1. Preimmune sera had no reactivity with the $F(ab')_2$ 4DC6. In addition, the responding patients' sera (post fourth injection) preabsorbed with normal mouse Ig demonstrated specific inhibition of binding of radiolabeled Ab1 antibody with Ab2, and there was no inhibition using preimmune sera. Although steric hindrance by Ab3 binding cannot be excluded in these assays, the results suggest the presence of true anti-anti-Id antibodies that share Ids with Ab1. Again, 3 of 4 patients were positive for Ab3 responses using this assay.

To determine whether Ab2 4DC6 immunized patient's sera bound specifically to semipurified gp37 antigen, the binding of patients' Ab3 sera to the gp37 antigen on the plate was tested by ELISA. Ab3 sera from patient 2, obtained after the fourth immunization, at different dilutions, reacted significantly with gp37 antigen, whereas preimmune sera Ab3 sera from patient 1 or Ab3 sera from one colon cancer patient treated with an unrelated Ab2 3H1 [36] showed marginal binding.

Next, the Ab3 serum was affinity purified through Ab2-Sepharose 4B column. Purified Ab3, which was predominantly IgG, isolated from patient 2 was compared with purified Ab1 for binding to the gp37 antigen using the fluorescent cytometry analysis. Purified Ab3 isolated from patient 2 demonstrated specific binding to the MOLT-4 cell line, which expresses cell surface gp37 antigen, without binding to the gp37 antigen-negative Raji cell line by immune flow cytometry. The Ab3 from patients 1 and 3 showed only marginal reactivity to MOLT-4 cells or semipurified gp37 antigen.

4.5. Cellular responses to anti-idiotype

Cellular immune responses were measured by the proliferation of peripheral blood mononuclear cells incubated with aluminum hydroxide-precipitated anti-Id antibody (4DC6) and its $F(ab')_2$ fragment. Aluminum hydroxide-precipitated unrelated anti-Id antibody 3H1 and its $F(ab')_2$ fragment were used as controls. Positive proliferative responses were seen in patients 2 and 3 that were somewhat comparable to the responses to the mitogen PHA. Preimmune cells had no proliferative response to the anti-Id Ab or its $F(ab')_2$, while postimmune cells had a significant response. There was also a minor but significant response to the isotype-matched 3H1 aluminum hydroxide-precipitated anti-Id Ab that was significantly less than that of the 4DC6 response; this finding probably represents a response to the non-Id components of the Ig molecule. Proliferative responses were first noted after the third injection and continued to increase with each ensuing injection. Flow cytometric analysis of the cultures demonstrated that more than 90% of the proliferating cells were CD4-positive T lymphocytes. The T-cell proliferative assay was not performed for patient 1, whereas patient 4 was anergic and did not even respond to PHA. We did not test T-cell prliferation in the presence of semipurified gp37 antigen due to a very limited supply and thus could not establish the antigen specificity of the cellular immune responses induced in the lymphocytes.

4.6. Toxicity and clinical responses

Toxicity was minimal, with only transient local reactions of mild erythema and mild to moderate induration at the injection site and mild fever and chills relieved by acetaminophen. The anti-Id treatment did not have any deleterious effect on hematopoietic cells or on renal or hepatic function.

Patients were monitored for disease activity at each vaccination visit. Patients 1 and 4 had extensive patch- and plaque-stage infiltrates, and patient 3 had tumor-stage mycosis fungoides. There were no SN2-positive circulating cells present in these patients. After four injections, the patients did not have objective responses. Patient 1 had a significant anti-anti-Id response but did not mount any significant anti-gp37 antibody response. This patient was lost to follow-up after the fourth injection. Patient 2 had discrete skin tumors as well as circulating lymphocytes that labeled with the SN2 Ab. This patient had no other measurable or detectable disease. After the second injection, there was marked induration at the injection site and a slight decrease in the size of the skin lesions. After the fourth injection, all nine skin lesions flattened to the surface of the skin. The decrease in the size of the tumors occurred as the titer of Ab3 in the sera rose during the first cycle of therapy. Numerous biopsies were obtained, and only one of the skin lesions demonstrated residual tumor cells. These cells did not stain with either Ab1 (SN2) murine mAb or Ab3 hyperimmune sera by immunoperoxidase assay. Circulating SN2-positive cells also disappeared. The patient was continued on monthly injections for an additional four injections (total of eight), and then the injections were discontinued. The tumors did not regrow, nor were there new tumors until six months after therapy was discontinued. At this time, there were no new tumors, but some of the original sites became thicker; the most significant growth was in the lesion that demonstrated residual lymphoma in the earlier biopsy. The Ab3 titer had declined, and anti-Id vaccine therapy was reinitiated with an additional nine injections. The titer of Ab3 increased, and there was a transient, partial clinical response followed by tumor growth. At this time, tumor cells did not react with the SN2 Ab1 or Ab3 hyperimmune sera by immunoperoxidase assay, and therapy was discontinued. Interestingly, circulating cells reactive with SN2 did not reappear.

The SN2 mAb identifies a highly restricted T-cell antigen, designated gp37, that is found on approximately 30% of patients' T cells with T-cell lymphoma and in 70% of children with T-acute lymphoblastic leukemia but is not found on normal T cells or other hematopoietic or nonhematopoietic tissues. We, therefore, felt this would be an ideal target antigen for an anti-Id vaccine. Tumors from all treated patients were gp37 antigen positive prior to the initial therapy. Three of four patients demonstrated an anti-anti-Id (Ab3) response to the anti-Id Ab, and two demonstrated specific Id T-cell responses. Only patient 2 mounted antitumor cell antibodies. Patient 2 had an excellent clinical response. We believe the clinical respose was related to the fact that this patient did not have cutaneous anergy and that he had the smallest tumor burden and the best immune response, including antitumor antibody response. We demonstrated binding of hyperimmune serum (Ab3), as well as purified Ab3, predominately IgG, to the gp37 antigen and the gp37-antigen-positive cell line MOLT-4. Unfortunately, we lost the pretherapy autologous tumor in a freezer thaw and therefore could not demonstrate binding. After 11 months, the patient's tumors began to regrow at some of the original tumor sites. Despite an excellent active immune response to retreatment with anti-Id antibody, the tumors only partially regressed and then began to regrow. They were gp37 antigen negative at that time, suggesting that the lack of response was secondary to the growth of gp37-antigen-negative variants. We ruled out the possibility that Ab3 blocked Ab1 binding by demonstrating the lack of binding of anti-human Ig or murine Ab2 to the tumor. Both reagents should have detected Ab3 if it were present on the tumor.

It was interesting that this anti-Id antibody was effective in eliciting immune responses despite the absence of a strong adjuvant. Aluminum hydroxide, although considered a weak adjuvant, was quite adequate in eliciting immune response. As noted in other studies, cross-linking of soluble determinants by aggregation or precipitation helped to increase antigenicity. Also, our mAb was a foreign protein and was injected as an intact Ig, and it is likely that the Fc portion of the murine Ig served as a carrier to help promote the immune responses. It was further interesting that our anti-Id antibody was able to stimulate an in vitro helper T-cell proliferative response in treated patients. The relative roles of patient 2's humoral and cellular immune responses in the clinical response are not known.

We believe our results demonstrate that anti-Id mAb can be effective in some patients. Because of the limited number of patients in this clinical trial, it is not possible to predict which patients will benefit from anti-Id vaccine therapy. Immunotherapy will likely be most effective in patients without cutaneous anergy who have minimal tumor burden.

5. Anti-idiotype vaccine therapy of human colorectal carcinoma

Adenocarcinoma of the colon is the second most common cancer, with over 150,000 new cases of cancer diagnosed annually in the United States each year. Although progress has been made in the adjuvant treatment of colorectal cancer, there continues to be a need for more effective therapy, since high-risk patients treated with adjuvant chemotherapy still have a high incidence (>50%) of recurrent disease.

The vast majority of colon cancer patients (>95%) express CEA, which was the focus for immunotherapy in this clinical trial. CEA is a 180-kDa cell surface glycoprotein that seems to have a role in cellular adhesion, cell-to-cell interactions, and possibly glandular differentiation [37,38]. CEA was first identified as a fetal antigen and re-expressed as a tumor-associated antigen. It is a member of a large family of glycoproteins that are expressed in fetal, normal, mature, and malignant tissues [38]. Several of the CEA-related glycoproteins in normal tissues share antigen cross-reactivity with CEA [39]. CEA itself is weakly antigenic. Numerous clinical trials have been undertaken to develop a therapeutic approach in tumors that expressed CEA using various labeled mAbs against CEA or related antigens. These murine monoclonal antibodies are employed to deliver radioactive isotopes or toxins to cells that express CEA, rather than to accomplish a purely immunologic effect. A direct immunologic approach to CEA-bearing tumors has been developed in our laboratory using an anti-Id vaccine, designated 3H1, that is the internal image of CEA. The aluminum hydroxide-precipitated anti-Id mAb 3H1 was used to treat colon cancer patients [40].

5.1. Selection of patients

All the patients had CEA-positive advanced colorectal carcinoma and had failed all other standard therapies. Baseline studies included a complete physical examination, chest radiography, computer axial tomography examination of the abdomen, serum CEA level, and routine blood counts and chemistries. All the patients had been off prior therapy for at least four weeks, and staging was repeated at the conclusion of therapy.

5.2. Treatment of patients

The patients were treated with either 1 mg, 2 mg or 4 mg of aluminum hydroxide-precipitated anti-Id antibody intracutaneously every other week for four injections. If the patients were stable at the end of the four injections, they were then continued with injections on a monthly basis and evaluated every three months. Patients were removed from study if they demonstrated growth of their tumor.

5.3. Humoral responses to anti-idiotype

The development of humoral immunity induced by immunization with alum-precipitated Ab2, 3H1 was assessed by testing sera obtained from patients before therapy and after each treatment with the vaccine. Hyperimmune sera (following the fourth injection of 3H1) from patients showed significant levels of total HAMA responses, including anti-iso/allo/and anti-anti-idiotypic antibodies against immunizing Ab2, 3H1, as determined by homogeneous sandwich RIA. Next, the sera from these immunized patients were checked for their ability to inhibit the binding of ^{125}I-labeled 8019 mAb (Ab1) to Ab2 3H1 on the plate by RIA or vice versa (inhibition of radiolabeled Ab2 binding to Ab1 on the plate). These reactions were performed in the presence of excess normal murine Ig to block human antibodies against isotypic and allotypic determinants. Seventeen out of 23 patients were positive for Ab3 responses by this assay.

5.4. Induction of anti-CEA antibodies by anti-Id 3H1

Next, we investigated whether 3H1 could induce an anti-CEA antibody response in immunized patients. For this, the crude sera obtained from patients after the fourth treatment were tested for the presence of antibody binding to radiolabeled purified CEA. For patients who received more than four injections, immune responses remained comparable or continued to increase in titer. A pure preparation of CEA was used to reduce the risk of obtaining false-positive results due to nonspecific binding. Immunization with 3H1 induced antibodies that bound to radiolabeled CEA. Thirteen of 23 patients developed anti-CEA antibodies in this phase 1b clinical trial.

To determine the reactivity with cell surface CEA, cultured CEA-positive human colon cancer LS174T cells were tested by immune flow cytometry. Crude sera from 3H1-immunized patients bound to LS174T cells and did not bind to human B-cell lymphoma cells, which do not express CEA. It had been previously shown that Ab1 8019 specifically immunoprecipitated the 180-kDa CEA by SDS-PAGE analysis. To confirm that the Ab3 induced by 3H1 was specific for the CEA molecule, the iodinated purified CEA preparation was immunoprecipitated by purified Ab3 preparations obtained from two patients as well as Ab1 and analyzed by SDS-PAGE. Both patients' Ab3 precipitated the same 180-kDa CEA band as that of murine Ab1 8019. There was no cross-reactivity when the iodinated CEA was reacted with purified Ab3 obtained from a patient treated with an unrelated Ab2 (4DC6).

We also compared the reactivities of Ab1 (8019) with that of patients' purified Ab3 by a sensitive immunoperoxidase assay on autologous and allogeneic colonic tumor specimens surgically removed from patients. The pattern of reactivity of Ab3 on autologous malignant colonic tissues was identical to that obtained with allogeneic tumor specimens. Ab1 8019 showed identical staining patterns, whereas there was no reactivity with control Ab3 obtained from a patient treated with an unrelated Ab2 (4DC6). Reactions with Ab1 or purified Ab3 resulted in the staining of both tumor cells as well as secreted mucinous materials. The staining was apical in glandlike structures and granular (cytoplasmic) in less differentiated areas. There was no reactivity of Ab1 and purified Ab3 on normal tissues from colon, cecum, duodenum, stomach, striated muscle, or smooth muscle.

5.5. Cellular immune responses to anti-idiotype

Cellular immune responses were measured by the proliferation of peripheral blood mononuclear cells incubated with aluminum hydroxide-precipitated anti-Id antibody 3H1 and aluminum hydroxide-precipitated control anti-Id antibody 4DC6. Positive proliferative responses were seen in 9 of 23 patients. All nine of these patients developed an Ab3 antibody response. Preimmune cells had no proliferative response to the anti-Id antibody, while postimmune cells had a significant response. Five of the responding patients (two treated with a 2-mg dose and three with a 4-mg dose) also showed T-cell proliferation in the presence of purified CEA, suggesting antigen-specific T-cell response. There was also a response to the isotype-matched 4DC6 Alu-Gel-precipitated anti-Id antibody; this response was significantly less than that of the 3H1 response, likely representing a response to the non-Id components of the murine Ig molecule. The difference in the response to 3H1-Alu-Gel compared with control 4DC6-Alu-Gel was significant, as was the response to CEA compared to BSA. There was no response to Alu-Gel itself. Flow cytometric analysis of the cultures demonstrated that more than 90% of the proliferating cells were CD4-positive T lymphocytes. The patients who were anergic for human antimouse antibody response also did not demonstrate any T-cell proliferative response.

5.6. Toxicity and clinical responses

Toxicity was minimal, with only local reactions at the injection site (mild erythema and induration) and mild fever and chills relieved by acetaminophen. The anti-Id treatment did not have any deleterious effect on hematopoietic cells or on renal or hepatic function.

Patients were monitored very closely for disease activity. All 23 patients eventually developed progressive disease.

5.7. Serial monitoring of circulating CEA

The CEA serum levels were recorded prior to immunization and determined after each immunization and then once monthly following completion of the immunization schedule. For this, patients' sera was heat inactivated to precipitate the Igs, which could theoretically interfere with monitoring assays involving murine mAb Ab1. CEA is heat stable and was measured in the clear centrifuged supernatant by routine assay. The serial monitoring of CEA correlated with disease progression, and all patients who clinically progressed had a rise in their serum CEA levels.

We have demonstrated that 13 of 23 patients injected with aluminum hydroxide-precipitated anti-Id 3H1 generated anti-CEA antibody by direct binding to radiolabeled purified CEA. None of these patients had preexisting antibody to CEA. We also demonstrated binding to autologous and allogeneic tumor as well as immunoprecipitation of purified CEA in selected patients. While the patients who did not generate a humoral immune response may have been truly anergic, it is possible that those who had elevated CEA levels generated small quantities of antibody that were bound to circulating CEA as immune complexes. Indeed, many patients had increasing levels of circulating immune complexes as determined by the Raji cell assay. Also, there is the possibility that some of the circulating anti-CEA antibodies may be bound to patients' tumor cell or are of low affinity. However, five of the patients still showed high binding of antibody to radiolabeled CEA, while four others showed somewhat modest binding. In future studies, we will stimulate patients' peripheral blood mononuclear cells in vitro with CEA or Ab2 for the induction of tumor-specific antibody.

Several patients demonstrated Id-specific T-cell proliferative responses of primarily CD4 T cells. Five of them also demonstrated CEA-specific T-cell proliferation in vitro. We believe the response observed in some patients against the purified CEA is based on the recognition of processed Id peptides, which have homology to the CEA sequence. In preliminary experiments, we have identified a peptide sequence region of CEA which has homology to a CDR of the light chain of our 3H1 anti-Id vaccine [41].

In summary, we have demonstrated specific active immunity to CEA in patients with advanced colorectal cancer treated with an anti-Id antibody that "mimics" CEA. In this phase 1b clinical trial, we could only accrue patients who failed conventional therapy. All of them had widespread advanced disease. The main purpose of this clinical trial was not to assess tumor response, but to determine the host's immunological response to the vaccine therapy. Some primary questions have been resolved. This anti-Id antibody can evoke an Ab3 as well as cellular immune response in patients, and any Ab3 so derived behaves like an Ab1-like antibody (Ab1'). The intensity of the response appeared to correlate positively with anti-CEA antibody (Ab1') and T-cell proliferative responses. Immune responses appeared independent of the level of circulating CEA. While there were too few patients to compare the 1-mg and the 2- and 4-mg doses, it is clear that patients were able to generate immunity at each of these doses. Toxicity was restricted to local cutaneous reactions lasting 24 to 48 hours, with mild fever and chills, and was relieved by acetaminophen.

Collectively, the immune responses in patients treated with an Id vaccine, which induced humoral and cellular responses against an otherwise nonimmunnogenic tumor antigen, justify follow-up clinical studies in patients with minimal tumor burden, as well as basic immunobiological studies to understand the mechanisms of the T-cell response at the clonal level. Such studies may lead to the development of second-generation idiotype vaccines consisting of cytokine–antibody fusion proteins [42] and idiotype-derived peptide vaccines [43].

6. Anti-idiotype vaccine therapy of breast cancer

We have initiated a phase Ib clinical trial for patients with advanced breast cancer with an anti-Id antibody, designated 11D10, which mimics a human milk fat globule (HMFG) membrane epitope. This 11D10 (Ab2) was raised against the anti-HMFG mAb MC-10 (Ab1). Patients were randomized to intracutaneous injections of 1, 2, 4, or 8 mg of 11D10 after it had been precipitated with aluminum hydroxide. Fifteen patients have thus far been entered into the trial, and the first 12 are evaluable for immune response [44]. Five out of 12 patients have generated significant levels of anti-anti-Id antibody (Ab3) that inhibited the binding of Ab2 to Ab1 and vice versa. Affinity-purified Ab3 from three patients' sera bound specifically to the purified HMFG antigen and immunostained the breast cancer tissue sections. The isotype of the antibody (Ab3/Ab1') was predominantly IgG. Peripheral blood lymphocytes (PBLs) isolated from 3 of 12 immunized patients showed in vitro Id-specific T-cell proliferative responses. The results suggest that anti-Id 11D10 can induce both humoral and cellular immune responses in some advanced breast cancer patients who were heavily pretreated. Toxicity was minimal, with only mild erythema and induration at the injection site. Future immunotherapy trials will employ breast cancer patients with minimal residual disease in the adjuvant setting.

7. Anti-idiotype vaccine therapy of melanoma

Disialoganglioside GD2 is expressed at high density on melanoma cells. Triggering an active immune response against GD2 with the use of an anti-Id mAb (Ab2) that is the internal image of GD2 offers a novel approach to the treatment of melanoma. We have generated and characterized an anti-Id mAb, designated 1A7, that mimics GD2 in biological and serological assays. Anti-Id 1A7 (Ab2) was raised against an anti-GD2 mAb, 14G2a (Ab1). We have initiated a phase 1b clinical trial for advanced melanoma patients with 1, 2, 4, and 8 mg of 1A7 mixed with 100 μg of the QS-21 adjuvant [45]. Five out of five patients treated thus far have generated anti-anti-Id antibodies (Ab3) that were capable of inhibiting the binding of Ab2 to Ab1 and vice versa. Also, affinity-purified Ab3 from 1A7 immunized patients' sera bound specifically to purified GD2 and inhibited the binding of Ab1 to GD2 or GD2-positive melanoma cell lines. The isotype of the GD2-specific antibody in the immunized patients' sera was mostly IgG. These antibodies demonstrated effective cell surface reactivity with tumor cells expressing GD2 by FACS analysis. Collectively, these data demonstrate that anti-Id 1A7 broke immune tolerance to GD2 and induced specific anti-GD2 antibodies in melanoma patients.

8. Conclusion

The anti-Id approach needs to be compared to other tumor therapies, established and experimental. A realistic assessment of the anti-Id therapy predicts that complete remission cannot be expected at the present time. However, evidence already exists that partial remission and responses are achieved with anti-Ids. Compared to chemotherapy, radiation therapy, or lymphokine therapy, the Id approach is a safer and less toxic form of treatment and might improve the quality of life in cancer patiens, which is sometimes compromised by more aggressive chemotherapy and/or radiation therapy. Furthermore, anti-Id therapy might be curative in the adjuvant setting.

Acknowledgment

This work was supported in part by the following grants from the National Institutes of Health (NIH): R01-CA47860; P01-CA57165; R01-CA60000; U01-CA65748; and R01-CA72018. We would like to thank Phyllis Burns for typing the manuscript.

References

1. Terry WD, Rosenberg SA (eds). 1982. Immunotherapy of Human Cancer. Amersterdam: Elsevier, North-Holland Biomedical Press.
2. Weigle WO. 1961. The immune response of rabbits tolerant to bovine serum albumin to the injection of other heterologous serum albumins. J Exp Med 114:111–125.
3. Tonegawa S. 1983. Somatic generation of antibody diversity. Nature 302:575–581.
4. Kunkel HG, Mannik M, Williams RC. 1963. Individual antigenic specificity of isolated antibodies. Science 140:1218–1219.
5. Oudin J, Michel M. 1963. A new allotype form of rabbit serum gammaglobulins, apparently associated with antibody function and specificity. CR Acad Sci (Paris) 257:805–808.
6. Williamson AR. 1976. The biological origin of antibody diversity. Annu Rev Biochem 45:467.
7. Stevenson GT, Glennie MJ. 1985. Surface immunoglobulin of B-lymphocytic tumors as a therapeutic target. Cancer Surv 4:213–244.
8. Lindenmann J. 1973. Speculations on idiotypes of homobodies. Ann Immunol Paris 124:171–184.
9. Jerne NK. 1974. Towards a network theory of the immune system. Ann Immunol Paris 125C:373–389.
10. Kennedy RC, Zhou EM, Lanford RE, Chan TC, Bona CA. 1987. Possible role of anti-idiotype antibodies in the induction of tumor immunity. J Clin Invest 80:1217–1224.
11. Freliner J, Sing A, Infante A, Fathman CG. 1984. Clonotypic antibodies which stimulate T cell clone proliferation. Immunol Rev 81:21–38.
12. Kaye JS, Porcelli S, Tite J, Jones B, Janeway CA Jr. 1983. Both a monoclonal antibody and antisera specific for determinants unique to individual cloned helper T cell lines can substitute for antigen and antigen-presenting cells in the activation of T cells. J Exp Med 158:836–856.
13. Paul WE, Bona C. 1982. Regulatory idiotopes and immune networks: a hypothesis. Immunol Today 3:230–234.
14. Kennedy RC, Dreesman GR, Butel JS, et al. 1985. Suppression of in vivo tumor formation induced by simian virus 40-transformed cells in mice receiving anti-idiotype antibodies. J Exp Med 161:1432–1439.
15. Nelson KA, Georege E, Swenson C, et al. 1987. Immunotherapy of murine sarcomas with auto-anti-idiotypic monoclonal antibodies which bind to tumor-specific T cells. J Immunol 138:2110–2117.
16. Raychaudhuri S, Saeki Y, Chen JJ, et al. 1987. Tumor-specific id vaccines. III. Induction of T helper cells by anti-id and tumor cell. J Immunol 139:3902–3910.
17. Raychaudhuri S, Saeki Y, Chen JJ, et al. 1987. Tumor-specific id vaccine IV: analysis of the network in tumor immunity. J Immunol 139:2096–2102.
18. Chen JJ, Saeki Y, Shi L, et al. 1989. Synergistic anti-tumor effects with combined 'internal image' anti-id and chemotherapy. J Immunol 143:1053–1057.
19. Raychaudhuri S, Köhler H, Saeki Y, Chen JJ. 1989. Potential role of anti-idiotype antibodies in active tumor immunotherapy. Crit Rev Oncol Hematol 9:109–124.
20. Chen JJ, Saeki Y, Köhler H. 1990. Idiotype matching: correlation of expression of protective idiotype in sera with survival of tumor mice. J Immunol 144:759–764.
21. Campbell MJ, Esserman L, Levy R. 1988. Immunotherapy of established murine B-cell lymphoma. Combination of id and cyclophosphamide. J Immunol 141:3227–3233.
22. Porgader A, Banerji R, Watanabe Y, Feldman M, Gilboa E, Eisenbach L. 1993. Anti-metastatic vaccination of tumor-bearing mice with two type of IFN-γ gene-inserted tumor cells. J Immunol 150:1458.
23. Herlyn D, Ross AH, Koprowski H. 1986. Anti-idiotype antibodies bear the internal image of a human tumor antigen. Science 232:101–102.
24. Herlyn D, Wettendorff M, Schmoll E, et al. 1987. Anti-idiotype immunization of cancer patients: modulation of the immune response. Proc Natl Acad Sci USA 84:8055–8059.
25. Herlyn D, Benden A, Kane M, et al. 1991. Anti-idiotype cancer vaccines: preclinical and clinical studies. In Vivo 5:615–624.

26. Mittelman A, Chen ZJ, Yank H, et al. 1992. Active specific immunotherapy in patients with melanoma. J Clin Invest 86:2136–2144.
27. Mittelman A, Chen ZJ, Yank H, et al. 1992. Human high molecular weight melanoma-associated antigen (HMW-MAA) mimicry by mouse anti-idiotypic monoclonal antibody MK2-23: induction of humoral anti-HMW-MAA immunity and prolongation of survival in patients with stage IV melanoma. Proc Natl Acad Sci USA 89:466–470.
28. Robins RA, Denton GWL, Hardcastle JD, Austin EB, Baldwin RW, Durrant LG. 1991. Antitumor immune response and interleukin2 production induced in colorectal cancer patients by immunization with human monoclonal anti-idiotypic antibody. Cancer Res 51:5425–5429.
29. Kwak LW, Campbell MJ, Cerwinski D, Hart S, Miller RA, Levy R. 1992. Induction of immune response in patients with B-cell lymphoma against the surface immunoglobulin idiotype expressed by their tumors. N Engl J Med 327:1209–1238.
30. Bhattacharya-Chatterjee M, Chatterjee SK, Vasile S, Seon BK, Köhler H. 1988. Idiotype vaccines against human T-cell leukemia. II. Generation and characterization of a monoclonal idiotype cascade (Ab1, Ab2 and Ab3). J Immunol 141:1398–1403.
31. Bhattacharya-Chatterjee M, Pride MW, Seon BK, Köhler H. 1987. Idiotype vaccines against human T-cell acute lymphoblastic leukemia (T-ALL). I. Generation and characterization of biologically active monoclonal anti-idiotopes. J Immunol 139:1354–1360.
32. Bhattacharya-Chatterjee M, Mukerjee S, Biddle W, Foon KA, Köhler H. 1990. Murine monoclonal anti-idiotype antibody as a potential network antigen for human carcinoembryonic antigen. J Immunol 145:2758–2765.
33. Chakraborty M, Mukerjee S, Foon KA, Ceriani R, Köhler H, Bhattacharya-Chatterjee M. 1995. Induction of human breast cancer-specific antibody response in cynomolgus monkeys by a murine monoclonal anti-idiotype antibody. Cancer Res 55:1525–1530.
34. Bhattacharya-Chatterjee M, Mrozek E, Mukerjee S, Ceriani RL, Köhler H, Foon KA. 1994. Anti-idiotype antibodies as potential therapeutic agents for human breast cancer. In Ceriani RL, ed. Proceedings of the 5th International Workshop on Breast Cancer Therapy and Immunology. New York: Plenum Press, pp. 387–401.
35. Sen G, Chakraborty M, Foon KA, Reisfeld RA, Bhattacharya-Chatterjee M. 1995. Murine monoclonal anti-idiotype antibody breaks tolerance and induces specific antibody response to human disialoganglioside GD2 in cynomolgus monkeys. Abstract presented at the 9th International Congress of Immunology, San Francisco CA, July 23–29, A5250, p. 885.
36. Foon KA, Oseroff AR, Vaickus L, et al. 1995. Immune responses in patients with T-cell lymphoma treated with an anti-idiotype antibody mimicking a highly restricted T-cell antigen. Clin Cancer Res 1:1285–1294.
37. Bebchimol S, Fuks A, Jothy S, et al. 1989. Carcinoembryonic antigen, a human tumor marker, functions as an intracellular adhesion molecule. Cell 57:327–334.
38. von Kleist S, Burtin P. 1979. Antigens cross-reacting with CEA. In Herberman RB, McIntire KR, eds. Immunodiagnosis of Cancer, vol. 9. New York: Marcel Dekkar, pp. 322–341.
39. von Kleist S, Chavanel G, Burtin P. 1972. Identification of an antigen from normal human tissue that cross-reacts with the carcinoembryonic antigen. Proc Natl Acad Sci USA 69:2492–2494.
40. Foon KA, Chakraborty M, John WJ, Sherratt A, Köhler H, Bhattacharya-Chatterjee M. 1995. Immune response to the carcinoembryonic antigen in patients treated with an anti-idiotype antibody vaccine. J clin Invest 96:334–342.
41. Pervin S, Sherratt A, Wang HT, Blalock EJ, Bhattacharya-Chatterjee M, Köhler H, Foon KA, Chatterjee SK. 1996. Proliferation of T-cells from colon cancer patients by peptides based on the structure of an anti-idiotype antibody mimicking CEA. Proc Am Assoc Cancer Res 37:473.
42. Tao MH, Levy R. 1993. Idiotype/granulocyte-macrophage colony-stimulating factor fusion protein as a vaccine for B-cell lymphoma. Nature 3362:755–758.
43. Williams WW, London SD, Weiner DB, Wadsworth S, Berzofsky JA, Robey F, Rubing DH, Greene MI. 1989. Immune response to a molecularly defined internal image idiotype. J Immunol 142:4392–4400.

5. Endocrine therapy of prostate cancer

Rick L. Bare and Frank M. Torti

1. Introduction

Cancer of the prostate is the most common neoplasm of adult men. In 1995, it was estimated that 244,000 men were diagnosed with prostate cancer and that 40,000 men died of this disease [1]. Although prostate-specific antigen (PSA) has greatly enhanced the early detection of prostate cancer, more than 50% of newly diagnosed prostate cancer patients already have advanced disease [2–6]. Up to 80% of these men will respond to hormonal ablation, yet the median survival of these patients is less than two years. Approximately 10% will live 10 years or longer [7,8].

2. The hypothalamic–pituitary–gonadal–prostatic axis

Huggins and Hodges first demonstrated the hormone responsiveness of prostate cancer in 1941 [9]. Theirs was the first work to demonstrate the hormone dependency of any human cancer. Since that time, the physiology of the endocrine pathways affecting the prostate have been well described. Testosterone supplied by the testes is the main androgen supporting the prostate. Testosterone accounts for approximately 95% of the circulating androgens [10]. The adrenal glands supply the remaining androgens in the form of androstenedione and dehydroepiandrosterone (the precursors of testosterone and dihydrotestosterone, respectively). Both the adrenal glands and the testes are under the control of the hypothalamus and anterior pituitary gland (figure 1). The hypothalamus releases leuteinizing hormone-releasing hormone (LHRH) and corticotropin-releasing factor (CRF). LHRH stimulates the anterior pituitary to release leuteinizing hormone (LH), which in turn stimulates the Leydig cells of the testes to produce testosterone. CRF also provides stimulus to the anterior pituitary to release adrenocorticotrophic hormone (ACTH). ACTH stimulates the production of cortisol and the adrenal androgens, androstenedione and dehydroepiandrosterone, by the adrenal cortex.

Circulating testosterone is converted to a more potent androgen,

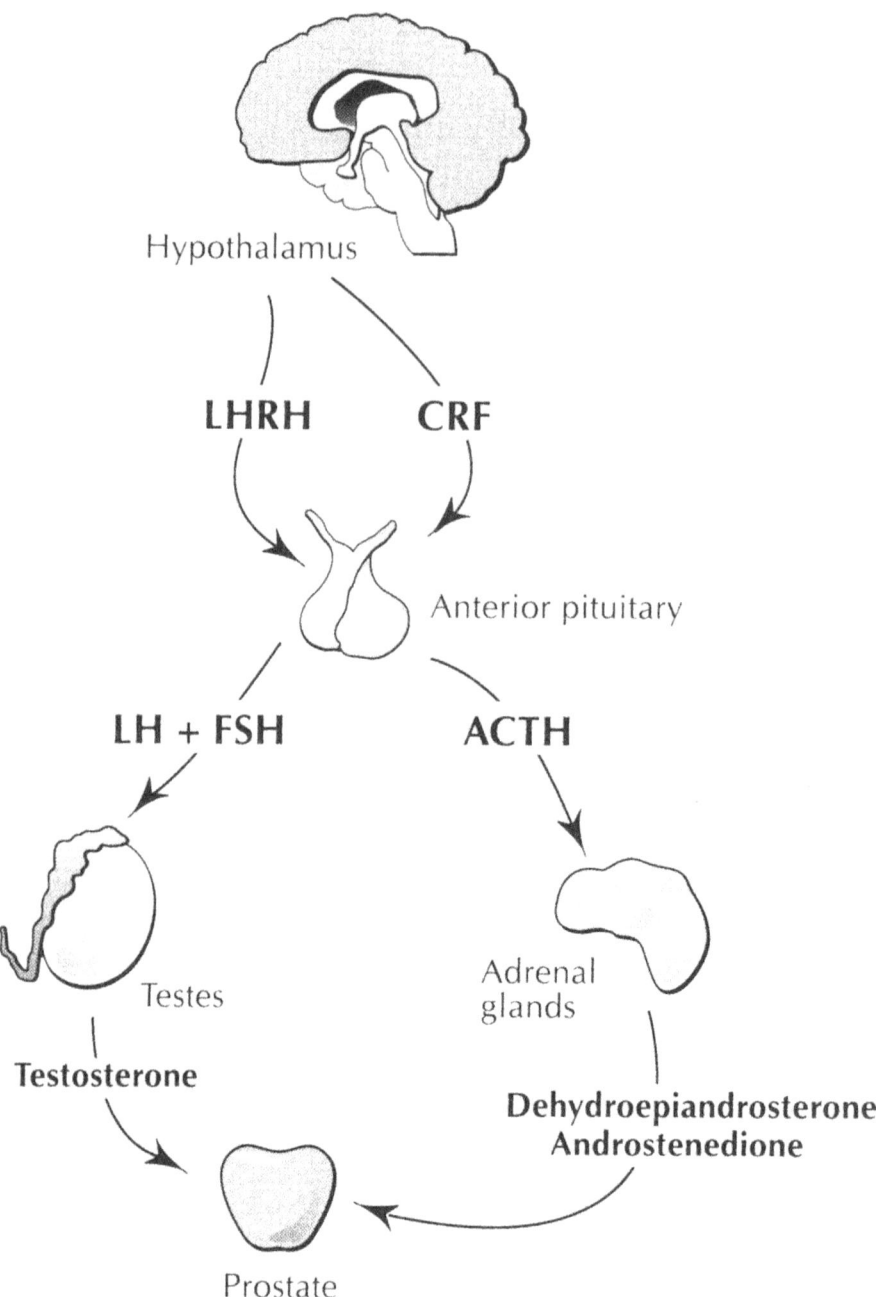

Figure 1. The hypothalamic–pituitary–gonadal axis. LHRH, leuteinizing hormone-releasing hormone; CRF, corticotropic-releasing hormone; LH, leuteinizing hormone; FSH, follicle stimulating hormone; ACTH, adrenocorticotrophic hormone.

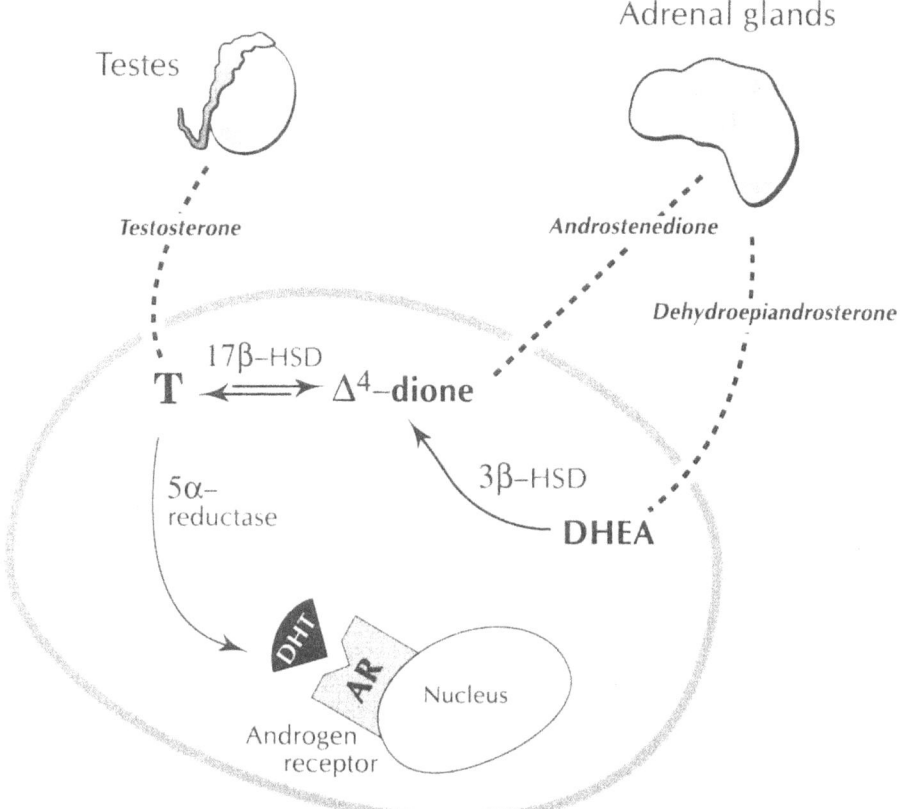

Figure 2. A prostate cell demonstrating dihydrotestosterone (DHT) production. 3β-HSD, 3-beta-hydroxysteroid dehydrogenase; Δ⁴-dione, androstenedione; T, testosterone; DHEA, dehydroepiandrosterone; 17β-HSD, 17-beta-hyroxysteroid dehydrogenase.

dihydrotestosterone, within the prostate. The enzyme responsible for this conversion is 5-alpha reductase (figure 2).

Androgen ablation can be carried out through a number of manipulations of the hypothalamic–pituitary–gonadal axis described above.

3. Methods of androgen deprivation

There are four basic methods for reducing androgen stimulation of the prostate (table 1):
1. Surgical castration
2. Medical suppression of gonadal function — medical castration
3. Antiandrogen blockade of prostatic androgen receptors
4. Inhibition of steroidogenesis

Table 1. Methods of androgen withdrawal[a]

Surgical castration	Medical castration	Antiandrogens	Inhibition of androgen biosynthesis

Bilateral orchiectomy	Estrogens
	  Diethystilbestrol
	  Estramustine phosphate
	  Conjugated estrogens
	  Chlortrianesene
	  Polyestradiol phosphate
	  Diethystilbestrol
	    diphosphate
	LHRH agonists
	  Leuprolide acetate
	  Goserelin
	(Steroidal antiandrogens)
		Nonsteroidal antiandrogens
		  Flutamide
		  Bicalutamide
		  Nilutamide
		Steroidal antiandrogens
		  Megestrol acetate
		  Cyproterone acetate
			Ketocomozole
			Aminoglutethamide
			Spironolactone
			(Steroidal antiandrogens)

[a] The steroidal antiandrogens have several sites of action.

3.1. Surgical castration

Bilateral orchiectomy remains the 'gold standard' for eliminating gonadal androgen secretion. This relatively simple outpatient procedure provides prompt reduction of circulating androgen levels within a few hours [11,12].

Another advantage is the relatively low cost compared with other methods of androgen ablation (table 1). The side effects include hot flashes, impotence, and loss of libido [13,14]. Surgical castration can be psychologically stressful for some men [15].

Adrenalectomy and hypophysectomy are no longer used routinely because of morbidity and limited clinical gain.

3.2. Gonadal suppression/medical castration

Medical castration may be accomplished with a variety of agents that ultimately inhibit luteinizing hormone (LH) stimulation of gonadal function. Estrogens were the first agents used in this capacity. They inhibit the release of LH from the anterior pituitary [16–19], thereby removing the stimulus for Leydig cells of the testis to produce testosterone.

Diethylstilbestrol (DES) is the most common estrogen used in the treatment of prostate cancer. Dosages of 1–5 mg have been well studied [20–25]. Some men attain castrate levels of serum testosterone with only 1 mg DES taken each day [22]. The first Veterans Administration Cooperative Urological Research Group (VACURG I) demonstrated the increased cardiovascular and thromboembolic risks of 5 mg DES over controls [23]. Other complications include gynecomastia, nausea, and edema [26]. Although fewer side effects are seen with the lower 1- and 3-mg doses (VACURG II), castrate levels of testosterone are not always achieved, particularly at the 1-mg dose [24,25]. Other estrogenic compounds include estramustine phosphate, conjugated estrogens, chlortrianesene (TACE), polyestradiol phosphate, and diethylstilbestrol diphosphate (Stilphostrol). All these agents have similar risk/benefit profiles [24,27–31].

The steroidal antiandrogens megestrol acetate and cyproterone acetate are progestational agents used in the treatment of prostate cancer. In addition to binding androgen receptors in prostate tissue, these agents inhibit LH secretion from the anterior pituitary and also inhibit steroidogenesis [32–35].

Megestrol acetate is given in a dose of 120 mg/day. Although castrate levels of testosterone can sometimes be achieved, a secondary rise in testosterone levels limits the clinical utility of this drug [36]. Advantages of megestrol acetate include reduced risks of gynecomastia and cardiovascular events, although there is no decrease in loss of libido. One major use of megestrol acetate in prostate cancer treatment is to control the hot flashes caused by androgen ablation. A dose of 20 mg twice daily is effective in reducing vasomotor hot flashes, with up to 70% of patients having complete resolution of symptoms [37,38].

Cyproterone acetate, another steroidal antiandrogen, has been studied extensively in Europe [32]. In addition to blocking the androgen receptors of the prostate, luteinizing hormone release is suppressed. The cardiovascular side effects of cyproterone acetate occur in approximately 10% of patients. The concomitant use of low-dose DES is required to prevent a secondary increase in serum testosterone level.

Leuteinizing hormone-releasing hormone(LRHH) analogues are now widely used in the treatment of advanced prostate cancer to produce indirect gonadal suppression. These agents are clinically equivalent to surgical castration both in side effects and in response rates [41–43]. LHRH is a decapeptide released naturally by the hypothalamus. These decapeptide analogues with substitutions of the sixth, ninth, and tenth amino acids have a much greater affinity for the pituitary receptors. Administration of high doses of these agents in a nonpulsatile fashion paradoxically suppressses gonadotropin release through chronic occupancy of receptor sites [44]. The initial flare of LH (and subsequently testosterone) lasts 1–2 weeks and can exacerbate pain. Spinal cord compression from spinal metastases and ureteral obstruction have been reported during this period. Antiandrogens have been used successfully to block this 'flare response' [45,46].

Two LHRH analogues are available for use in the United States. Both are available in depot forms that require monthly administration, and both are now available in longer-lasting depot forms that reduce the required administration to every three months. Lupron (Leuprolide) depot, produced by TAP Pharmaceuticals, is administered intramuscularly, and Zoladex (Goserelin), produced by Zeneca Pharmaceuticals, is administered subcutaneously. Zoladex is currently the least expensive of the two, though both are very

Table 2. Approximate patient costs of androgen withdrawal therapies

Therapy	Cost[a]/month	Cost/year
Lupron[b]	$496	$5952
Zoladex[b]	$358	$4296
Casodex	$289	$3468
Eulexin[c]	$149	$1788
Orchiectomy[d]	$5167	

[a] Average of retail and hospital-based pharmacy prices, Winston-Salem, NC, USA (March 1996).
[b] Allowable Medicare charges in North Carolina, USA (March 1996).
[c] Dose of 125 mg T.i.d.
[d] Average cost at North Carolina Baptist Hospital, Winston-Salem, North Carolina, USA (March 1996).

expensive compared to other hormone therapies (table 2). In addition to the flare phenomenon (and costs), side effects such as hot flashes and impotence are observed [41,47].

3.3. Antiandrogens

In addition to the steroidal antiandrogens (cyproterone acetate and megestrol acetate) described previously, there are several nonsteroidal antiandrogens to discuss.

Flutamide is a potent nonsteroidal antiandrogen that inhibits the uptake and binding of testosterone and dihydrotestosterone to nuclear receptors [48–50]. Side effects are mainly related to the gastrointestinal system. Diarrhea is most common. Severe hepatotoxicity occurs rarely. Gynecomastia, rash, and depression are less common. Flutamide has been used as monotherapy in patients wishing to maintain potency [51–53]. More commonly, flutamide is used in combination with orchiectomy or LHRH analogues. The dose is 125–250 mg po three times daily with an approximate patient cost of $150–$300 per month (depending on dose; see table 1).

Bicalutamide is another nonsteroidal pure antiandrogen that recently received FDA approval. The current recommended dosage is 50 mg per day. There is apparently less toxicity, though there is certainly no cost advantage. Casodex has also been studied as monotherapy for advanced prostate cancer. Soloway et al. reported the results of an open-label multicenter North American trial of daily 50 mg Bicalutamide (Casodex) [54]. Of 150 patients studied, the overall objective response rate was 70%. Breast pain and gynecomastia developed in up to 76% of patients. Because of suboptimal effects on PSA levels, the use of Casodex as monotherapy for advanced prostate cancer does not appear warranted.

Nilutamide (Anandron) is a third nonsteroidal antiandrogen that appears to have equal potential to flutamide and bicalutamide in monotherapy and combination therapy trials [55,56].

3.4. Inhibition of steroidogenesis

Several agents inhibit adrenal and gonadal steroidogenesis. Ketoconazole is an antifungal agent that, when given in doses of 1200–1600 mg per day, can reduce circulating testosterone to castrate levels within four hours. There is inhibition of cytochrome P-450-dependent enzymes, including 12-hydroxylase and 17,20-desmolase. Side effects include severe hepatitis (rare but occasionally fatal), decreased libido, lethargy, and gynecomastia [57,58]. Although this agent may be equivalent to orchiectomy in its ability to rapidly lower circulating testosterone, it is ineffective in maintaining castrate levels [59]. This drug should be considered a treatment of choice in patients with impending spinal cord compression and bleeding dyscrasias (or other comorbidities) that preclude surgical castration.

Aminoglutethamide inhibits desmolase and cytochrome P-450-dependent enzymes responsible for the conversion of cholesterol to pregnenolone, thus inhibiting both adrenal and gonadal production of steroids [60–62]. Concomitant glucocorticoid administration is required. Otherwise, the resultant increase in ACTH levels will override the effects of aminoglutethimide.

Spironolactone also inhibits steroidogenesis through blockade of 17-alpha-hydroxylase, thus decreasing production of the androgens (testosterone, dehydroepiandrosterone, and androstenedione) [63,63]. Decreased libido, gynecomastia, and diarrhea and reported with its use. Rarely, agranulocytosis can occur. This drug is not commonly used in prostate cancer treatment.

4. Prognostic factors in metastatic prostate cancer

For treatment planning, it may be beneficial to have information indicating which patients may respond best to hormone therapy.

Primary tumor stage and grade are potential prognostic indicators. However, tumor found on biopsy is not always indicative of the grade of the tumor as a whole [65]. Also, metastatic sites of disease often are less differentiated than the primary tumors. Extent of disease as determined by bone scan has been catagorized by Soloway et al. [66]. They found that patients with less than six lesions on bone scan at the time of diagnosis have significantly better two-year survival rates than patients with more extensive disease [67].

Contrary to its potential predictive value with other malignancies, *performance status* may not be a clinically useful prognostic indicator in prostate cancer patients. Most of these men enjoy good performance status at the time of diagnosis.

Several laboratory evaluations may be useful in predicting outcome of treatment. Some studies indicate that elevated prostatic acid phosphatase (PAP) levels at diagnosis indicate a worse prognosis [68–69], while others dispute this finding [70–72].

Prostate-specific antigen (PSA) levels have been shown to correlate with response to androgen deprivation therapy [73–76]. Pretreatment PSA levels may be inversely proportional to survival. Killian et al. [74] report that higher pretreatment PSA levels correlate with higher recurrence rates and decreased time to progression. Others have been unable to correlate prognosis with pretreatment PSA levels [70,71,77].

Serum *alkaline phosphatase* levels have been shown by Chodak et al. to be the most significant prognostic indicator of survival [78].

Serum *testosterone* levels may also have prognostic value in predicting response to androgen ablation. Patients with low pretreatment serum testosterone levels have lower survival rates than those with higher pretreatment levels [67,78–84].

Almost every factor found to have prognostic significance in some studies of metastatic prostate cancer treatment has been found to have no prognostic potential by others. Therefore, there are no prognostic indicators to determine who should or should not be treated with androgen deprivation.

5. Maximum androgen blockade

The theoretical appeal of suppressing both testicular and adrenal androgens has led to the development of multiple therapeutic combinations. Surgical maximum androgen ablation combines orchiectomy and adrenalectomy or hypophysectomy. Adrenalectomy and/or hypophysectomy are procedures no longer used except in rare instances in the treatment of prostate cancer [85–89]. In the early 1980s, there were a number of studies comparing orchiectomy alone with orchiectomy and adrenal androgen suppression or blockade [90–93].

Labrie et al. studied combining an antiandrogen (flutamide) with an LHRH agonist (leuprolide) [90]. Their report of 97% response rates and 89% two-year survivals led to a large-scale study designed by the National Cancer Institute [93]. This project enlisted a total of 617 patients with advanced (D_2) prostate cancer. The patients were randomized in a double-blind fashion to receive leuprolide plus placebo or leuprolide plus flutamide. There was a significant increase in progression-free survival — 16.5 versus 13.9 months — in the patients receiving flutamide ($p < 0.01$). Survival was also increased to 35.6 months (flutamide group) versus 28.3 months (leuprolide alone) ($p < 0.01$) [93]. The many randomized trials that followed have now undergone meta-analysis by the Prostate Cancer Trialists Collaboration Group [94]. The Group identified 25 trials comparing castration (surgical or medical with LHRH analogues) versus maximum androgen blockade (MAB), castration plus antiandrogens. Individual patient data were available in 22 of these trials for a total of 5710 patients. Median follow-up was 40 months. Deaths were reported in 3283 of these 5710 patients (57%). Mortality rates were 58% for castration alone and 56% for MAB. The five-year survival estimate was 22.8% for the castration-alone group and 26.2% for the MAB group, with no statistically significant difference. (figure 3). The Group concludes that there is no available evidence at this time demonstrating a survival advantage to MAB over castration alone. Although references supported by meta-analysis are not as certain as for single research studies, this analysis again raises the question of the use of combined hormone treatments.

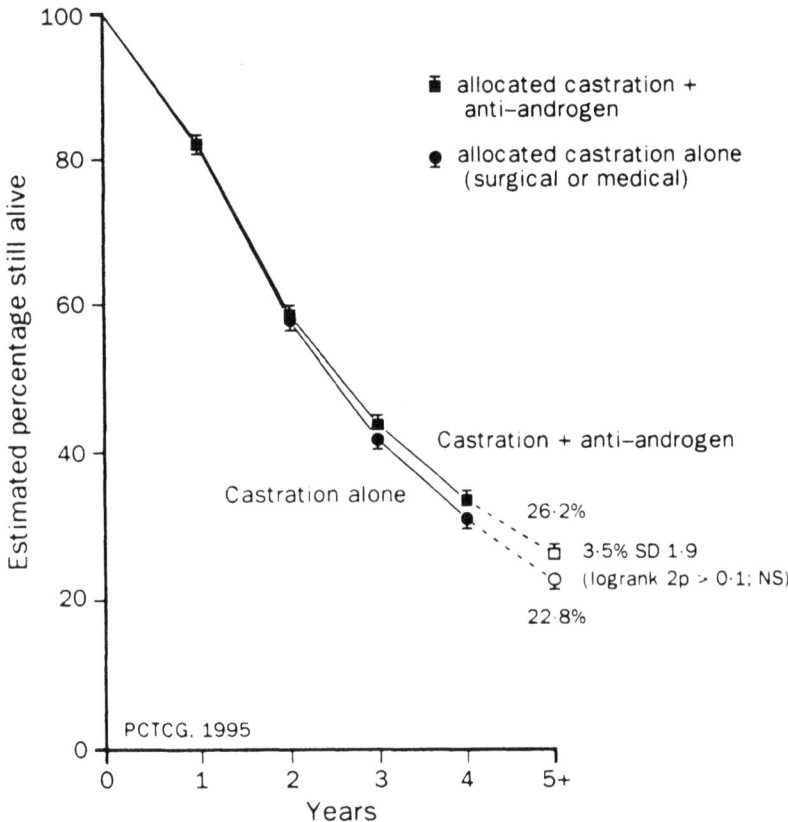

Figure 3. Survival in 22 randomized prostate cancer trials: MAB vs. castration alone (5710 patients, 3283 deaths). In the first year, there were 475 deaths out of 2512 person-years in the MAB group (logrank O-E = −6.0, variance = −196.1, NS) versus 498 of 2561 in the controls. In the second year there were 594 of 1778 (−0.5, 212.5, NS) versus 606 of 1787. After year 2, there were 525 of 1911 (−34.1, 206.5, 2 $p < 0.02$) versus 587 of 1774. From the Prostate Cancer Trialists' Collaborative Group. 1995. Lancet 346:265–269. Reprinted with permission.

5.1. Timing of therapy (early versus delayed versus intermittent androgen withdrawal)

No definitive randomized studies have addressed the impact of early versus delayed androgen deprivation therapy on the overall survival of patients with advanced prostate cancer. Indirectly, the Veterans Administration Cooperative Urological Research Group (VACURG) produced some data comparing the timing of therapy in their first study [23]. This study compared castration, 5 mg DES/day, and castration plus 5 mg DES/day versus placebo. Placebo was not adequately studied, however, because patients eventually progressed and received hormonal or castration therapy at relapse. Therefore, the comparison was viewed as early versus delayed therapy. There was no impact on overall survival, though progression was delayed with early therapy. Because no definitive studies are available to direct the timing of hormonal therapy, timing is currently an individual choice of the patient and physician. Quality-of-life issues should weigh heavily in this decision. Many fully informed patients may choose no treatment until they are symptomatic from their disease.

To balance this controversy, intermittent androgen suppression is being investigated in the treatment of metastatic prostate cancer. Klotz et al. used intermittent DES to treat 19 patients [95]. DES was stopped when a clinical response was noted and reinitiated when disease progressed. Impotence induced by therapy was reversed in 9 of 10 men upon withdrawal of DES therapy. No adverse effects on survival were noted. More recently, Goldenberg et al. used intermittent total androgen blockade to treat 47 patients [96]. Treatment was interrupted when nadir PSA levels were reached and restarted when PSA levels rose to 10–20 ng/mL. This cycle was repeated until D_3 disease developed. The off-treatment periods were associated with recovery of potency in men with therapy-induced dysfunction. Their preliminary results indicate no negative effects on survival or time to progression.

5.2. Antiandrogen withdrawal

Patients who demonstrate PSA progression while being treated with maximum androgen blockade may benefit from withdrawal of the antiandrogen. Dupont et al. studied 40 patients with progressive metastatic prostate cancer despite total androgen blockade (medical or surgical castration and flutamide) [97]. Flutamide was discontinued, and 30 patients responded with decreasing PSA levels. Seventeen patients demonstrated PSA decreases to the normal range. Nieh demonstrated a similar response to withdrawal of casodex (bicalutamide) in three patients [98].

Akakura et al. reported declining PSA levels in two patients upon withdrawal of a steroidal antiandrogen, chlormadinone acetate [99]. The decline in PSA levels noted with antiandrogen withdrawal is associated with no change in testosterone or adrenal androgen levels.

Sartor et al. demonstrated a flutamide withdrawal response when combined with administration of aminoglutethamide [100]. Though the etiology of the flutamide withdrawal phenomenon remains speculative, Sartor's group proposes that proliferation of cancer cells containing mutant androgen receptors occurs during prolonged flutamide exposure. Furthermore, these mutant receptors are felt to aberrantly recognize flutamide metabolites and nonandrogenic steroids as androgenic stimuli. Dupont et al. suggest that flutamide therapy may increase sensitivity to androgens with prolonged therapy [97].

Whatever the cause of this phenomenon, antiandrogenic withdrawal should be considered a viable treatment modality in patients developing hormone refractory disease.

5.3. 5-Alpha-reductase inhibitors combined with antiandrogens

As monotherapy, 5-alpha reductase inhibitors have little efficacy in the treatment of advanced prostate cancer [101]. The nuclear receptor binding dihydrotestosterone (DHT) also binds testosterone (with lower affinity), explaining the marginal effect of finasteride treatment in this disease.

Likewise, flutamide and bicalutamide have limited efficacy as monotherapy for advanced prostate cancer [54,102], presumably because the increased serum testosterone levels associated with antiandrogen therapy result in higher levels of DHT. Thus there is increased competition for the androgen receptors, overriding the antiandrogen blockade.

In an effort to decrease the side effects of androgen derivation therapy and to achieve regression of disease, Fleshner and Trachtenberg treated 22 advanced prostate cancer patients with combination flutamide and finasteride [103]. Since neither drug decreases testosterone levels, 86% of these men maintained sexual function. The initial mean PSA level of 42.9 ng/mL was reduced to 3.6 ng/mL and 2.9 ng/mL at 3 and 6 months, respectively. Those results were maintained at two-years follow-up. This regimen appears less effective than the combination of LHRH agonists and flutamide in reducing serum PSA to undetectable levels. However, it remains to be tested whether survival is similar with these two therapies. Patients may be willing to accept this therapy in exchange for fewer side effects.

5.4. Neoadjuvant hormonal therapy prior to radical prostatectomy

A challenging problem for urologic surgeons is clinical understaging of prostate cancer compared to pathologic stage. Up to two thirds of patients with clinically localized stage B tumors are found to have capsular penetration or positive surgical margins on sectioning the surgical specimen [104–108]. These patients are felt to be at higher risk of recurrence and progression of disease [105]. Because castration is known to cause involution of metastatic prostate cancer, possibly through triggering apoptosis and suppressing cellular proliferation [109], there is increasing interest in neoadjuvant hormone therapy as a means of decreasing positive surgical margin rates.

The results of several studies indicate a significant decrease in positive surgical margins in patients treated with three month of neoadjuvant androgen ablation [110–112]. The most common regimen contains an LHRH agonist and an antiandrogen. Labrie et al. enrolled 161 patients in the first randomized trial of neoadjuvant androgen ablation prior to radical prostatectomy [110]. Those patients assigned to the neoadjuvant treatment arm received three months of Lupron and flutamide. They determined that neoadjuvant therapy resulted in a decrease in positive surgical margins from 33.8% to only 7.8%. Similar results were reported by Soloway et al. in a multi-institutional randomized prospective study comparing radical prostatectomy alone versus radical prostatectomy preceded by three months of Lupron and flutamide [111]. They report capsular penetration in 47% in the pretreatment group versus 78% in the control arm. Positive surgical margins were found in only 18% of the neoadjuvant therapy group versus 48% of controls.

Though most investigators agree that preoperative androgen withdrawal results in a significant decrease in serum PSA and prostate volume, many have not been able to demonstrate significant decreases in cancer-positive surgical margin rates [113–117].

Oesterling et al. reviewed 22 patients with stage B or C disease who underwent preoperative androgen withdrawal [116]. There were no demonstrable differences in tumor size, stages, or DNA ploidy over appropriately matched controls. Similarly, Pummer et al. demonstrated no histopathologic changes as an effect of androgen deprivation, although serum PSA levels were significantly reduced [117].

Theoretically, androgen ablation-induced decreases in prostate volume would facilitate surgical extirpation. However, in this respect, Macfarlane et al. [113] and Soloway et al. [116] demonstrated no advantage to androgen ablation. There were no differences in blood loss or operative time.

Though the potential exists to decrease cancer-positive surgical margin rates with preoperative androgen withdrawal, longer follow-up is needed to document any survival advantage.

5.5. Neoadjuvant hormonal therapy prior to radiation therapy

Recently, there has been renewed interest in neoadjuvant hormonal therapy for prostate cancer patients treated with radiation. Initial studies met with little success. Some studies indicated decreased survival rates with the addition of neoadjuvant hormonal therapy [118]. Recent studies, however, have demonstrated possible benefit from the combined therapy. Zelefsky et al. conducted a study that attempted to reduce the volume of normal tissues subjected to radiation therapy by using neoadjuvant hormonal therapy to reduce prostate volume [119]. Twenty-two patients with bulky disease were treated with three months of neoadjuvant maximum androgen blockade (leuprolide and flutamide). Dose–volume histogram calculations for all normal tissue structures were determined from simulation and conformal treatment planning before and after neoadjuvant hormonal therapy. Decreases in the volume of rectal wall, bladder, and small bowel receiving radiation were demonstrated. This group feels that neoadjuvant hormonal therapy is useful in optimizing the geometry of the target volume in relation to the adjacent normal tissues. Forman et al. concur with these findings in their study of 20 patients with stage T_1 and T_2 disease treated with three months neoadjuvant leupolide followed by irradiation [120. They believe this regimen will lead to improvement in the therapeutic ratio by reducing the morbidity of treatment.

Hanks et al. (Radiation Therapy Oncology Group) randomized patients with clinical T_2C, T_3, or T_4 disease to receive either two months of neoadjuvant and concomitant Goserelin (Zoladex) plus flutamide or radiation alone [121]. They demonstrated significant decreases in local failure rate at three years as well as significant increases in the number of patients having PSA of less than 4.0 ng/mL at three years in the neoadjuvant hormone therapy group. Disease-free survival was also significantly increased in the hormone therapy group at three years.

As with neoadjuvant hormonal therapy and surgery, the results here are promising, but overall survival benefits are yet to be determined.

6. Summary

Endocrine therapy is effective treatment for patients with metastatic prostate cancer. Most patients will benefit from androgen withdrawal in terms of symptomatic relief and delay in progression of disease. It does not, however, cure patients with metastatic prostate cancer. This finding emphasizes the need for the development of effective nonendocrine therapies.

References

1. Wingo PA, Tong T, Bolden S. 1995. Cancer statistics. Cancer 45:8.
2. Lang PH. 1993. The next era for prostate cancer: controlled clinical trials. JAMA 269:95–96.
3. Catalona WJ, Smith DS, Ratliff TL, Dodds KM, Coplen DE, Yuan JJ, Petros JA, Andriole GE. 1991. Measurement of prostate-specific antigen in serum as a screening test for prostate cancer. N Engl J Med 324:1156–1161.
4. Brawer MK, Chetner MP, Beatie J, Buchner DM, Vessella RL, Lange PH. 1992. Screening for prostatic carcinoma with prostate specific antigen. J Urol 147:841–851.
5. Richie JP, Catalona WJ, Ahmann FR, et al. 1993. Effect of patient age on early detection of prostate cancer with serum prostate-specific antigen and digital rectal examination. Urology 42:365–374.
6. Catalona WJ, Smith DS, Ratliff TL, Basler JW. 1993. Detection of organ confined prostate cancer is increased through prostate-specific antigen-based screening. JAMA 270:948–954.
7. Murphy GP, Beckley S, Brady MF, et al. 1983. Treatment of newly diagnosed metastatic

prostate cancer patients with chemotherapy agents in combination with hormones versus hormones alone. Cancer 51:1264–1272.
8. Resnick MI, Grayhack JT. 1978. Treatment of stage IV carcinoma of the prostate. Urol Clin North Am 5:141–161.
9. Huggins C, Hodges CV. 1941. Studies in prostate cancer 1: the effect of castration on serum phosphotases in metastatic carcinoma of the prostate. Cancer Res 1:293–297.
10. Walsh PC. 1975. Physiologic basis for hormonal therapy in carcinoma of the prostate. Urol Clin North Am 2:125.
11. Grayhack JT, Keeler TC, Kozlowski JM. 1987. Carcinoma of the prostate: hormonal therapy. Cancer 60 (Suppl):589–601.
12. Maatman TJ, Gupta MK, Montie JE. 1985. Effectiveness of castration versus intravenous estrogen therapy in producing rapid endocrine control of metastatic cancer of the prostate. J Urol 133:620.
13. Ellis WJ, Grayhack JT. 1963. Sexual function in aging males after orchiectomy and estrogen therapy. J Urol 89:895.
14. Eaton AC, McGuire N. 1983. Cyproterone acetate in treatment of post-orchiectomy hot flushes. Lancet 2:1336.
15. Cassileth BR, Soloway MS, Vogelzang NJ, et al. 1989. Patients choice of treatment in state D prostate cancer. Urology 33 (Suppl 5):57–62.
16. Dodds EC, Goldberg L, Lawson W, et al. 1938. Oestrogenic activity of certain synthetic compounds. Nature 141:247–248.
17. Griffiths K, Davies P, Eaton CL, et al. 1988. Cancer of the prostate. Endocrine factors. In Clark JR, ed. Oxford Reviews of Reproductive Biology, vol. 9. Oxford, England: Oxford University, pp. 192–259.
18. Griffiths K, Davis P, Easton CL, et al. 1992. Endocrine factors in the initiation, diagnosis and treatment of prostatic cancer. In Voigt KD, Knabbe C, eds. Endocrine Dependent Tumors. New York: Raven, pp. 83–130.
19. Piva F, Motta M, Marini L. 1979. Regulation of and hypothalamic and pituitary function; long, short, and ultra short feedback loops. In DeGroot LJ, ed. Endocrinology. New York: Grune and Stratton, pp 21–33.
20. Grayhack JT, Keeler TC, Kozlowski JM. 1987. Carcinoma of the prostate: hormonal therapy. Cancer 60:589–601.
21. Citrin DL, Kies MS, Wallemark CB, et al. 1985. A phase II study of high-dose estrogens (diethylstilbestrol diphosphate) in prostate cancer. Cancer 56:457–460.
22. Beck PH, McAnich JW, Goebel JL, Sutzmann RE. 1978. Plasma testosterone in patients receiving diethylstilbestrol. Urology 11:157–160.
23. Veterans Administration Cooperative Urological Research Group. 1967. Treatment and survival of patients with cancer of the prostate. Surg Gynecol Obstet 124:1011–1017.
24. Blackard CE. 1975. The Veterans' Administration Cooperative Urological Research Group studies of carcinoma of the prostate: a review. Cancer Chemother Rep 59:225–227.
25. Byar DP. 1973. Proceedings 1973. The Veterans Administration Cooperative Urological Research Group's studies of cancer of the prostate. Cancer 32:1126–1130.
26. Glashan RW, Robinson MRG. 1981. Cardiovascular complications in the treatment of prostatic carcinoma. Br J Urol 53:624–627.
27. Benson RC Jr, Gill GM. 1986. Estramustine phosphate compared with diethylstilbestrol: a randomized, double blind, crossover trial for stage D prostate cancer. Am J Clin Oncol 9:341.
28. Benson RC Jr, Gill GM, Cummings KB. 1983. A randomized double blind, crossover trial of diethylstilbestrol (DES) and estramustine phosphate (Emcyt) for stage D prostatic carcinoma. Semin Oncol 10 (Suppl 3):43.
29. Benson RC, Wear JB, Gill GM. 1979. Treatment of stage D hormone-resistant carcinoma of the prostate with estramustine phosphate. J Urol 121:452–454.
30. Baba S, Janetschek G, Pollow K, Hahn K, Jacobi GH. 1982. The effects of chlorotrianisene (Tace) of kinetics of 3H-testosterone metabolism in patients with carcinoma of the prostate. Br J Urol 54 (4):393–398.

31. Rohlf PL, Flocks RH. 1969. Stilphosterol therapy in 100 cases of prostatic carcinoma. J Iowa Med Soc 59:1096.
32. Rost A, Schmidt-Gollwitzer M, Hantelman W, et al. 1981. Cyproterone acetate, testosterone, LH, FSH, and prolactin levels in plasma after intramuscular application of cyproterone acetate in patients with prostatic cancer. Prostate 2:315.
33. Geller J, Albert JD. 1983. Endocrine therapy; predictors of response to prostatic cancer. Semin Urol 1:191.
34. Geller J, Albert JD. 1983. Comparison of various hormonal therapies for prostatic carcinoma. Semin Oncol 10:34.
35. Geller J, Albert J, Geller S, et al. 1976. Effects of megestrol acetate (Megace) on steroid metabolism and steroid-protein binding in the human prostate. J Clin Endocrinol Metab 43:1000.
36. Geller J, Albert J, Yen SSC. 1978. Treatment of advanced cancer of the prostate with megestrol acetate. Urology 12:537.
37. Loprinzi CL, Michalak JC, Quella SK. et al. 1994. Megestrol acetate for the prevention of hot flashes. N Engl J Med 331:347–352.
38. Smith JA Jr. 1994. A prospective comparison of treatments for symptomatic hot flashes following endocrine treatment for carcinoma of the prostate. J Urol 152:132.
39. Smith RB, Walsh PC, Goodwin EW. 1973. Cyproterone acetate in the treatment of advanced carcinoma of the prostate. J Urol 110:106.
40. Jacobi GH, Altwein JE, Kurth KH, et al. 1980. Treatment of advanced prostatic cancer with parenteral cyproterone acetate; a phase III randomised trial. Br J Urol 52:208.
41. Soloway MS. 1988. Efficacy of buserelin in advanced prostate cancer and comparison with historical controls. Am J Clin Oncol 11 (Suppl) 1:529–532.
42. The Leuprolide Study Group. 1984. Leuprolide versus diethylstilbestrol for metastatic prostate cancer. N Engl J Med 311:1281–1286.
43. Klioze SS, Miller MF, Spiro TP. 1988. A randomized comparative study of buserelin with DES/orchiectomy in the treatment of stage D2 prostate cancer patients. Am J Clin Oncol 2 (Suppl):S5176–S5182.
44. Corbin A. 1982. From contraception to cancer. A review of the therapeutic applications of LHRH analogues as antitumor agents. Yale J Biol Med 55:27–47.
45. Labrie F, Dupont A, Belanger A, Lachance R. 1987. Flutamide eliminates the risk of disease flare in prostatic cancer patients treated with a luteinizing hormone-releasing hormone agonist. J Urol 138:804–806.
46. Kuhn JM, Billebaud R, Navrail H, et al. 1989. Prevention of the transient adverse effects of a gonadotropin-releasing hormone analogue (buserelin) in metastatic prostatic carcinoma by administration of an antiandrogen (nilutamide). N Engl J Med 321:413–418.
47. Crawford ED, Eisenberger MA, McLeod DG, et al. 1989. A controlled trial of leuprolide with and without flutamide in prostatic carcinoma. N Engl J Med 321:419–424.
48. Neri RO, Kassem N. 1984. Biological and clinical properties of antiandrogens. In Bresciani F, ed. Progress in Cancer Research and Therapy, vol. 31. New York: Raven Press, p. 507.
49. Neri R, Florance K, Koziol P, et al. 1972. A biological profile of a nonsteroidal antiandrogen SCH 13521 (4'-nitro-3'trifluoromethylisobutyranlide). Endocrinology 91:427–437.
50. Knuth UA, Hano R, Nieschlag E. 1984. Effect of flutamide or cyproterone acetate on pituitary and testicular hormones in normal men. J Clin Endocrinol Metab 59:963–969.
51. Sogani PC, Vagaiwala MR, Whitmore WF Jr. 1984. Experience with flutamide in patients with advanced prostate cancer without prior endocrine therapy. Cancer 54:744–750.
52. Lund F, Rasmussen F. 1988. Flutamide versus stilboestrol in the management of advanced prostatic cancer — a controlled prospective study. Br J Urol 61:140–142.
53. Jacobo E, Schmidt JD, Weinstin SH, et al. 1976. Comparison of flutamide (SCH-13521) and diethylsilbestrol in untreated advanced prostatic cancer. Urology 8:231–234.
54. Soloway MS, Schellhammer PF, Smith JA Jr, Chodak GW, Vogelzan NJ, Kennealey GT. 1995. Bicalutamide in the treatment of advanced prostatic carcinoma: a phase II

noncomparative multicenter trial evaluating safety, efficacy and long-term endocrine effects of monotherapy. J Urol 154:2110–2114.
55. Namer M, Amiel J, Toubol J. 1988. (RU23908) associated with orchiectomy in stage D prostate cancer. Preliminary results of a double blind study. Am J Clin Oncol 31:719–729.
56. Raynaud JP, Bonne C, Meguilewsky M, Lefebvre FA, Belanger A, Labrie F. 1984. The pure antiandrogen RU 23908 (Anandron) a candidate of choice for the combined antihormonal treatment of prostatic cancer: a review. Prostate 5:299–311.
57. Trachtenberg J, Pont A. 1984. Ketoconazole therapy for advanced prostate cancer. Lancet 2:433–435.
58. Pont A, Williams PL, Azhar S, et al. 1982. Ketoconazole blocks testosterone synthesis. Arch Intern Med 142:2137–2140.
59. Vanuytsel L, Ang KK, Vantongelen K, et al. 1987. Ketoconazole therapy for advanced prostatic cancer: feasibility and treatment results. J Urol 137:905.
60. Cash R, Brough AJ, Cohen MNP, et al. 1967. Aminoglutethiamide (Elipten-Ciba) as an inhibitor of adrenal steroidogenesis: mechanism of action and therapeutic trial. J Clin Endocrinol Metab 27:1239.
61. Blankenstin MA, Bakker GH. 1985. Rational for suppression of adrenal steroidogenesis in advanced prostatic cancer. Prog Clin Biol Res 185A:161.
62. Sanford EJ, Drago JR, Rohner TJ Jr, et al. 1976. Aminoglutethimide medical adrenalectomy for advanced prostatic carcinoma. J Urol 115:174.
63. Baba S, Murai M, Jitsukawa S, et al. 1978. Antiandrogenic effects of spironolactone; hormonal and ultrastructural studies in dogs and men. J Urol 119:375.
64. Walsh PC, Siiteri PK. 1975. Suppression of plasma androgens by spironolactone in castrated men with carcinoma of the prostate. J Urol 114:254.
65. Garnett JE, Oyasu R, Grayhack JT. 1984. The accuracy of diagnostic biopsy specimens in predicting tumor grades by Gleason's classification of radical prostatectomy specimens. J Urol 131:690.
66. Soloway MS, Hardeman SW, Hickey D, Raymond J, Todd B, Soloway S, et al. 1988. Stratification of patients with metastatic prostate cancer based upon extent of disease on initial bone scan. Cancer 61:195–202.
67. Soloway MS. 1990. The importance of pretreatment testosterone and other prognostic variables in the response to androgen deprivation therapy. Prog Clin Biol Res 350:141–148.
68. Maatman TJ, Gupta MK, Montie JE. 1984. The role of serum prostatic acid phosphatase as a tumor marker in men with advanced adenocarcinoma of the prostate. J Urol 132:58.
69. Ercole CJ, Lange PH, Mathisen M, Chiou RK, Reddy PK, Vsseela RL. 1987. Prostate specific antigen and prostatic acid phosphatase in the monitoring and staging of patients with prostatic cancer. J Urol 138:1181–1184.
70. Matzkin H, Lewyshon O, Ayalon D, Braf Z. 1989. Changes in prostate specific markers under chronic gonadotropin releasing hormone analogue treatment of stage D prostate cancer. Cancer 63:1287–1291.
71. Siddall JK, Hetherington JW, Cooper EH, et al. 1986. Biochemical monitoring of carcinoma of prostate treated with an LHRH analogue. Br J Urol 56:676–687.
72. Matzkin H, Ebert P, Todd B, van der Zwaag R, Soloway MS. 1992. Prognostic significance of changes in prostate specific markers in endocrine treatment of stage D2 prostate cancer. Cancer 70:2302–2309.
73. Kuriyama M, Wang MC, Lee CL, et al. 1987. Use of human specific antigen in monitoring prostate cancer. Cancer Res 41:3874–3876.
74. Killian CS, Yang N, Enrich LJ, et al. 1985. Prognostic importance of prostate specific antigen for monitoring patients with stages B2 to D1 prostate cancer. Cancer Res 45:886–891.
75. Smith JA, Crawford ED, Lange PH, et al. 1991. PSA correlation with response and survival in advanced carcinoma of the prostate. J Urol 145:384A.
76. Cooper EH, Armitage TG, Robinson MRG, et al. 1990. Prostatic specific antigen and the prediction of prognosis in metastatic prostatic cancer. Cancer 66:1025–1028.

77. Arai Y, Yoshiki T, Yoshida O. 1990. Prognostic significance of prostate specific antigen in endocrine treatment for prostatic cancer. J Urol 144:1415–1419.
78. Chodak GW, Vogelzang NJ, Caplan RJ, Soloway MS, Smith JA. 1991. Independent prognostic factors in patients with metastatic (stage D2) prostate cancer. JAMA 265:618–621.
79. Soloway MS, Ishikawa S, van der Zwang R, Todd B. 1989. Prognostic factors in patients with advanced prostate cancer. Urology 33 (Suppl):53–56.
80. Harper ME, Pierrepooint CG, Griffiths K. 1984. Carcinoma of the prostate; relationship of pretreatment hormone levels to survival. J Clin Oncol 20:477–482.
81. Robinson MRG, Thomas BS. 1971. Effect of hormonal therapy on plasma testosterone levels in prostatic carcinoma. Br Med J 4:391–394.
82. Adlercreutz H, Rannikko S, Kairento AL, Karonen SL. 1981. Hormonal pattern in prostatic cancer: correlation with primary response to endocrine treatment. Acta Endocrinol (Copenh) 98:634–640.
83. Hickey DP, Todd B, Soloway M. 1986. Pretreatment testosterone levels; significance in androgen deprivation therapy. J Urol 136:1038–1040.
84. Eriksson A, Carlstrom K. 1988. Prognostic value of serum hormone concentrations in prostatic cancer. Prostate 13(3):249–256.
85. Huggins C, Scott WW. 1945. Bilateral adrenalectomy in prostate cancer. Ann Surg 122:1031–1041.
86. Harrison JH, Thorn GW, Jenkins D. 1953. Total adrenalectomy for reactivated carcinoma of the prostate. N Engl J Med 248:86–92.
87. Brendler H. 1973. Adrenalectomy and hypophysectomy for prostatic cancer. Urology 2:99–102.
88. Morales PA, Brendler H, Hotchkiss RS. 1955. Role of the adrenal cortex in prostate cancer. J Urol 73:399.
89. Silverberg GD. 1977. Hypophysectomy in the treatment of disseminated prostate carcinoma. Cancer 39:1727.
90. Labrie F, Dupont A, Belanger A, et al. 1982. New hormonal therapy in prostatic carcinoma: combined treatment with an LHRH agonist and an antiandrogen. Clin Invest Med 5:267–275.
91. Labrie F, Dupont A, Belanger A, et al. 1983. New approach in the treatment of prostate cancer: complete instead of partial withdrawal of androgens. Prostate 4:579–594.
92. Labrie F, Dupont A, Belanger A. 1985. A complete androgen blockade in the treatment of prostate cancer. In de Vita VT, Hellman S, Rosenberg SA, eds. Important Advances in Oncology. Philadelphia: JB Lippincott. 193.
93. Crawford ED, Eisenberg MA, McLeod DG, et al. 1989. A controlled trial of leuprolide with and without flutamide in prostatic carcinoma. N Engl J Med 321:419–424.
94. Prostate Cancer Trialists' Collaborative Group. 1995. Maximum androgen blockade in advanced prostate cancer: an overview of 22 randomised trials with 3283 deaths in 5710 patients. Lancet 346:265–269.
95. Klotz LH, Herr HW, Morse MJ, Whitmore WF Jr. 1986. Intermittent endocrine therapy for advanced prostate cancer. Cancer 58:2546–2550.
96. Goldenberg SL, Bruchowsky N, Gleave ME, Sullivan LD, Akakura K. 1995. Intermittent androgen suppression in the treatment of prostate cancer: a preliminary report. Urology 45:839–844.
97. Dupont A, Gomez JL, Cusan L, Koutsillieris M, Labrie F. 1993. Response to flutamide withdrawal in advanced prostate cancer in progression under combination therapy. J Urol 150:908–913.
98. Nieh PT. 1995. Withdrawal phenomenon with the antiandrogen casodex. J Urol 153:1070–1072.
99. Akakura K, Akimoto S, Ohki T, Shimazaki J. 1995. Antiandrogen withdrawal syndrome in prostate cancer after treatment with steroidal antiandrogen chlormadinone acetate. Urology 45:700–705.

100. Sartor O, Cooper M, Weinberger M, Headlee D, Thibault A, Tompkins A, Steinberg S, Figg WD, Linehan WM, Myers CE. 1994. Surprising activity of flutamide withdrawal, when combined with aminoglutethimide, in treatment of 'hormone-refractory' prostate cancer. J Natl Cancer Inst 86:222–227.
101. Presti JC, Fair WR, Andriole G, et al. 1992. Multicenter randomized double blind, placebo controlled study to investigate the effect of finasteride (MK-906) on stage D prostate cancer. J Urol 148:1201–1204.
102. Newling DWW. 1989. The use of flutamide as monotherapy in the treatment of advanced prostate cancer. In Murphy GP, Khoury S, eds. Therapeutic Progress in Urological Cancers. New York: Alan R. Liss, pp. 117–121.
103. Fleshner NE, Trachtenberg J. 1995. Combination of finasteride and flutamide in advanced carcinoma of the prostate; effective therapy with minimal side effects. J Urol 154:1642–1646.
104. Rosen MA, Goldstone L, Lapin S, Wheeler T, Scardino PT. 1992. Frequency and location of extracapsular extension and positive surgical margins in radical prostatectomy specimens. J Urol 148:331.
105. Lange PH, Narayan P. 1983. Understaging and undergrading of prostate cancer; argument for postoperative radiation as adjuvant therapy. Urology 21:113.
106. Bigg SW, Kavoussi LR, Catalona WJ. 1990. Role of nerve sparing radical prostatectomy for clinical stage B2 prostate cancer. J Urol 144:1420.
107. Anscher MS, Prosnitz LR. 1987. Postoperative radiotherapy for patients with carcinoma of the prostate undergoing radical prostatectomy with positive surgical margins, seminal vesicle involvement and/or penetration through the capsule. J Urol 138:1407.
108. Jones EC. 1990. Resection margin status in radical retropubic prostatectomy specimens: relationship to type of operation, tumor size, tumor grade and local tumor extension. J Urol 144:89.
109. Westin P, Stattin P, Damber JE, Bergh A. 1995. Castration therapy rapidly induces apoptosis in a minority and decreases cell proliferation in a majority of human prostatic tumors. Am J Pathol 146:1368–1375.
110. Labrie F, Dupont A, Cusan L, et al. 1993. Downstaging of localized prostate cancer by neoadjuvant therapy with flutamide and lupron; the first controlled and randomized trial. Clin Invest Med 16:499–509.
111. Soloway MS, Sharifi R, Wajsman Z, McLeod D, Wood DP Jr, Puras-Baez A. 1995. Randomized prospective study comparing radical prostatectomy alone versus radical prostatectomy preceded by androgen blockade in clinical stage B2(T2bNXMO) prostate cancer. The Lupron Depot Neoadjuvant Prostate Cancer Study Group. J Urol 154:424–428.
112. Gleave ME, Goldenberg SL, Jones EC, Bruchovsky N, Sullivan LD. 1996. Biochemical and pathological effects of 8 months of neoadjuvant androgen withdrawal therapy before radical prostatectomy in patients with clinically confined prostate cancer. J Urol 155:213–219.
113. Macfarlane MT, Abi-Aad W, Stein A, Danella J, Belldegrun A, deKernion JB. 1993. Neoadjuvant hormonal deprivation in patients with locally advanced prostate cancer. J Urol 150:132–134.
114. Aprikian AG, Fair WR, Reuter VE, Sogani P, Herr H, Russo P, Sheinfeld J. 1994. Experience with neoadjuvant diethylstilboestrol and radical prostatectomy in patients with locally advanced prostate cancer. Br J Urol 74:630–636.
115. Narayan P, Lowe BA, Carroll PR, Thompson IM. 1994. Neoadjuvant hormonal therapy and radical prostatectomy for clinical stage C carcinoma of the prostate. Br J Urol 73:544–548.
116. Oesterling JE, Andrews PE, Suman VJ, Zincke H, Myers RP. 1993. Preoperative androgen deprivation therapy: artificial lowering of serum prostate specific antigen without downstaging the tumor. J Urol 149:779.
117. Pummer K, Crawford ED, Daneshgari F, Andros B, Pfister S, Miller GJ. 1994. Hormonal pretreatment does not affect the final pathologic stage in locally advanced prostate cancer. Urology 44:38.
118. Ray GR, Cassady R, Bagshaw MA. 1973. Definitive radiation therapy of carcinoma of the prostate: a report on 15 years of experience. Radiology 106:407.

119. Zelefsky MJ, Leibel SA, Burman CM, Kutcher GJ, Harrison A, Happersett L, Fuks Z. 1994. Neoadjuvant hormonal therapy improves the therapeutic ratio in patients with bulky prostatic cancer treated with three-dimensional conformal radiation therapy. Int J Radiat Oncol Biol Phys 29:755–761.
120. Forman JD, Kumar R, Haas G, Montie J, Porter AT, Mesina CF. 1995. Neoadjuvant hormonal downsizing of localized carcinoma of the prostate; effects on the volume of normal tissue irradiation. Cancer Invest 13:8–15.
121. Hanks GE, Hanlon A, Schultheiss T, Corn B, Shipley WU, Lee WR. 1994. Early prostate cancer: the national results of radiation treatment from the Patterns of Care and Radiation Therapy Oncology Group studies with prospects for improvement with conformal radiation and adjuvant androgen deprivation. J Urol 152:1775–1780.

6. Endocrine therapy of endometrial cancer

Samuel S. Lentz

1. Introduction

Endometrial carcinoma is the most common gynecologic malignancy, with approximately 34,000 new cases diagnosed yearly in the United States. It is the fourth most common cancer in American women and accounts for approximately 4000 deaths per year, as noted by the American Cancer Society. The majority of cases, approximately 75%, are confined to the uterus at the time of diagnosis and have a relatively good prognosis. However, a significant number of patients present annually for treatment with advanced or recurrent disease.

The etiologic association of steroid hormones and endometrial carcinoma was first suggested by early animal data in which continuous exogenous estrogen exposure was shown to exert a potentially carcinogenic effect on the endometrium [1]. Additionally, clinical findings of endometrial hyperstimulation by unopposed estrogen either endogenously or exogenously solidified the evidence of a positive association between estrogen and endometrial hyperplasia and carcinoma. Clinical situations such as polycystic ovarian disease, hormonally active ovarian neoplasms (including theca cell and granulosa cell tumors), as well as hormone replacement therapy with unopposed estrogen are associated with an increased risk of endometrial carcinoma.

The hormonal effects on the endometrium are exerted through interaction with hormone receptors that bind to the specific hormone in the cytosol for transport to the nucleus, where the translational effects on DNA are seen. The effects of estrogens are stimulatory, with the initiation of protein synthesis important in cell proliferation. Also, these effects include an increase in the estrogen and progesterone receptor proteins. For progestins, there are similar cytosol transport proteins with entry into the nucleus and binding to DNA. This is followed by a decrease in cell protein synthesis, including estrogen and progesterone receptors, as well as inhibition of mitosis and promotion of cellular differentiation. This process is seen in the normal endometrium and, as is anticipated, the level of receptors vary with the menstrual cycle. Martin et al. evaluated the receptor levels in normal endometrium. As seen in premenopausal women (figure 1), the amount of estrogen receptor (ER) is low in the

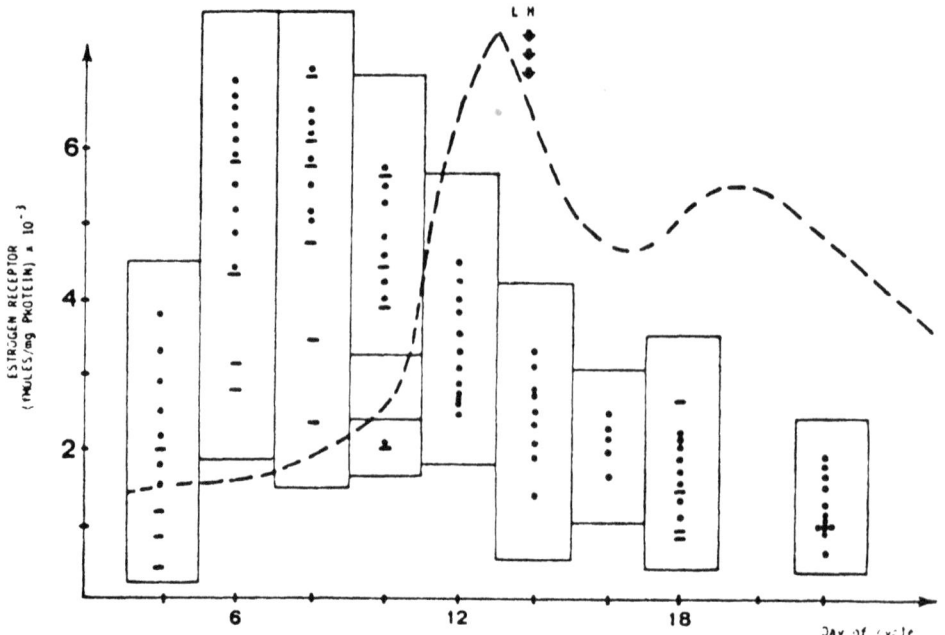

Figure 1. Cytoplasmic estrogen receptor levels in normal endometrium during the cycle. Two buffers were used to prepare cytosol: GTEM buffer (•) and sucrose buffer (−). The dotted line represents the variation in circulating estradiol. The LH peak is shown. The squares are for the confidence interval of the date of biopsies (±1 day) and of receptor content (±SEM).

beginning of the cycle, increasing to a maximum of 5820 + 250 fmoles/mg protein on day 8. The lowest levels are seen in the luteal phase, namely, 1320 + 150 fmoles/mg protein on day 22. Figure 2 indicates again low levels of progesterone receptors (PRs) at the initiation of the cycle (437 + 50 fmoles/mg protein on day 4) and a maximum level (3015 + 120 fmoles/mg protein on day 12) with subsequent decreases to levels seen at the beginning of the cycle. Also, in the postmenopausal woman, levels of receptors reflect the influence of estrogen stimulation. Without estrogen stimulation, ER levels were low at 110 + 50 fmoles/mg protein, and PR not measurable. Under the influence of estrogens, ERs and PRs are increased in the postmenopausal endometrium [2].

This normal physiologic effect of endogenous progesterone to inhibit the proliferative effects of estrogens led to its therapeutic use. This antiproliferative effect of progesterone on the endometrium prompted the initial use by Kistner in 1959 in the reversal of a preinvasive endometrial lesion [3]. The use of progestin therapy has been directed toward three different clinical situations that will be addressed in this chapter. Also, the issue of hormone replacement therapy in patients previously treated for endometrial cancer will be discussed.

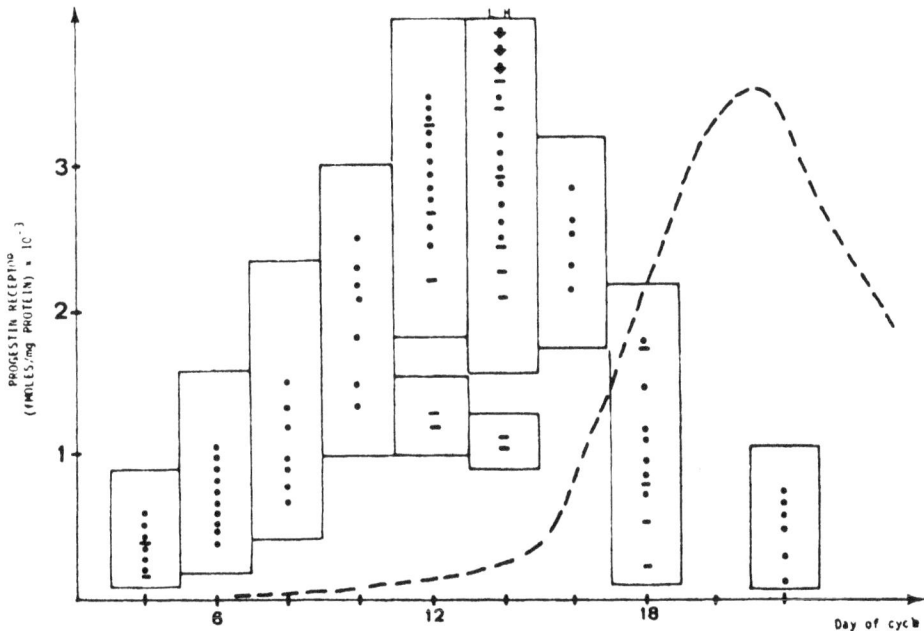

Figure 2. Cytoplasmic progestin receptor levels in normal endometrium during the cycle. Two buffers were used to prepare cytosol: GTEM buffer (•) and sucrose buffer (−). The dotted line represents the variation in circulating progesterone. The LH peak is shown. The squares are for the confidence interval of the date of biopsies (±1 day) and of receptor content (±SEM).

2. Primary therapy for early disease

Histologically it is difficult, at times, to distinguish severe endometrial hyperplasia from well-differentiated adenocarcinoma. It is recognized that hyperplastic lesions can be reversed with progestin therapy. Endometrial carcinoma is typically a postmenopausal disease; however, approximately 5% of cases are in patients under 40 years of age. Andrews initially described the progestin therapy in a group of patients with endometrial carcinoma associated with Stein–Leventhal syndrome [4]. Farhi et al. reported on the successful use of progestin therapy, in three patients under 25 years of age with well-differentiated endometrial carcinoma who were interested in preserving fertility [5]. Extreme care and close follow-up must be used in these exceptional and rare cases if primary hormonal therapy is used. For example, a study by Gitsch et al. reported on 17 premenopausal patients with endometrial carcinoma in whom synchronous ovarian malignancies were found in 29.4% and 29% had stage III or IV disease. Ten of these patients had well-differentiated lesions; however, results were not stratified according to grade [6]. Berek and Hacker suggested, in very young patients with well-differentiated carcinoma, a two-month trial of progestin therapy followed by repeat curettage. If no disease is found with subsequent evaluation, conservative therapy may be continued [7]. In general, primary hormone therapy for endometrial cancer cannot be condoned except in the debilitated patient who is not a surgical or radiation candidate. Also, care must be exercised in treating the patient with severe atypical endometrial hyperplasia with progestins. The diagnosis, whether by curettage or biopsy, may not be reflective of the extent of disease. Janicek and Rosenshein found carcinoma in 43% of the uterine specimens removed with a preoperative diagnosis of atypical hyperplasia based on curettage or office biopsy. Myometrial invasion was present in 89% with 37% having stage IC disease. In addition, 21% had grade 2 or higher lesions [8].

3. Adjuvant therapy for early disease

Despite the generally good prognosis associated with surgical stage I (table 1), endometrial carcinoma, five-year survival rates of approximately 75% may be seen in some subgroups. This finding has led to the consideration of adjuvant hormone therapy in some patients with early disease. Although the role of progestin therapy has been proven in advanced or recurrent disease, the use in the adjuvant setting has not been established. To date, available studies have not shown any consistent benefit to progestin use in the adjuvant setting [9–11]. Vergote et al., using biweekly injections of 1000 mg of hydroxyprogesterone caproate in 1148 patients with clinical stage I and II endometrial cancer, found in high-risk patients (poorly differentiated, deeply invasive, poor histologic subtype) a better disease-free survival in the treatment group; however, the crude survival was not different [12]. No randomized, prospec-

Table 1. 1988 FIGO surgical staging for endometrial carcinoma

Staging

Stage Ia	G123	Tumor limited to endometrium
Stage Ib	G123	Invasion to less than one half the myometrium
Stage Ic	G123	Invasion to more than one half the myometrium
Stage IIa	G123	Endocervical glandular involvement only
Stage IIb	G123	Cervical stromal invasion
Stage IIIa	G123	Tumor invades serosa and/or adnexa, and/or positive peritoneal cytology
Stage IIIb	G123	Vaginal metastases
Stage IIIc	G123	Metastases to pelvic and/or para-aortic lymph nodes
Stage IVa	G123	Tumor invasion of bladder and/or bowel mucosa
Stage IVb		Distant metastases including intra-abdominal and/or inguinal lymph nodes

Histopathology — degree of differentiation
Cases of carcinoma of the corpus should be classified (or graded) according to the degree of histologic differentiation, as follows:
G1 = 5% or less of a nonsquamous or nonmorular solid growth pattern
G2 = 6%–50% of a nonsquamous or nonmorular solid growth pattern
G3 = More than 50% of a nonsquamous or nonmorular solid growth pattern

tive analysis of progestin therapy versus placebo has been performed in surgically stage I patients, nor will it likely be done due to the large number of patients and extended follow-up that would be required.

4. Advanced or recurrent disease hormonal therapy

4.1. Progestins

The initial report by Kelley and Baker reviewed the use of the progestational agents, progesterone or hydroxyprogesterone caproate (Delalutin), in the treatment of metastatic endometrial carcinoma, with an observed response rate of 29% [13]. Subsequently, other studies noted response rates in approximately one third of the cases. Kauppila reviewed a total of 1068 patients treated in 17 different trials with either medroxyprogesterone acetate, megestrol acetate, or hydroxyprogesterone caproate and found an overall response rate of 34% [14]. In this review, the average duration of response was 16–28 months, and the average survival time was 18–33 months.

Other studies have shown a somewhat less optimistic response rate (table 2). Thigpen reported the Gynecologic Oncology Group (GOG) data using medroxyprogesterone acetate (MPA) 50 mg orally, three times daily in patients with advanced or recurrent endometrial carcinoma. Of 219 patients with measurable disease, there was an 8% complete response and a 6% partial response. Fifty-two percent of the patients had stable disease for at least one month, while 34% developed progressive disease within one month. The median survival was 10.4 months [15]. A subsequent dose–response study comparing oral MPA 200 mg/day versus 1000 mg/day found response rates of 26% and 18%, respectively [16]. Podratz reported on the use of various progestational agents in the treatment of endometrial carcinoma at the Mayo Clinic, noting an objective overall response rate of 11.2% and a survival at five years of only 8% [17]. This finding is in agreement with Piver's 15.8% response

Table 2. Response rates in progestin therapy

Study [ref]	Dose	Route	Overall response
MPA (Provera, Upjohn)			
Thigpen [15]	150 mg/day	Oral	14%
Thigpen [15]	200 mg/day	Oral	26%
	1000 mg/dL	Oral	18%
Piver [18]	1 g/wk	Intramuscular	18%
Megestrol acetate (Megace, Bristol-Myers Oncology)			
Podratz [17]	320 mg/day	Oral	11%
Hydroxyprogesterone caproate (Delalutin, Squibb)			
Podratz [17]	1–3 g/wk	Intramuscular	9%
Piver [18]	1 g/wk	Intramuscular	14%

rate [18]. The differences observed between studies may to some degree be related to a large number of high-grade lesions (47%) as seen in the data by Podratz, as well as large numbers of receptor-negative tumors in the initial GOG study (42%). In addition, the definition of objective response as used by Podratz, namely, duration for at least three months, was not as strict in some of the prior, more optimistic reports.

As alluded to above, there does not appear to be an appreciable difference in response between the various types of progestational agents when different studies are compared [14]. Podratz found objective response rates of 11%, 9%, and 12% for megestrol, hydroxyprogesterone, and medrogestone, respectively, in his retrospective review [17]. Priver et al. found no significant difference in responses between medorxyprogesterone acetate and hydroxyprogesterone caproate administered intramuscularly [18].

Route of administration and dose–response have been evaluated with MPA by the GOG. Sall et al. measured serum blood levels in 22 patients with advance or recurrent endometrial carcinoma who had been randomized to receive either MPA 50 mg orally three times daily or MPA 300 mg weekly intramuscularly. Serum levels were measured immediately after administration and subsequently on a weekly basis, with a consistently higher level noted in the group receiving oral MPA [19]. Although response rates were not evaluated in this study, the results summarized in Kauppila's review in which the response rates were similar for oral and intramuscular MPA (41% and 32%, respectively) suggest the oral route of MPA to be the preferred method of administration [14].

Dose–response analysis has not produced consistent results. A GOG phase III trial evaluated oral MPA at two dose levels, 200 mg/day and 1000 mg/day, as noted above. Two hundred and seventy-eight evaluable patients were randomized, with a 26% response rate in the low-dose arm and 18% in the high-dose arm, differences not statistically significant; however, results appeared to favor the low-dose level [16]. The dose response of three different levels of megestrol was evaluated in a nonrandomized study by Geisler [20]. Although the response rates of 48% and 43% at the two higher dose levels — 160 and 80 mg/day respectively — were better than the 14% response rate seen at the 40 mg/day dosage, this finding was not statistically significant.

Of interest, the serum levels of high-dose MPA, when used in doses of approximately 1 g orally per day, are similar to the levels achieved with megestrol at the standard dose of 160 mg/day [21]. Thus, regarding dose response, the above data would suggest that significantly high-dose progestin therapy would necessitate a drug such as megestrol in the 800-mg-daily dose range. High-dose progestins may have alternate mechanisms of antitumor activity exclusive of their primary function of receptor binding. Blossey et al. showed in breast cancer patients that MPA also exerted its antitumor activity in a dose-related fashion by interference with the hypothalamopituitary adrenal axis, thereby suppressing adrenal steroid secretion [22]. Muss et al., in a phase III trial, compared high-dose MA (800 mg/day) with the standard

160 mg/day dosage in recurrent breast cancer patients who failed to respond to prior endocrine therapy. A significant improvement was observed in response rates, progression-free survival, and overall survival for patients who received the high-dose regimen [23]. A recent GOG phase II study evaluated this high-dose regimen (MA, 800 mg/day) in patients with advanced or recurrent hormonally naive endometrial cancer. The overall response rate was 24%, which was no different than that seen in prior studies with lower standard dosages. Thus, at least in endometrial cancer, dose intensification does not appear to improve outcome [24].

Response rates of endometrial carcinoma to progestin therapy appear to be related to several clinical and pathologic factors (table 3). Clearly, a relationship of response to grade has been delineated with higher responses seen in well-differentiated tumors. Early studies, as delineated by Kohorn, noted a 50% response rate to progestin therapy in grade 1 lesions and 15% in grade 3 neoplasms [25]. Although the overall response rates were lower, Podratz confirmed the inverse correlation of grade to response with a 20.5% response in low-grade lesions and only a 1.4% response in high-grade lesions [17]. The interrelationship of grade and receptor expression was noted by Creasman with estrogen and progesterone positivity seen in 70%, 55%, and 41% of the well-, moderately, and poorly differentiated lesions, respectively [26]. With the degree of differentiation an inadequate predictor of response, a more sensitive correlation was observed between hormone receptor positivity and response to progestin therapy. Kauppila reviewed five studies and noted the presence or absence of cytosolic progesterone receptors in 105 patients to have an 86% predictability of response, with 89% of PR-positive tumors hormone sensitive in comparison to only 17% in PR-negative tumors. A similar though less reliable relationship was seen with estrogen receptors, where only 64% of the ER-positive tumors responded to progestin therapy versus 11% of the ER-negative tumors [14]. Similar findings were seen in the GOG data, in which a 40% response was seen in ER-positive, PR-positive tumors but only a 12% response in ER-positive, PR-negative and ER-negative, PR-negative tumors [15]. As seen from the above, the presence of progesterone receptors appear to be a better predictor of response to hormonal therapy than the presence of estrogen receptors. In addition, studies suggest that the presence of cytosol progesterone receptors is a positive independent predictor of survival [27,28].

Table 3. Predictors of response to hormonal therapy

Histological grade
Receptor status (progesterone)
Disease recurrence in prior field of radiation
Tumor burden
Time from diagnosis to treatment
Recurrence versus primary metastatic disease

With PR positivity more predictable than ER positivity, both in predicting response to hormone therapy and as an independent predictor of survival, the significant PR level considered positive has not been clearly defined in endometrial cancer. The cutoff level is somewhat empiric, based on breast cancer data, and variable from study to study. The significant value may differ depending on whether the outcome parameter is based on response to hormonal therapy or simply is used as an independent predictor of survival as noted above. For instance, in the study by Ingram et al. cited above, where the PR was found to be an independent prognosticator of survival, the cutoff value of 100 fmoles/mg of protein was noted to be significant [28]. Chambers et al. found a PR level of greater than 50 fmoles/mg to be of prognostic significance in predicting survival, while others have observed PR levels of greater than 15 fmoles/mg to be prognostic [29,30]. On the other hand, when the response to hormonal therapy is evaluated, the level of PR considered as the positive cutoff has generally been lower but variable, ranging from 5 fmoles/mg to 50 fmoles/mg [15,31–33]. Certainly, the degree of response appears to be directly proportional to the level of PR positivity. For example, Ehrlich et al., who considered PR levels greater than 50 fmoles/mg to be positive, noted an 88% response to progestin therapy in PR-positive tumors and only a 6% response in PR-negative tumors [33]. However, Quinn et al., using 5 fmoles/mg as a cutoff for positive PR, noted only a 22% response in PR-positive lesions versus no responses in PR-negative lesions [31].

Other factors appear to influence response to hormonal therapy. Early studies suggested higher response rates in patients with pulmonary metastasis than in those with nonpulmonary metastasis, although in the analysis by Reifenstein, response was not influenced by the site of disease provided that the recurrence was not in the field of prior radiation [34–36]. It is reasonable to speculate that a decreased tumor response in a prior radiation field would be, in part, due to a decreased blood supply to the area and thus diminished drug delivery. In evaluating survival factors, Podratz noted that, in addition to low histologic grade, minimal tumor burden ($10\,\text{cm}^3$ or less) and long interval before hormone treatment had a positive association with improved survival. Contrary to some earlier reports, no significant difference in survival was noted in association with the site of metastasis; however, the effect of prior radiation was not addressed [17]. Age also has been considered prognostic of response, with older patients having a lower response; however, this outcome is likely related to an increased proportion of high-grade lesions in older individuals [37–39]. Response with recurrent lesions has been noted to be better than that seen in primary advanced disease; however, this finding, at least to some degree, is probably related to tumor burden as noted above [40].

4.2. Tamoxifen

Tamoxifen, a nonsteroidal antiestrogen, has been evaluated in endometrial carcinoma based on prior experience with breast cancer. Its use either as a

Table 4. Response rates in antiestrogen therapy

Study [ref]	Dose	Route	Overall response
Single agent			
Moore (pooled data) [43]			
Tamoxifen (Novadex, ICI Pharma)	20–40 mg/day	Oral	22% (0%–53% range)
Combination hormone therapy			
Carlson [50]			
Tamoxifen	20 mg/day	Oral	33%
MPA	250 mg/wk	Intramuscular	
Rendina [51]			
Tamoxifen	40 mg/day	Oral	35%
MPA	250 mg/wk	Intramuscular	
Pandya [53]			
Tamoxifen	20 mg/day	Oral	19%
Megestrol	160 mg/day	Oral	

single agent or combined with other hormonal therapy is related to its ability to inhibit the binding of estradiol to the estrogen receptor [41] and to increase progesterone receptors, as has been seen in endometrial carcinoma [42]. Moore reviewed eight studies using tamoxifen (20–40 mg/day) in endometrial carcinoma, and a pooled overall response rate of 22% was seen [43] (table 4). The response rates have been widely variable. Bonte et al. noted overall response rates of 53% in 17 patients treated with 40 mg/day [44]. The GOG data reported by Slavik, however, had no responses in 19 patients resistant to prior hormone and/or chemotherapy receiving tamoxifen at 20 mg/day [45]. Edmonson et al. found an overall response of 21% in patients without prior hormone therapy and 0% response in those patients deemed progesterone refractory [46]. The variable response rates along with the data by Edmonson suggests that, like progestin therapy, response to tamoxifen is more likely to be observed in patients with low-grade tumors, in those with hormone receptor positivity, and in those who have had prior response to progestin therapy. The use of tamoxifen therapeutically in endometrial carcinoma is perhaps tempered by the concern of tamoxifen-induced endometrial neoplasia in patients receiving the drug for breast cancer. Several studies confirm an increased risk of endometrial cancer in this group of patients. Fornander et al. noted a 6.4-fold increase in the risk of endometrial cancer in patients receiving tamoxifen 40 mg/day, and Fisher et al., in the NSABP B-14 trial, found the relative risk for endometrial cancer to be 7.5 in the tamoxifen-treated group compared to a placebo [47,48].

It is known that progestin therapy leads to downregulation of the progesterone receptor, which is considered at least partially responsible for the short duration of response [49]. Based on this information, studies of combination hormonal therapy, predominately using tamoxifen, have attempted to reverse this receptor downregulation (table 4). Carlson et al. studied receptor levels in

25 untreated patients before and after tamoxifen administration, noting an increase in PR positivity posttreatment to 84% compared to 52% pretreatment. An overall response rate of 33% in hormone-naive patients treated with concurrent tamoxifen and MPA was similar to that seen with single-agent progestin therapy [50]. Rendina et al. noted similar results in patients failing prior hormone therapy who were treated with tamoxifen and MPA, with no significant difference seen with regard to prior hormone response status [51]. However, Kline et al., in a group of patients with poorly differentiated lesions, had a response rate of only 5% in 20 patients treated with sequential tamoxifen and MPA [52]. Pandya et al. compared single-agent megestrol to megestrol and tamoxifen, with no benefit found with combination therapy (response rates were 20% and 19%, respectively) [53]. Thus, at present, it would appear that overall responses are similar to those seen with single-agent progestin therapy and that response is inversely related to grade. The GOG presently is involved in a phase II study using continuous tamoxifen with intermittent medroxyprogesterone acetate as a potential means to increase the magnitude and lengthen the duration of response with continued upregulation of the progesterone receptors using tamoxifen. A recently completed GOG trial of alternating megace and tamoxifen therapy in advanced or recurrent endometrial cancer is presently being analyzed.

4.3. Other hormonal treatment

Other therapeutic hormonal modalities have been utilized on a limited basis (table 5). Gonadotropin-releasing hormone (GnRH) agonists have received a great deal of attention in the treatment of various gynecologic disorders. Kullander, recently reviewing the use of GnRH analogues in the treatment of endometrial carcinoma, referenced the first reported use of gonadotropin-releasing hormone for endometrial carcinoma in a 36-year-old premenopausal patient with a well-differentiated lesion [54]. Gallagher et al. evaluated GnRH response in 17 postmenopausal patients with recurrent endometrial carcinoma. All patients showed gonadotropin suppression and an overall response rate of 35% [55]. Based on these data, the GOG is presently evaluating the use of goserelin acetate in the treatment of recurrent or refractory endometrial cancer. The specific mechanism responsible for this response is not thoroughly known but probably is associated with diminished endogenous estrogen levels

Table 5. Other hormonal modalities

GnRH analogues
Clomiphene citrate
Aminoglutethimide
RU-486 (mifepristone)
Androgens

as well as a direct effect on endometrial cancer cells, since GnRH binding sites have been demonstrated [56].

Clomiphene citrate has been shown to reverse endometrial hyperplastic changes as well as carcinoma confined to the uterus [57,58]. The aromatase inhibitor, aminoglutethimide, has been used more extensively in breast carcinoma, where the major mechanism of action appears to be blocking the conversion of androgen to estrogens in peripheral tissues and inhibition of adrenal steroid secretion. Use of aminoglutethimide in endometrial carcinoma is limited and appears to offer no advantage over conventional progestin therapy, with response rates of 22% as reported in the review by Kauppila [14]. RU-486 (mifepristone), a synthetic steroid with both antiprogesterone and antiglucocorticoid activities, has been used predominantly as an abortifactant; however, recent data suggest potential use in endometriosis and uterine leiomyomata [59–61]. Although specific information regarding the use of RU-486 in endometrial carcinoma is not available, limited data on the use of other similar antiprogestins in xenotransplanted endometrial carcinoma suggest no significant tumoricidal effect in comparison to medroxyprogesterone acetate and tamoxifen [62]. Finally, there are no clinical data regarding the use of androgens in the treatment of endometrial carcinoma. Concerns regarding the use of androgens include significant side effects as well as peripheral conversion to estrogens, resulting in a potential stimulatory rather than inhibitory effect. Interestingly, Gentola found the synthetic androgen methyltrienolone to inhibit the growth of grade II endometrial adenocarcinoma in vitro while seeing no inhibitory effect from testosterone or dihydrotestosterone [63].

5. Combination therapy

5.1. Cytotoxic agents and hormones

To enhance response rates, combination therapy with cycotoxic agents and hormones has been evaluated. Phase II studies using multiagent chemotherapy and progestational agents have generally reported response rates in the range of 50% [64–66]. To date, only two randomized prospective studies have been done in patients with recurrent or metastatic endometrial carcinoma, both with response rates similar to those seen with single-agent cytotoxic regimens (table 6). Horton et al. reported the Eastern Cooperative Oncology Group (ECOG) results with responses of 16% and 27% in the two treatment groups, a difference that overall was not statistically significant [67]. There was some indication that survival was longer in ambulatory patients treated with megestrol, cyclophosphamide, and doxorubicin; however, this regimen was associated with greater hematologic toxicity. The GOG study randomized 295 patients with advanced or recurrent endometrial cancer to

Table 6. Combination cytotoxic and hormonal therapy response rates

Study [ref]	Drug and dosage		Cycle	Overall response
Horton [67]	Megestrol	240 mg/day	—	27%
	Cyclophosphamide	400 mg/m^2	Monthly	
	Doxorubicin	40 mg/m^2	Montly	
	versus			
	Megestrol	240 mg/day	—	16%
	Cyclophosphamide	250 mg/m^2	Monthly	
	Doxorubicin	30 mg/m^2	Monthly	
	5-Fluorouracil	300 mg/mg^2/day × 3 day	Monthly	
Cohen [68]	Megestrol	180 mg/day × 8 wk	—	38%
	Melphalan	7 mg/m^2/day × 4 day	Every 3 wk	
	5-Fluorouracil	525 mg/m^2/day × 4 day	Every 3 wk	
	versus			
	Megestrol	180 mg/day × 8 wk	—	36%
	Cyclophosphamide	400 mg/m^2	Every 3 wk	
	Doxorubicin	40 mg/m^2	Every 3 wk	
	5-Fluorouracil	400 mg/m^2	Every 3 wk	

one of two regimens: 1) melphan, 5-fluorouracil, and megestrol acetate or 2) adriamycin, 5-fluorouracil, cyclophosphamide, and megestrol acetate. The objective response rates of the 257 evaluable patients with measurable disease was approximately 37% in both groups, which is not significantly higher than that seen with adriamycin alone [68]. At present, hormones in combination with chemotherapeutic agents do not appear to enhance response rates, although no randomized trial with and without hormonal therapy has been performed.

5.2. Radiation therapy and hormones

Although prospective data are lacking, studies suggest a synergistic relationship between progestins and radiation therapy [67–71]. The potential for progestins to enhance radiosensitivity in endometrial carcinoma was investigated in vitro by Huber et al. [72]. The addition of MPA to tissue cultures increased the sensitivity of endometrial adenocarcinoma cells to radiation. This effect of MPA was thought to be potentially related to its ability to prolong the radiosensitive late G_2 phase of the cell cycle, as shown by Hustin [73]. Thus, progestins may have a role in conjunction with radiation in the treatment of recurrent or advanced disease.

6. Hormone replacement therapy in endometrial cancer

Since the majority of patients with endometrial cancer have early-stage disease and survive without recurrence, an ancillary hormone question revolves around the physiologic rather than therapeutic use of hormones to prevent the acute and long-term hypoestrogenic effects. Certainly, if one peruses the 1995 *Physician's Desk Reference* with regard to estrogen use, a prominent contraindication listed is a history of endometrial cancer. This concern is based primarily on data correlating unopposed estrogen with the induction of endometrial hyperplasia and carcinoma. Interestingly, in a review of the bibliography related to this general class of drugs, the latest reference given is 1976, with no specific study listed substantiating this warning [74]. There is no prospective, randomized study addressing this issue; therefore, the physician must address the safety of estrogen replacement for patients who have a previous history of endometrial cancer by using only limited retrospective analysis and some educated, logical assumptions. Creasman et al. reported the experience at Duke, in which 221 patients after completion of therapy for stage I endometrial carcinoma were placed, in a nonrandomized fashion, on estrogen replacement. Although only 47 patients received estrogens and the majority received vaginal preparations, after controlling for known risk factors, the estrogen-treated group had a significantly longer disease-free survival [75]. Other studies have subsequently substantiated Creasman's results [76,77]. Lee et al. followed 44 patients with low-risk stage I endometrial cancer (grade 1 or 2, less than 50% myometrial invasion, absence of metastasis) for a minimum of two years on oral estrogens. There was no difference in recurrence between the estrogen users and low-risk nonusers. Furthermore, eight deaths occurred in the nonuser group, of which five were secondary to myocardial infarctions [78]. The ACOG Committee Opinion, August 1993, states that women with a history of endometrial carcinoma without factors predictive of recurrence are candidates for estrogen replacement [79]. The benefits of alleviating the acute symptoms of hypoestrogenism, such as hot flushes and vaginal atrophy, in addition to the long-term protection against osteoporosis and cardiovascular disease must be addressed. As noted above, there are nearly 4000 deaths in the U.S. annually from endometrial carcinoma in contrast to 450,000 deaths in postmenopausal women from cardiovascular disease as well as 40,000 deaths from hip fractures related to osteoporosis. Nevertheless, the issue will remain until a proper prospective, randomized study to answer the question is conducted.

7. Conclusions

There appear to be limited indications for the use of hormonal therapy in the primary therapy of endometrial carcinoma. Such therapy would involve predominantly those patients who are not candidates for either surgery or radiation. Also, there are no data to support hormonal therapy for endometrial cancer in the adjuvant setting.

Hormone therapy, although initially promising, has not substantially altered long-term survival for patients with recurrent or metastatic endometrial carcinoma. Currently, one can anticipate an overall response with hormonal therapy of approximately 25% regardless of the specific agent, without consideration of other prognostic factors; however, if the lesion is PR positive, the response rate approaches 70%–80%. At present, even if the initial fresh tissue was not analyzed for receptors, immunohistochemical methods can be used on paraffin-imbedded archival tissue for both ERs and PRs. As noted by Soper et al., this method may be more accurate in that contamination by receptor-positive nontumor tissue is obviated [80]. This method of receptor analysis also allows for evaluation of small samples such as those obtained with fine-needle aspiration. Of interest, Runowicz et al., using the dextran-coated charcoal technique, noted differences in receptors levels based on location. Using greater than 19 fmoles/mg for ER positivity and 30 fmoles/mg for PR positivity, in the primary tumor 70% and 60% of cases were positive for ER and PR, respectively, whereas in the metastatic sites 63% were ER positive and only 25% PR positive [81]. This finding may explain the lack or variability of response noted in patients with a receptor-positive primary tumor. Also, despite the fact that fewer grade 3 endometrial cancers have measurable levels of PR, determination of these levels would be potentially important. Chambers et al. reported in grade 3 lesions a five-year survival rate of 48% and 20%, respectively, for hormone receptor-rich versus receptor-poor lesions [82]. If not performed on the fresh tissue at diagnosis, immunohistochemical analysis could be used either on archival tissue or on fresh biopsy material.

With no obvious advantage of parenteral over oral administration, patients are generally treated with either oral medroxyprogesterone acetate (200 mg/day) or megestrol acetate (160–320 mg/day). Megestrol acetate would appear perhaps preferable to MPA because of its better gastrointestinal absorption and higher serum levels. In clinical situations in which progestin therapy is contraindicated, such as deep venous thrombosis or pulmonary embolism, the use of tamoxifen (20 mg twice daily) may be considered. Major advantages of hormonal therapy include its high therapeutic index and tolerance, which is generally unaffected by prior treatment. In addition, as an added benefit, recent data suggests that progestins, specifically megestrol acetate, may be useful in the treatment of cancer cachexia, a problem not uncommonly seen in patients with advanced disease [83,84]. Although not clearly defined, it is empirically considered necessary to treat patients for at least three months to see maximum response as outlined by Kohorn in his review of SGO data [25]. Also, the duration of therapy has not been adequately addressed; however, treatment is generally maintained as long as response is seen. The major problems with this treatment modality are predictability of response and achieving a sustained response. To address these issues will require the use of current information in conjunction with enhanced hormone receptor data as well as knowledge at the molecular level involving growth factors and oncogenes. Clinically useful information will also require further prospective, randomized studies in which recognized independent prognostic variables are appropriately considered.

Finally, use of physiological estrogen replacement in patients with a history of low-risk endometrial carcinoma may be considered; however, these patients must be adequately informed of the lack of prospective data.

References

1. Meissner WA, Sommers SC, Sherman G. 1957. Endometrial hyperplasia, endometrial carcinoma, and endometriosis produced experimentally by estrogen. Cancer 10:500–509.
2. Martin PM, Rolland PH, Gammerre M, Serment H, Toga M. 1979. Estradiol and progesterone receptors in normal and neoplastic endometrium: correlations between receptors, histopathological examinations and clinical responses under progestin therapy. Int J Cancer 23:321–329.
3. Kistner RW. 1959. Histological effects of progestins on hyperplasia and carcinoma in situ of the endometrium. Cancer 12:1106–1122.
4. Andrews WC, Andrews MC, 1960. Stein–Leventhal syndrome with associated adenocarcinoma of the endometrium. Am J Obstet Gynecol 80:632–636.
5. Farhi DC, Nosanchuk J, Silverberg SG. 1986. Endometrial adenocarcinoma in women under 25 years of age. Obstet Gynecol 68:741–745.
6. Gitsch G, Hanzal E, Jensen, D, Hacker NF. 1995. Endometrial cancer in premenopausal women 45 years and younger. Obstet Gynecol 85(4):504–508.
7. Berek JS, Hacker NF, eds. 1994. Practical Gynecologic Oncology, 2nd ed. Baltimore, MD: Williams & Wilkins, p. 311.
8. Janicek MF, Rosenshein NB. 1994. Invasive endometrial cancer in uteri resected for atypical endometrial hyperplasia. Gynecol Oncol 52(3):373–378.
9. DePalo G, Mersom M, Del Vecchio M, et al. 1985. A controlled clinical study of adjuvant medroxyprogesterone acetate (MPA) therapy in pathological stage I endometrial cancer with myometrial invasion. Proc Am Soc Clin Oncol 4:121.
10. Lewis GC Jr, Slack HN, Mortel R, Bross IDJ. 1974. Adjuvant progestogen therapy in the primary definitive treatment of endometrial cancer. Gynecol Oncol 2:368–376.
11. MacDonald RR, Thorogood J, Maston MK. 1988. A randomized trial of progestogens in the primary treatment of endometrial carcinoma. Br J Obstet Gynaecol 95:166.
12. Vergote I, Kjorstad K, Abeler V, Kolstad P. 1989. A randomized trial of progestogen therapy in early endometrial cancer. Cancer 64:1011.
13. Kelley RM, Baker WH. 1961. Progestational agents in the treatment of carcinoma of the endometrium. N Engl J Med 264:216–222.
14. Kauppila A. 1984. Progestin therapy of endometrial, breast and ovarian carcinoma. Acta Obstet Gynecol Scand 63:441–450.
15. Thigpen T, Blessing J, DiSaia P, et al. 1986. Oral medroxyprogesterone acetate in advanced or recurrent endometrial carcinoma: results of therapy and correlation with estrogen and progesterone receptor levels. The Gynecologic Oncology Group experience. In Baulier EE, Iacobelli S, McGuire WW, eds. Endocrinology and Malignancy. Parthenow Publishers, pp. 446–454.
16. Thigpen T, Blessing J, Hatch K, et al. 1991. A randomized trial of medroxyprogesterone acetate (MPA) 200 mg versus 1000 mg daily in advanced or recurrent endometrial carcinoma: a Gynecologic Oncology Group (GOG) study (abstract). J Clin Oncol 10:185.
17. Podratz KC, O'Brien PC, Malkasian GD, et al. 1985. Effects of progestational agents in treatment of endometrial carcinoma. Obstet Gynecol 66:106–110.
18. Piver MS, Barlow JJ, Lurain JR, et al. 1980. Medroxyprogesterone acetate (Depo-Provera) vs. hydroxyprogesterone caproate (Delalutin) in women with metastatic endometrial adenocarcinoma. Cancer 45:268–272.
19. Sall S, DiSaia P, Morrow CP, et al. 1979. A comparison of medroxyprogesterone serum concentrations by the oral or intramuscular route with persistent or recurrent endometrial carcinoma. Am J Obstet Gynecol 135:647–650.

20. Geisler HE. 1973. The use of megestrol acetate in the treatment of advanced malignant lesions of the endometrium. Gynecol Oncol 1:340–344.
21. Miller AA, Bechter R, Schmidt CG. 1988. Plasma concentrations of medroxyprogesterone acetate and megestrol during long-term follow-up in patients treated for metastatic breast cancer. J Cancer Res Clin Oncol 114:186–190.
22. Blossey HC, Wander HE, Koebberling J, et al. 1984. Pharmacokinetic and pharmacodynamic basis for the treatment of metastatic breast cancer with high-dose medroxyprogesterone acetate. Cancer 54:1208–1215.
23. Muss HB, Case LD, Capizzi RL, et al. 1990. High- versus standard-dose megestrol acetate in women with advanced breast cancer: a phase III trial of the Piedmont Oncology Association. J Clin Oncol 8:1797–1805.
24. Lentz SS, Brady MF, Major FJ, Reid GC, Soper JT. 1996. High-dose megestrol acetate in advanced or recurrent endometrial carcinoma: a Gynecologic Oncology Group Study. J Clin Oncol 14:357–361.
25. Kohorn KI. 1976. Gestagens and endometrial carcinoma. Gynecol Oncol 4:398–411.
26. Creasman WT, Soper JT, McCarty KS Jr, et al. 1985. Influence of cytoplasmic steroid receptor content on prognosis of early stage endometrial carcinoma. Am J Obstet Gynecol 151:922–932.
27. Erhlich CE, Young PCM, Stehman FB, et al. 1988. Steroid receptors and clinical outcome in patients with adenocarcinoma of the endometrium. Am J Obstet Gynecol 158:796–807.
28. Ingram SS, Roseman J, Heath R, et al. 1989. The predictive value of progesterone receptor levels in endometrial cancer. Int J Radiat Oncol Biol Physiol 17:21–27.
29. Chambers JT, MacLusky N, Eisenfield A, et al. 1988. Estrogen and progestin receptor levels as prognosticators for survival in endometrial cancer. Gynecol Oncol 31:65–77.
30. Creasman WT, Soper JT, McCarty KS, et al. 1985. Influence of cytoplasmic steroid receptor content on prognosis of early stage endometrial carcinoma. Am J Obstet Gynecol 151:922–932.
31. Quinn MA, Cauchi M, Fortune D. 1985. Endometrial carcinoma: steroid receptors and response to medroxyprogesterone acetate. Gynecol Oncol 21:314–319.
32. Creasman WT, McCarty KS, Barton TK, et al. 1980. Clinical correlates of estrogen and progesterone-binding proteins in human endometrial adenocarcinoma. Obstet Gynecol 55:363–370.
33. Ehrlich CE, Young PCM, Cleary RE. 1981. Cytoplasmic progesterone and estradiol receptors in normal, hyperplastic, and carcinomatous endometria: therapeutic implications. Am J Obstet Gynecol 141:539–546.
34. Kennedy BJ. 1963. Progestogens in the treatment of carcinoma of the endometrium. Surg Gynecol Obstet 127:103–114.
35. Malkasian GD, Decker DG, Mussey E, et al. 1971. Progestogen treatment of recurrent endometrial carcinoma. Am J Obstet Gynecol 110:15–23.
36. Reifenstein EC. 1974. The treatment of advanced endometrial cancer with hydroxyprogesterone caproate. Gynecol Oncol 2:377–414.
37. Bonte J, Decoster JM, Ide P, et al. 1978. Hormonoprophylaxis and hormonotherapy in the treatment of endometrial adenocarcinoma by means of medroxyprogesterone acetate. Gynecol Oncol 6:60–75.
38. Ng A, Reagan J. 1970. Incidence and prognosis of endometrial carcinoma by histologic grade and extent. Obstet Gynecol 35:437–443.
39. Wade ME, Kohorn EI, Morris JMcL. 1967. Adenocarcinoma of the endometrium; evaluation of preoperative irradiation and factors influencing prognosis. Am J Obstet Gynecol 99:869–876.
40. Deppe G. 1982. Chemotherapeutic treatment of endometrial carcinoma. Clin Obstet Gynecol 25:93–99.
41. Jordan VC, Hoerner S. 1975. Tamoxifen and the human carcinoma 85 estrogen receptor. Eur J Cancer 11:205–206.

42. Schwartz PE, MacLusky N, Naftolin F, et al. 1983. Tamoxifen-induced increase in cytosol progestin receptor levels in a case of metastatic endometrial cancer. Gynecol Oncol 16:41–48.
43. Moore TD, Phillips PH, Nerenstone SR, et al. 1991. Systemic treatment of advanced and recurrent endometrial carcinoma: current status and future directions. J Clin Oncol 9:1071–1088.
44. Bonte J, Ide P, Billiet G, et al. 1981. Tamoxifen as a possible chemotherapeutic agent in endometrial adenocarcinoma. Gynecol Oncol 11:140–161.
45. Slavik M, Petty WM, Blessing JA, et al. 1984. Phase II clinical study of tamoxifen in advanced endometrial adenocarcinoma: a Gynecologic Oncology Group study. Cancer Treat Rep 68:809–811.
46. Edmonson JH, Krook JE, Hilton JF, et al. 1986. Ineffectiveness of tamoxifen in advanced endometrial carcinoma after failure of progestin treatment. Cancer Treat Rep 70:1019–1020.
47. Fornander T, Cedermark B, Mattsson A, et al. 1989. Adjuvant tamoxifen in early breast cancer: occurrence of new primary cancers. Lancet 21:117–120.
48. Fisher B, Costantino JP, Redmond CK, et al. 1994. Endometrial cancer in tamoxifen-treated breast cancer patients: findings from NSABP B-14. J Natl Cancer Inst 86:527–537.
49. Mortel R, Levy C, Wolff JC, et al. 1981. Female sex steroid receptors in postmenopausal endometrial carcinoma and biochemical response to an antiestrogen. Cancer Res 41:1140–1147.
50. Carlson JA, Allegra JC, Day TG, et al. 1984. Tamoxifen and endometrial carcinoma: alterations in estrogen and progesterone receptors in untreated patients and combination hormonal therapy in advanced neoplasia. Am J Obstet Gynecol 149:149–153.
51. Rendina GM, Donadio C, Fabri M, et al. 1984. Tamoxifen and medroxyprogesterone therapy for advanced endometrial carcinoma. Eur J Obstet Gynecol Reprod Biol 17:285–291.
52. Kline RC, Freedman RS, Jones LA, et al. 1987. Treatment of recurrent or metastatic poorly differentiated adenocarcinoma of the endometrium with tamoxifen and medroxyprogesterone acetate. Cancer Treat Rep 71:327–328.
53. Pandya KJ, Yeap BY, Davis TE. 1989. Phase II study of megestrol and megestrol + tamoxifen in advanced endometrial carcinoma: an Eastern Cooperative Oncology Group study (abstract). Proc Annee Meet Am Assoc Cancer Res 30:A1037.
54. Kullander S. 1992. Treatment of endometrial cancer with GnRH analogs. Recent Results Cancer Res 124:69–73.
55. Gallagher CJ, Oliver RT, Oram DH, et al. 1992. Gonadotropin-releasing hormone analog treatment for recurrent progestogen-resistant endometrial cancer (abstract). Proc Annee Meet Am Soc Clin Oncol 11:A704.
56. Pahwa GS, Kullander S, Vollmer G, et al. 1991. Specific low affinity binding sites for gonadotropin releasing hormone in human endometrial carcinomata. Eur J Obstet Gynecol Reprod Biol 41:135–142.
57. Kistner RW. 1965. Induction of ovulation with clomiphene citrate (Clomid). Obstet Gynecol Surv 20:873–900.
58. Wall JA, Franklin RR, Kaufman RH. 1964. Reversal of benign and malignant changes with clomiphene. Am J Obstet Gynecol 88:1072–1085.
59. Baulieu EE. 1989. Contragestion and other clinical applications of RU 486, an antiprogesterone at the receptor. Science 245:1351–1357.
60. Kettel LM, Murphy AA, Mortola JF, et al. 1989. Endocrine responses to long-term administration of the antiprogesterone RU-486 in patients with pelvic endometriosis. Fertil Steril 56:402–407.
61. Murphy AA, Kettel LM, Morales AJ, et al. 1993. Regression of uterine leiomyomata in response to the antiprogesterone RU 486. J Clin Endocrinol Metab 76:513–517.
62. Distler W, Vering A. 1992. Antigestagene-pharmakologie und anwendungsperspektiven. Gynakologe 25:226–230.
63. Gentola GM. 1985. Inhibition of endometrial carcinoma cell cultures by a synthetic androgen. Cancer Res 45:6264–6267.

64. Deppe G, Jacobs AJ, Bruckner H, et al. 1981. Chemotherapy of advanced and recurrent endometrial carcinoma with cyclophosphamide, doxorubicin, 5-fluorouracil, and megestrol acetate. Am J Obstet Gynecol 140:313–316.
65. Lovecchio JL, Averette HE, Lichtinger M, et al. 1984. Treatment of advanced or recurrent endometrial adenocarcinoma with cyclophosphamide, doxorubicin, cis-platinum, and megestrol acetate. Obstet Gynecol 63:557–560.
66. Fung Kee Fun M, Krepart GV, Lotocki RJ, et al. 1991. Treatment of recurrent and metastatic adenocarcinoma of the endometrium with cisplatin, doxorubicin, cyclophosphamide, and medroxyprogesterone acetate. Obstet Gynecol 78:1033–1038.
67. Horton J, Elson P, Gordon P, et al. 1982. Combination chemotherapy for advanced endometrial cancer. Cancer 49:2442–2445.
68. Cohen CJ, Bruckner HW, Deppe G, et al. 1984. Multidrug treatment of advanced and recurrent endometrial carcinoma: a Gynecologic Oncology Group Study. Obstet Gynecol 63:719–726.
69. Mussey E, Malkasian GD. 1966. Progestogen treatment of recurrent carcinoma of the endometrium. Am J Obstet Gynecol 94:78–85.
70. Karlstedt K. 1971. Progesterone treatment for local recurrence and metastases in carcinoma corpus uteri. Acta Radiol (Stockholm) 10:187–192.
71. Wentz WB. 1985. Progestin therapy in lesions of the endometrium. Semin Oncol 12 (Suppl 1):23–27.
72. Huber H, Husslein P, Michalica W, et al. 1984. Radiosensitizing effect of medroxyprogesterone acetate on endometrial cancer cells in vitro. Cancer 54:999–1001.
73. Hustin J. 1976. Morphology and DNA content of endometrial cancer under progesterone treatment. Acta Cytol 20:556–558.
74. Physicians' Desk Reference. Oradel, NJ: Medical Economics Co., 1995.
75. Creasman WT, Henderson D, Hinshaw W, et al. 1986. Estrogen replacement therapy in the patient treated for endometrial cancer. Obstet Gynecol 67:326–330.
76. Baker DP. 1990. Estrogen-replacement therapy in patients with previous endometrial carcinoma. Compr Ther 16(1):28–35.
77. Hutchinson-Williams KA, Gutmann JN. 1991. Estrogen replacement therapy (ERT) in high-risk cancer patients. Yale J Biol Med 64:607–626.
78. Lee RB, Burke TW, Park RC. 1990. Estrogen replacement therapy following treatment for stage I endometrial carcinoma. Gynecol Oncol 36:189–191.
79. ACOG Committee Opinion, Number 126, August 1993.
80. Soper JT, Segreti EM, Novotny DB, et al. 1990. Estrogen and progesterone receptor content of endometrial carcinomas: comparison of total tissue versus cancer component analysis. Gynecol Oncol 36:363–368.
81. Runowicz DC, Nuchtern LM, Braunstein JD, Jones JG. 1990. Heterogeneity in hormone receptor status in primary and metastatic endometrial cancer. Gynecol Oncol 38:437–441.
82. Chambers JT, Merino M, Kohorn EI, et al. 1988. Estrogen and progesterone receptor levels as prognosticators for survival in endometrial cancer. Gynecol Oncol 31:65.
83. Aisner J, Tcheckmedyian NS, Tait N, et al. 1988. Studies of high-dose megestrol acetate: potential applications to cachexia. Semin Oncol 12 (Suppl 1):76–78.
84. Feliu J, Gonzales-Baron M, Berrocal A, et al. 1992. Usefulness of megestrol acetate in cancer cachexia and anorexia. A placebo-controlled study. Am J Clin Oncol 15:436–440.

7. Phytochemicals for the prevention of breast and endometrial cancer

J. Mark Cline and Claude L. Hughes, Jr.

1. Introduction

Observations of dietary and cultural differences in the spectrum of tumor types and incidence underlie the growing interest in the role of phytochemicals in cancer prevention. The relatively lower risk of breast and endometrial cancer in some Asian populations compared to Western women is well documented [1–3] (figure 1). The observation that the risk of breast cancer increases in Asian immigrants to the U.S. [4] and in urban subpopulations within Japan [5] suggests that epigenetic factors are responsible for the difference. American-born children of Asian immigrants have a 60% higher risk of developing breast cancer [4] relative to Asian immigrants born in Asia. This finding may reflect degree of assimilation into Western habits and/or a risk factor exerting an adverse effect during development. The increase in breast cancer that occurs in Asians who consume typically 'Western' foods also implicates diet as a cause for the lower incidence of breast cancer [5]. Asian diets typically contain less fat and a higher proportion of vegetables, including soy products, when compared to Western diets. Demographic evidence for a role of diet in endometrial cancer is not as well explored; however, epidemiologic and animal studies indicate a protective effect of vegetable intake [6,7].

Phytochemicals with potential anticancer properties span a wide range of chemical types and activities (table 1; figure 2). Additionally, their presence, concentration, and bioavailability in any of the thousands of plant species used by humans is variable and incompletely documented. Nonetheless, there is considerable epidemiologic evidence for diminution of breast and uterine cancer risk by phytochemicals (table 2). Biochemical, in vitro, and in vivo studies support the hypothesis that natural plant products and purified plant-derived compounds exert valuable protective effects on normal cells and inhibit the growth of tumor cells, potentially leading to prevention of tumor initiation and progression (tables 1 and 3). These effects have led to the development of both dietary and pharmaceutical chemopreventive strategies, but these approaches have not been thoroughly explored or exploited. The purpose of this chapter is to support further development of chemopreventive

Kenneth A. Foon and Hyman B. Muss (eds), BIOLOGICAL AND HORMONAL THERAPIES OF CANCER. Copyright © 1998. Kluwer Academic Publishers, Boston. All rights reserved.

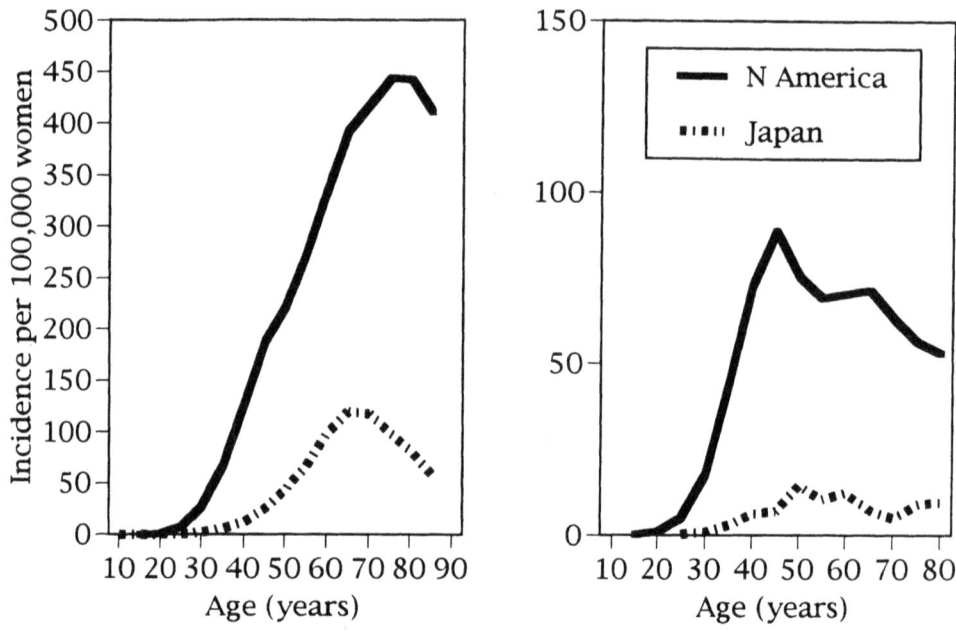

Figure 1. Incidence of breast (left panel) and endometrial (right panel) cancers as a function of age in North American (solid lines) and Japanese (dashed lines) women. Reprinted with permission from [3].

Table 1. Specific phytochemical classes with chemopreventive properties

Phytochemical type	Examples	Mechanisms of anticancer activity	References
Carotenoids	Beta-carotene	Induction of differentiation Antioxidant Antiproliferative Antiangiogenic	[8–13]
Vitamin C	Ascorbic acid	Antioxidant Induction of differentiation	[14–17]
Vitamin E	—	Antioxidant	[16,18]
Folic acid	—	Prevention of DNA hypomethylation Inhibition of oncogene expression	[19,20]
Selenium	—	Antioxidant	[21]
Fiber	Polysaccharides, cellulose, hemicellulose, pectin, gums, mucilages, lignin	Modulation of estrogen metabolism Binding of carcinogens Lowering of bile acids	[22–25] [26–28]
Organosulfur compounds and derivatives			
Dithiolthiones	—	Antioxidant Induction of phase II enzymes	[29–31]

Table 1. (Continued)

Phytochemical type	Examples	Mechanisms of anticancer activity	References
Glucosinolates and indoles	Glucobrassicin (3-indolylmethyl glucosinolate), sinigrin (2-propenyl glucosinolate, indole-3-carbinol	Induction of phase II enzymes Inhibition of estradiol metabolism Inhibition of DNA adduct formation	[32–34]
Isothiocyanates and thiocyanates	Sulforaphane Benzyl ITCs Phenyl ITCs	Inhibition of DNA methylation Induction of phase II enzymes Inhibition of estradiol metabolism	[17,29,30]
Allium compounds	Alliin Diallyl sulfide	Induction of GST and microsomal monooxygenases Antiproliferative	[35]
Coumarins	Coumestrol	Induction of phase II enzymes Inhibition of estradiol metabolism	[36,37]
Flavonoids	Quercetin Kaempferol Nobiletin Tangeretin Rutin	Antioxidant Phase I enzyme modulation	[38–41]
Protease inhibitors	Bowman–Birk inhibitor Other serine protease inhibitors	Epoxide scavenging Inhibition of proteolysis by tumor cells Inhibition of transformation?	[42,43]
Sterols	Beta-sitosterol Campesterol Stigmasterol	Modulation of endogenous steroidogenic pathways	[44]
Isoflavones	Genistein Daidzein Kievitone	Weak estrogen agonists Tyrosine kinase inhibition Topoisomerase inhibitors Angiogenesis inhibition Elevation of sex hormone-binding globulin	[24,45–54]
Lignans	Secoisolariciresinol Matairesinol	Weak estrogen agonists Aromatase inhibition Elevation of sex hormone-binding globulin	[24,54]
Saponins		Antiproliferative Cell surface effects	[55]
Inositol hexaphosphate		Inhibition of proliferation	[56,57]
Terpenes	d-limonene 18β glycirrhizic acid Kawheol palmitate	Induction of GST Induction of tumor differentiation Modulation of growth factor effects G-protein modification Anti-initiating effects	[58–61] [60] [61]
Polyphenols	Ellagic acid Epigallocatechin gallate Cucurmin	Antioxidant Induction of phase II enzymes Inhibition of DNA methylation Inhibition of DNA topoisomerase Cyclooxygenase inhibition	[51,62–65]

Table 2. Epidemiologic studies of anticancer effects of plant foods or specific phytochemicals in breast and uterus

Author, year, location	Site	Study type	Food or phytochemical	Odds ratio (95% CI) or stated effect[a]
Graham, 1982, New York	B	Case–control	Cruciferous vegetables	1.0
Zemla, 1984, Poland	B	Case–control	Raw vegetables	0.7 (NS)
Katsouyanni, 1986, Greece	B	Case–control	Vegetables	↓ ($p < 0.001$)
			Fruit	↓ ($p < 0.1$)
			Squash	↓ ($p < 0.1$)
			Raw cabbage	↓ ($p < 0.1$)
			Cucumbers	0.9 (0.7–1.0)
			Carrots	0.8 (0.6–1.0)
			Lettuce	0.8 (0.6–1.0)
			Vegetable index	0.2 (0.1–0.4)
Hirayama, 1986, Japan	B	Cohort	Miso soup	↓
LaVecchia, 1986, Italy	U	Case–control	Green vegetables	0.3 (0.2–0.4)
			Carrots	NS
			Fruit	0.4 (0.3–0.7)
Zemla, 1986, Poland	U	Case–control	Raw vegetables	0.4 ($p < 0.001$)
LaVecchia, 1987, Italy	B	Case–control	Green vegetables	0.4 (0.3–0.5)
			Fresh fruit	
Hislop, 1988, British Columbia	B	Case–control	Yellow vegetables	0.9 (0.5–1.7)
			Carrots	0.4 (0.2–0.8)
			Green vegetables	1.0 (0.6–1.6)
van't Veer, 1990, Netherlands [66]	B	Case–control	Cereals	0.42 (0.19–0.92)
			Fiber	0.55 (0.26–1.17)
			Beta-carotene	0.63 (0.31–1.26)
			Vegetables	0.63 (0.30–1.32)
Barbone, 1993, USA [6]	U	Case–control	Carotene	0.4 (0.2–0.8)
Hunter, 1993, USA [67]	B	Case–control	Vitamin C	1.03 (0.87–1.21)
			Vitamin E	0.99 (0.83–1.19)
Levi, 1993 Switzerland [15]	B	Case–control	Green vegetables	0.4 ($p < 0.05$)
			Cruciferous vegetables	0.5 ($p < 0.05$)
			Onions	0.4 ($p < 0.01$)
			Pears	0.5 ($p < 0.05$)
			Beta-carotene	0.4 ($p < 0.01$)
			Vitamin C	0.7 (NSD)
Levi, 1993 Italy, Switzerland [68]	U	Case–control	Beta-carotene,	0.49 ($p < 0.01$)
			Vitamin C	0.46 ($p < 0.01$)
			Vegetables	0.38 ($p < 0.01$)
			Fresh fruit	0.45 ($p < 0.01$)
			Whole grains	0.43 ($p < 0.01$)
Potischman, 1993, USA [69]	U	Case–control	Cereals and grains	0.6 (0.4–1.1)
			Fiber	0.7 (0.4–1.3)
			Folate-rich foods	0.9 (0.6–1.6)
			Cruciferous vegetables	0.8 (0.5–1.3)
			Vitamin C	1.3 (0.7–2.2)

Table 2. (Continued)

Author, year, location	Site	Study type	Food or phytochemical	Odds ratio (95% CI) or stated effect[a]
Rohan, 1993, USA [25]	B	Cohort	Fiber	0.68 (0.48–1.00)
			Vitamin E	0.96 (0.63–1.45)
			Vitamin C	0.88 (0.62–1.26)
			Beta-carotene	0.77 (0.53–1.10)
Shu, 1993, China [70]	U	Cohort	Vegetables	1.4 ($p = 0.39$)
			Cruciferous vegetables	1.1 ($p = 0.67$)
			Allium	0.7 ($p = 0.12$)
			Fruits	0.7 ($p = 0.25$)
			Fiber	1.1 ($p = 0.70$)
			Carotene	1.3 ($p = 0.72$)
			Vitamin C	1.1 ($p = 0.78$)
Baghurst, 1994, Australia [27]	B	Case–control	Fiber	0.48 (0.30–0.76)
Willett, 1994, USA [71]	B	Cohort	Fiber	1.14 (0.86–1.15)
Dorant, 1995, Netherlands [35]	B	Cohort	Onions	0.95 (0.61–1.47)
			Leeks	1.08 (0.79–1.48)
			Garlic	0.87 (0.58–1.31)
Negri, 1996 Italy [72]	B	Case–control	Beta-carotene	0.84
			Vitamin E	0.75
			Vitamin C	NS

[a] p values are χ^2 for trend.
Adapted from [29].

Table 3. General mechanisms of cancer chemoprevention by phytochemicals

Type of activity	Compounds	Reference
Anti-initiating		
Inhibition of carcinogen formation	Ascorbic acid, alpha tocopherols, phenols	[17]
Blockage of carcinogenic reactions	Phenols, terpenes, indole-3-carbinol, ellagic acid	[17,40]
Enhancement of carcinogen degradation	Isothiocynates, indoles	[17,40]
Antioxidant/electrophile scavenging	Alpha tocopherol, carotenoids	[9,17,40]
Arachidonic acid inhibitors	Flavonoids, carotenoids	[73]
Antipromoting		
Topoisomerase inhibitors	Genistein	[51]
Modulation of sex steroid activity	Coumestrol, genistein, daidzein, phloretin, formononetin, biochanin A, indole-3-carbinol	[45] [33]
Antiproliferative agents	Genistein, carotenoids	[48,74,75]
Angiogenesis inhibitors	Genistein	[52]
Antioxidants	Beta-carotene, ascorbic acid	[10,16]
Differentiation-inducing agents	Beta-carotene/vitamin A, genistein	[11,76]
Aromatase inhibitors	Lignans, flavonoids	[54]
Tyrosine kinase inhibitors	Genistein	[47,49]
Apoptosis inducers	Genistein	[52]
Invasion inhibitors	Protease inhibitors	[43]

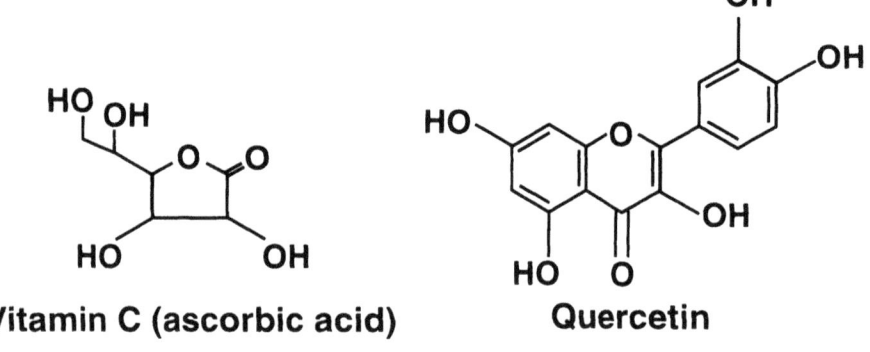

Figure 2. Structures of selected phytochemicals with anticarcinogenic properties.

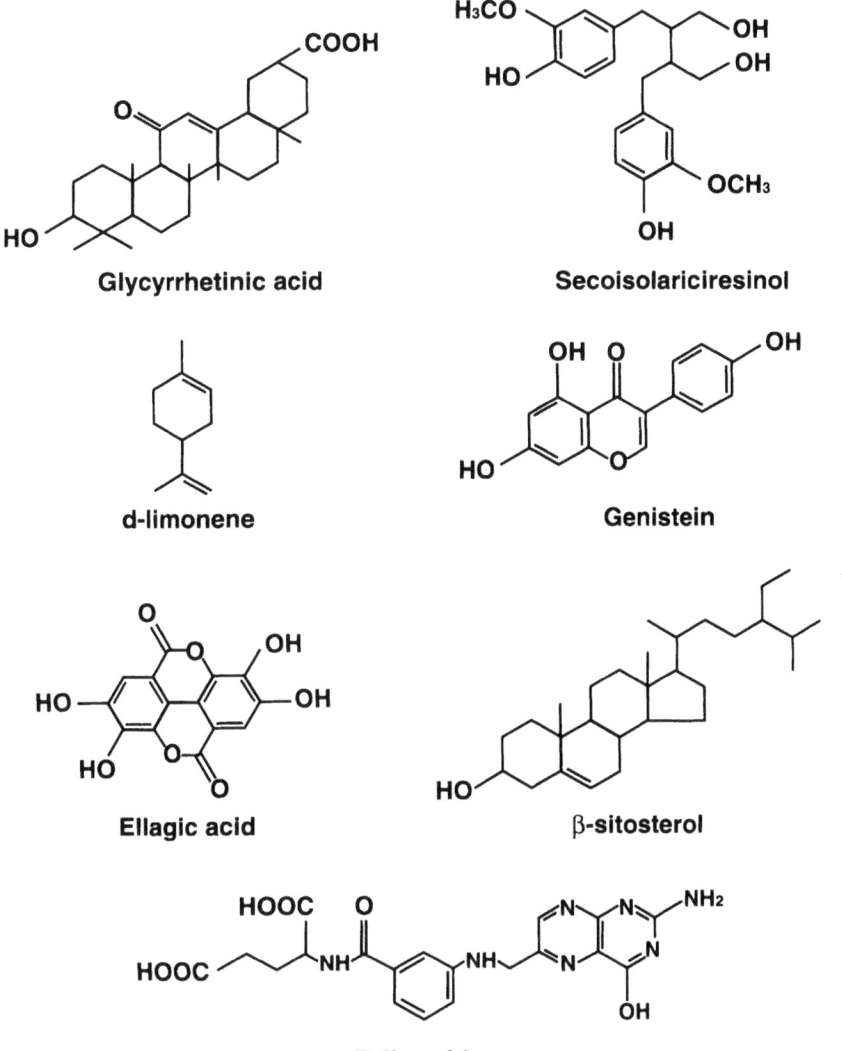

Figure 2. (Continued)

strategies by summarizing the currently available evidence regarding potential anticancer activity of phytochemicals in the breast and endometrium.

2. Epidemiology

Broad evidence for a protective effect of phytochemicals has come from case–control and cohort studies of the effects of vegetable and fruit intake on cancer risk, and this topic has been the subject of several reviews [14,29,30,77]. Several studies have specifically examined the effects of vegetable and fruit intake on breast cancer risk. For the most part, these studies indicate a protective effect of vegetable intake, particularly for vegetables that are rich in carotenoids (table 2). Estimates of specific phytochemical consumption have provided further data regarding their protective effects (table 2). Beta-carotene intake has been associated with lower breast cancer risk in several studies (table 3) ([8,66]; reviewed in [10]). Similarly, higher dietary fiber intake has been associated with lower risk of breast cancer in several epidemiologic studies (reviewed in [23]; see also [2,25,27]), with the notable exception of the Nurses Health Study [71]. The effect of vitamin C is less clear. Rohan et al. found a negative association between intake and breast cancer risk, but other studies have shown no effect (reviewed in [16,78]). A comparison of breast cancer patients with omnivorous and vegetarian women by Adlercreutz [79] revealed that their urinary excretion of enterolactone, a metabolite of dietary fiber-associated lignans, is half that of healthy omnivores and one sixth that of vegetarians. This finding provides indirect evidence for the role of dietary fiber or absorption of fiber-associated metabolites in breast cancer prevention. Beta-carotene and vitamin C intake via vegetable and fruit consumption correlate with more favorable prognostic indices in breast cancers (e.g., more abundant estrogen and progesterone receptors and a greater degree of histologic tumor differentiation) [80] and longer survival in breast cancer patients [81].

The effect of dietary phytochemical consumption on endometrial cancer risk is less well explored. Levi et al. [68] found a strong negative association between beta-carotene and vitamin C intake and endometrial cancer risk among Swiss women, but no clear effect was seen in similar studies in China [70] and the U.S. [69]. Barbone et al. [6] demonstrated a protective effect of carotene intake on endometrial cancer. Zheng et al. [82] found a weak negative correlation between endometrial cancer and plant food intake in the Iowa Women's Health Study.

3. Experimental evidence for anticancer effects — pathophysiology and general preventive mechanisms

In general, mechanisms of cancer chemoprevention are based either on prevention of initiation (the genetic event leading eventually to expression of the neoplastic phenotype) or on inhibition of promotion (exogenous influences on the initiated cell leading to proliferation or gene expression that cause the neoplasm to develop). These general mechanisms of action are outlined below and in table 3, and have been the subject of a number of excellent reviews [17,73,83]. Some compounds, such as carotenoids and isoflavones, are pleiotropic, exerting protective effects by a number of differing mechanisms. In addition to these identified mechanisms, further prospects for more effective, specific prevention of endometrial and breast cancer will derive from our growing understanding of the normal tropic stimuli for those tissues. Regulation of normal breast and endometrial growth have been well reviewed recently [84–87]. The merging of these two fields into the study of modulating effects of phytochemicals on growth factor expression and activity is a relatively new endeavor, with work to date primarily limited to the effects of phytoestrogenic compounds and retinoids (see below). Other exciting possibilities are suggested by consideration of the known regulatory factors for each tissue (table 4). A number of new avenues for exerting antiproliferative/chemopreventive effects are possible.

Table 4. Endogenous regulators of breast and endometrium

Regulator	Effect on breast[a]	Effect on endometrial epithelium[b]	Phytochemical effects
Amphiregulin	↑	—	
Epidermal growth factor	↑	↑	Receptor modulation (folic acid) [20]
Insulin-like growth factor I	↑	↑	Decreased proliferative responses (d-limonene) [88]
Insulin-like growth factor II	↑	↑	
Acidic fibroblast growth factor	↑	↑	
Basic fibroblast growth factor	↑	↑	
Estradiol	↑	↑	Competitive inhibition, differentiation (phytoestrogens) [45,89] Differentiation, receptor induction (vitamin C, retinoids) [80]
Mammastatin	↓	—	
Mammary-derived growth factor 1	↓	—	
Mammary-derived growth inhibitor	↓	—	
Platelet-derived growth factor	↑	↑[c]	
Transforming growth factor α	↑	↑	Decreased responses (retinoids) [74]
Transforming growth factor β	↓	↑,↓	Potentiation of inhibitory effect (phytoestrogens) [75], (d-limonene) [88]
Müllerian inhibiting factor	—	↓	
Tumor necrosis factor α	—	↓	
Progesterone	↑	↓	Differentiation, receptor induction (phytoestrogens) [90] Vitamin C, retinoids [80]
Relaxin	↑	—	[91]
Prolactin	↑	—	

[a] From [85].
[b] From [86].
[c] Stimulatory for stromal cells.

3.1. Prevention of tumor initiation

Compounds that prevent initiating events include antioxidants, electrophile scavengers or inducers of endogenous scavenging systems, inducers of xenobiotic-metabolizing enzymes, and agents that inhibit formation of endogenous oxidants. Such agents are divided into those that prevent formation of carcinogens and those that prevent the carcinogen from interacting with DNA [17]. Carcinogen formation can potentially be blocked by
- impeding intestinal formation of carcinogens from dietary precursors [92]
- inhibiting metabolic activation of carcinogens [17,83]
- impeding formation of endogenous reactive products of inflammation (e.g., inhibitors of arachidonic acid metabolism [93])

Carcinogens can be inhibited from interacting with DNA by
- enhancing metabolic conjugation/deactivation of carcinogens [17,83]
- direct scavenging of reactive molecules (in the case of antioxidant phytochemicals) [16]
- inhibiting DNA binding by carcinogens [94]
- increasing fidelity of DNA repair (e.g., protease inhibitors) [73]

A brief consideration of the major classes of anti-initiating agents follows.

3.1.1. Antioxidants. Antioxidants found in plants include vitamin E, the carotenoids, flavonoids, phenols, isoflavones, selenium, and others [30,95]. The anticancer effects of such compounds derive in part from their ability to scavenge reactive electrophilic compounds that might produce DNA damage. Dorgan and Schatzkin [16] reviewed the epidemiologic and experimental evidence for anticancer effects of carotenoids, vitamin E, vitamin C, and selenium; evidence of a protective effect was considered most convincing for the carotenoids. The most profound antioxidant effect of dietary phytochemicals may be indirect, by induction of endogenous antioxidant systems (see below).

3.1.2. Enzyme inducers. A number of plant-derived agents induce phase I (oxidation, reduction, or hydrolysis) [96] and phase II (conjugating) xenobiotic metabolizing enzymes [97]. Most notable among these are the indole-containing compounds derived from cruciferous vegetables, such as the glucosinolates and indole-3-carbinol [32], although a broad range of similar and unrelated compounds are similarly active. It is noteworthy that phase I enzyme induction can either 1) decrease the amount of carcinogen present by converting it to a less reactive metabolite or 2) convert a procarcinogen into a carcinogen [40,96,98]. Fiala et al. [40], in a review of dietary anticarcinogens, pointed out that similar compounds (for example, phenolic flavonoids) may have differing effects on the formation of carcinogens, with some inhibiting and some accelerating the formation of reactive nitroso compounds from nitrites.

3.1.3. Inhibitors of arachidonic acid metabolism. The role of arachidonic acid metabolism in carcinogenesis has recently become a topic of interest in the field of chemoprevention. Some nonsteroidal and steroidal inhibitors of inflammation have anticarcinogenic effects, as do plant-derived inhibitors of lipoxygenase (flavonoids and carotenoids) [73]. Arachidonic acid inhibitors such as nonsteroidal anti-inflammatory drugs decrease risk of colorectal cancer; however, the evidence is less clear for breast and endometrium [99]. Mechanistically, inhibition of prostaglandin H synthase and lipoxygenase decreases local inflammation with its associated formation of reactive oxygen species and other mutagens such as malondialdehyde [93]. Additionally, the process of liberation of arachidonic acid from membranes, a critical signal transduction event, may play a role in carcinogenesis [73].

3.2. Blockers of tumor promotion

Compounds that inhibit promotion are typically those that impede proliferation of the initiated cell or those that enhance cell loss from proliferating cellular populations.

3.2.1. Inducers of apoptosis. Derangement in the expression of genes regulating apoptosis is an early feature in the development of many neoplasms, leading to loss of the normal balance of cell division and cell loss. Phytochemicals that exert differentiating and antiproliferative effects, such as retinoids and genistein, also are inducers of apoptosis [100,101].

3.2.2. Antiproliferative agents. Several compounds with demonstrated anticancer activity, such as glycyrrhetinic acid and genistein, modulate signal transduction by alteration of kinase or phospholipase activity [73]. Also, modulation of the effects of growth factor action is a feature of several cancer-inhibiting phytochemicals or their metabolites. Some examples of this type of effect are the following:
- The isoflavone genistein inhibits dioxin-induced downregulation of the inhibitory growth factor transforming growth factor-β (TGF-β) in hepatoma cells, presumably by its tyrosine kinase-inhibiting activity [75].
- Retinol inhibits the TGF-α-induced proliferative response of T47D breast carcinoma cells [74].
- Retinoic acid decreases insulin-like growth factor-1 (IGF-1)-mediated c-*fos* induction in breast carcinoma cells [102].

3.2.3. Modulation of tumor gene expression. In addition to the known antimutagenic and growth factor-mediated effects on tumor gene expression, various phytochemicals have been shown to impede genetic alterations associated with increased cancer risk. Such effects include ensuring adequacy of DNA methylation (folic acid) [20], inhibition of oncogene expression (retinoids) [103], and binding to topoisomerase II [51].

3.2.4. Inducers of differentiation. Lamartiniere et al. [89,104] demonstrated that genistein given to neonatal or juvenile rats decreases the incidence of DMBA-induced mammary gland neoplasms, and additionally accelerates the normal pattern of mammary gland differentiation. In this instance, the effects are similar to those of neonatally administered estrogen, which in the hormonal milieu of early development is a differentiating agent [105]. However, genistein also exerts a differentiating effect outside the developmental setting; the mechanistic basis of this phenomenon may lie in its tyrosine kinase- or topoisomerase-inhibiting activity [106]. A variety of phytochemicals induce differentiation in the HL-60 leukemia cell system [107]. A few, such as d-limonene and related terpenes, induce differentiation of mammary gland tumors in rats [60,108].

3.2.5. Modulators of hormone activity. The widely used but imprecise term *phytoestrogen* includes many nonsteroidal plant-derived compounds with structural or functional similarities to estrogen, including isoflavones, lignans, phytic acids, and others (reviewed in [109]). A family of isoflavone compounds constitute the major phytoestrogens in soy products. Most isoflavones act as weak estrogens in vitro — for example, in the stimulation of alkaline phosphatase activity by endometrial cells [110]. Lignans, diphenolic compounds associated with plant fiber (e.g., secoisolariciresinol), also may act as weak estrogens [111,112]. Urinary excretion of active phytoestrogen-derived compounds indicates that these dietary compounds are bioavailable and absorbed. Setchell et al. [113] measured urinary excretion of the phytoestrogen metabolite equol after a 40-g oral dose of soy isolate and demonstrated a 1000-fold increase in some subjects. Subsequently, Adlercreutz et al. [114] demonstrated a 20- to 30-fold difference in baseline urinary equol excretion between Asian and Western women, a finding that is of considerable interest in light of the differences in breast and endometrial cancer incidence in these populations. Women consuming diets higher in grain fiber and isoflavones also have higher concentrations of serum sex-hormone-binding globulin (SHBG) and a lower percentage of free estradiol in serum [24,111]. Diphenolic phytoestrogen compounds also inhibit aromatase activity [54] and 17β-hydroxysteroid oxidoreductase type 1 [37], thus potentially diminishing formation of estradiol from other steroids. In the rat model of mammary carcinogenesis induced by DMBA, soy products decrease the incidence of neoplasms (reviewed in [47]). Data from our laboratory indicate a lack of tumor promotion in soy-protein-fed rats. Specifically, in animals fed a diet containing 13 mg of isoflavones per kilogram body weight, no tumors occurred, compared to an average of three tumors per rat for those animals given conjugated equine estrogens plus medroxyprogesterone acetate (Cline et al., unpublished data).

Martin [115] postulated that phytoestrogens might promote tumor growth because of their proliferation-inducing effect on MCF-7 mammary carcinoma cells and their relatively low affinity (27% of estradiol) for SHBG. This finding is in contrast to the demonstrated anticancer activity of genistein. Further work by Mäkelä et al. [116] has shown that genistein, coumestrol, biochanin A, and zearalenol all failed to inhibit estradiol-induced cell proliferation in MCF-7 cells, and in some cases further increased proliferation rates in a receptor-dependent manner. This finding implies that the anticancer effects of these compounds are not based on competitive inhibition at the estrogen receptor. Furthermore, Peterson et al. [48] demonstrated receptor independence of the antiproliferative effect of genistein in mammary carcinoma cell lines.

3.2.6. Protease inhibitors. The most abundant protease inhibitors in plants are the serine protease inhibitors specific for trypsin, chymotrypsin, elastase, and other mammalian proteolytic enzymes. The most extensively studied of the protease inhibitors is the soybean Bowman–Birk inhibitor (BBI), which was initially described as an inhibitor of intestinal proteolytic enzymes in livestock but was subsequently found to exert a variety of anticancer effects in vitro and in vivo (reviewed in [42]) (figure 3). The major anticancer effect of protease inhibitors may lie in their potential inhibition of tumor invasion in the early stages of tumorigenesis [43].

3.2.7. Angiogenesis inhibitors. In mature, differentiated tissues, angiogenesis is required only infrequently — for example, during wound healing and other reparative processes. An exception to this generality is in the female reproductive tract, where neovascularization of the endometrium and corpora lutea occurs regularly. Tumor angiogenesis is a vital step in tumor progression and presents an opportunity for preventive or therapeutic intervention [117]. Genistein and retinoids are both inhibitors of angiogenesis [12,52].

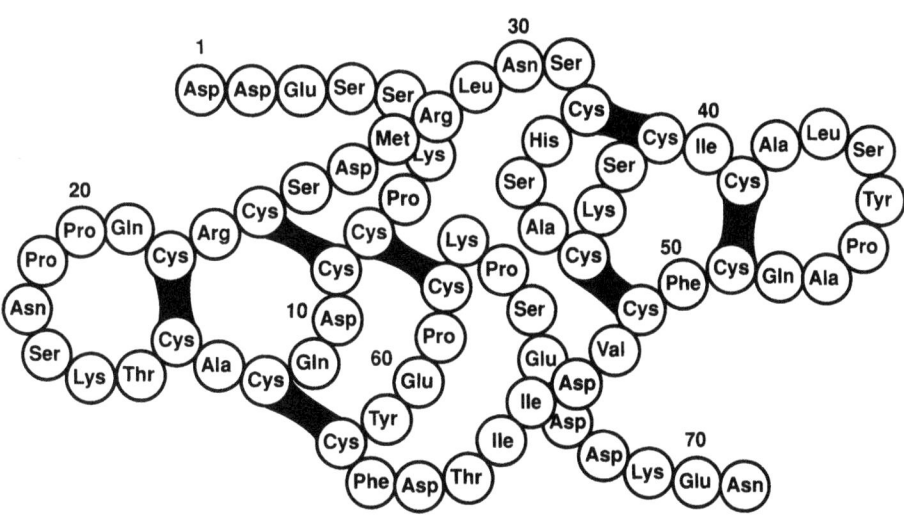

Bowman-Birk inhibitor

Figure 3. Structure of the Bowman–Birk inhibitor, a protease inhibitor found in soybeans.

4. Experimental evidence for anticancer effects — specific compounds

Phytochemicals with known or potential anticancer activity fall into several chemical classes (table 1), which to some degree are predictive of their effects. We have summarized the structures of selected representative compounds in figure 2. The anticancer effects of specific substances in animal models are listed in table 5. The reader also is referred to the thorough reviews of animal chemoprevention trials by E1-Bayoumy [78] and Dragsted et al. [118].

4.1. Carotenoids/retinoids

Plant carotenoids include beta-carotene, lutein, lycopene, and other compounds derived from a variety of green and yellow vegetables and fruits. These compounds are antioxidants [9,13] and act as precursors for vitamin A synthesis, which can modulate the effects of growth factors such as TGF-α and IGF-I, as mentioned above. Retinoids derived from carotenoids are morphogenic hormones during development [119]; retinoid receptor proteins are widely distributed in normal tissues and modulate a number of growth- and differentiation-associated events [11,120]. Retinoids inhibit oncogene expression in a number of tumor cell lines in vitro [103] and induce cell differentiation in lymphoid and epithelial tumor cell lines [11]. Retinoids also inhibit tumor development in a number of rat and mouse models [78,121,122]. Recent work by Swisshelm et al. [76] indicates that the normal morphogenetic and differentiating effects of retinoids may be ineffective in tumor cells due to a loss of retinoic acid receptors.

4.2. Vitamin C

Vitamin C (ascorbic acid) is present in green and yellow fruits and vegetables. It is a potent antioxidant and prevents the formation of carcinogenic nitrosamines [17]. There is little evidence, however, for anticarcinogenic effects in rodent models of mammary or endometrial neoplasia. A review of the literature in 1994 identified only equivocal evidence for chemopreventive activity in rodent models of chemically induced mammary carcinogenesis [78]. A single study of endometrial carcinogenesis examined the effect of vitamin C on uterine sarcomas induced in mice by 1,2-dimethylhydrazine/estradiol dipropionate; in this study, the incidence of endometrial sarcomas was markedly decreased [123].

4.3. Vitamin E

The effect of tocopherols on carcinogenesis is not profound, and many studies have found no effect on the development of chemically induced mammary neoplasms in rodents (reviewed in [78]). Ip [124] found that vitamin E supplementation inhibited the increased incidence of mammary neoplasms induced

Table 5. Animal studies of the anticarcinogenic effects of phytochemicals in breast and uterus

Plant product or compound	Effect on tumorigenesis
Mammary tumors	
Allium derivatives	↓
Beta-carotene	↓
Beta-sitosterol	→
Caffeine/coffee	→
Carotenoids	↓
Catechin	↓
Chlorogenic acid	→
Coumarin	↓
Cruciferous vegetables	↓
Curcumin	↓
d-Limonene	↓
Dithiolthiones	↓
Dried green coffee	↓
Ellagic acid	→
Fiber	↓
Flavonoids	→
Folic acid	→
Garlic	↓
Genistein	↓
Glucosinolates and indoles	↓
Glycirrhizic acid	↓
Indole-3-carbinol	↓
Inositol hexaphosphate	→
Isoflavones	↓
Isothiocynates and thiocynates	↓
Kahweol palmitate	↓
Lignans	→
Orange oil	↓
Polyphenols	↓
Protease inhibitors/Bowman–Birk	↓
Quercetin	→
Rosemary extract	↓
Saponins	→
Selenium/organoselenium compounds	↓
Soy products	↓
Vitamin C	→
Vitamin E	→
Endometrial tumors	
Indole-3-carbinol	↓
Vitamin C	↓

by a high polyunsaturated-fat diet in the rat DMBA model; however, a chemopreventive effect of vitamin E alone was not seen.

4.4. Selenium-containing foods

Experimental diets rich in selenium (Brazil nuts, garlic, and onions) inhibit mammary carcinogenesis in the rat DMBA model. Selenium-fertilized garlic is more protective in the rat DMBA model than is selenium-poor garlic [21]. Inorganic selenium is also clearly chemopreventive in rodent chemical carcinogenesis assays [78], but its utility is limited by its toxicity. There is some evidence that organoselenium compounds, such as those derived from alliums, are more strongly chemopreventive than selenium in Brazil nuts or inorganic supplements (reviewed in [21]). As is the case for vitamin E, the beneficial effects of selenium are found primarily in animals fed a diet high in polyunsaturated fats (reviewed in [16]).

4.5. Folic acid

Folic acid is abundant in fruits and vegetables, and therefore intake of folic acid is correlated with lower cancer rates. In animals fed a diet deficient in compounds acting as methyl group donors, folic acid prevents DNA hypomethylation and its associated elevations in c-myc, c-fos, c-Ha-ras, and EGFR gene expression [20]. In theory, this effect would be chemopreventive. However, data from animal studies do not clearly support a chemopreventive role for folic acid [19].

4.6. Fiber

The anticancer effects of fiber on colon and mammary gland in humans and animal models have been reviewed by Weisburger [22]. In rodent models, as in women, high dietary lignan intake modulates estrogen metabolism and excretion [24]. Arts et al. [26] and Kendall and Cohen [28] demonstrated a protective effect of a high-fiber diet on NMU-induced mammary carcinomas in rats, which was accompanied by an increase in fecal estrogen excretion, interpreted as interruption of enterohepatic recycling of estrogens.

4.7. Coumarins

Coumarins have been found to inhibit carcinogenesis in animal models and are inducers of phase II enzymes such as glutathione-S-transferase [36]. Coumestrol is a potent inhibitor of 17 beta-hydroxysteroid oxidoreductase type 1 in vitro [37]. This enzyme converts estrone to 17 beta-estradiol; therefore, its inhibition may reduce estrogen-dependent tumor promotion. In the DMBA model, coumarin and hydroxycoumarin decreased tumor size but not multiplicity [125], implying an antiprogression effect.

4.8. Organosulfur compounds

Glucosinolates comprise a large group of compounds derived from cruciferous vegetables, which exert a number of potentially chemopreventive effects (for reviews, see [32,126]). Glucosinolates induce production of hepatic mixed-function oxidases, leading to the accelerated metabolism of xenobiotics. Cruciferous vegetables and purified indole-3-carbinol inhibit chemically induced mammary gland neoplasms in rats [127] and spontaneous mammary tumors in mice [128]. Indole-3-carbinol also decreases the incidence of spontaneous endometrial tumors in the endometrial carcinoma-prone Donryu rat strain [7]. The mechanistic basis for cancer prevention by indole-3-carbinol may lie in its induction of xenobiotic-metabolizing enzymes, for example, aryl hydrocarbon hydroxylase [127]. Indole-3-carbinol also alters estradiol metabolism. In women, Bradlow et al. [33] demonstrated that indole-3-carbinol increased the circulating ratio of 2-OH-estrone to estradiol. Isothiocyanates and thiocyanates (benzyl-, phenyl-, and norbornyl-) are cruciferous vegetable-derived sulfur-containing compounds that inhibit chemically induced rodent mammary tumors [78,126]. The potential for chemoprevention by isothiocyanates has been recently reviewed by Hecht [128]. Potential chemopreventive activities of these type of compounds include prevention of carcinogen activation [128] and induction of phase II enzymes [129]. The isothiocyanate sulforaphane is a selective phase II enzyme inducer that acts without induction of phase I enzymes [129]. Organic sulfur-containing compounds found in garlic and onions are known to exert anti-initiating effects, possibly through induction of GST and microsomal monooxygenases and antiproliferative effects (reviewed in [130]). Allium-derived organosulfur compounds inhibit proliferation in a canine mammary carcinoma cell line [131]. However, work examining a specific effect of allium-derived compounds on reproductive tract is lacking.

4.9. Flavonoids

Flavonoids, such as quercetin, kaempferol, and others, have antioxidant properties in general. They may either inhibit or induce hepatic mixed-function oxidases, making effects on xenobiotic metabolism difficult to generalize. Quercetin and kaempferol have been reported to inhibit cytochrome P450 [40]. The 'estrogenicity' of plant flavonoids is similarly variable; kaempferol is an estrogen receptor agonist in MCF-7 cells, inducing expression of PS2 protein, whereas quercetin is not [38]. The cancer-preventive potential of plant flavonoids has in the past been considered minimal [39], although another review presents a more optimistic view [41].

4.10. Bowman–Birk and other protease inhibitors

In vitro, Bowman-Birk inhibitor (BBI) prevents radiation-induced cell transformation [132] and prevents nuclear binding of the estrogen receptor complex in MCF-7 breast carcinoma cells [133]. Most reports of anticancer activity attributable to the BBI in animal models have been in colon carcinogenesis studies, where profound inhibitory effects are seen (reviewed in [42]). However, BBI inhibits proteolysis by fibroblasts and breast carcinoma cells in vitro [43], and BBI is widely distributed in tissues after oral administration in mice [134]; thus, antitumor effects may be more widespread.

4.11. Sterols

Phytosterols include many plant-derived substances, including beta-sitosterol, campesterol, stigmasterol and others. Evidence for the chemopreventive activity of plant sterols has come primarily from epidemiologic studies of colon carcinogenesis [135]. However, there also is substantial evidence from animal studies that beta-sitosterol has endocrine-modulating and estrogenic effects. Mechanistically, it is likely that plant sterols alter steroid metabolism by virtue of their structural similarity to mammalian sterols (reviewed in [44]).

4.12. Isoflavones

Isoflavones appear to possess a plethora of potentially anticarcinogenic properties. Genistein, daidzein, biochanin A, formononetin, and their conjugates constitute the major isoflavones in widely consumed plants. The most extensively studied isoflavone is the soy derivative genistein (figure 1). Genistein binds with approximately 1/250th of the affinity of estradiol to the estrogen receptor [45]. Several investigators have shown that in the absence of estrogen, isoflavones have weakly estrogenic effects, whereas in the presence of estrogen, they may exert an antagonistic effect [46,136]. This finding suggests a competitive, estrogen receptor-mediated mechanism. However, the generality of this phenomenon has not been shown for all tissues, and particularly not for the mammary gland. It may be that the weak estrogenicity of genistein has little to do with its breast cancer-protective effects [137]. Genistein has antiproliferative effects in MCF-7 breast cancer cells without respect to their estrogen receptor positivity [48]. This effect is, therefore, presumably not dependent on the receptor and may be mediated by genistein's potent inhibition of tyrosine kinase activity [49]. Genistein is also an inhibitor of DNA topoisomerase [50], which may be an integral part of its differentiation-inducing properties [106]. It is also an antioxidant [138], and induces apoptosis in breast cancer cell lines in vitro [100]. Furthermore, genistein also has antiproliferative and antiangiogenic effects on vascular endothelial cells in vitro [52], leading to the hypothesis that its antiangiogenic properties may be responsible for the relatively indolent nature of breast carcinomas in Asian women. Another isoflavone, kievitone (derived from red kidney beans), has shown similar and possibly more potent antiproliferative effects in MCF-7 cells stimulated by a variety of growth factors, although kievitone appears to have less potent tyrosine kinase activity [53].

4.13. Saponins

Saponins are amphophilic glycoside compounds abundant in legumes and a variety of herbaceous plants such as ginseng [139]. The potential anticancer effects of saponins were recently reviewed by Rao and Sung [55]; however, data relevant to mammary and endometrial cancer prevention are lacking.

4.14. Inositol hexaphosphate (phytic acid)

In vitro, phytic acid inhibits proliferation of MCF-7 cells at concentrations greater than 1 mM [56]. Thompson and Zhang [57] found that dietary phytic acid supplementation (1.2%) induced lower proliferation indices in the ducts and terminal end buds of the mammary glands of rats, a finding that correlated positively with colonic proliferation in the same animals. Phytic acid also inhibits mammary tumor development in the DMBA model [56,140]. Potential anticancer effects of phytic acid have been recently reviewed by Shamsuddin [56].

4.15. Terpenes

The monoterpene d-limonene inhibits initiation of chemically induced mammary carcinomas in rats [78,141]. Studies with orange oil also have shown a protective effect [59]. This effect for d-limonene and the related monoterpene sobrerol has been attributed to the induction of hepatic GST and UDPGT enzymes [58]. An initiation-blocking effect is seen in the case of DMBA-induced tumors, because DMBA requires metabolic activation; for the direct carcinogen NMU, the effect is absent [60]. D-limonene induces regression of chemically induced mammary neoplasms in rats, reputedly by the induction of cell differentiation [60]. Regression is associated with induction of a more differentiated tumor phenotype [60] and increased concentrations of the inhibitory growth factor TGF-β and IGF-II receptor in the regressing mammary carcinoma cells [88]. In a study by Crowell et al. [108], sobrerol had greater anticancer effects than d-limonene in the DMBA tumor-promotion model. In the same study, these investigators found that anticancer activity correlated with degree of hydroxylation of terpenes [108]. More recent work by this group indicates that perillyl alcohol and related metabolites of limonene are potent inhibitors of G-protein isoprenylation and that this event may be critical in the observed inhibition of cell proliferation and induction of a differentiation [61]. This and other findings relevant to mammary carcinogenesis were reviewed recently by Gould [142]. Kahweol palmitate and other coffee-bean-derived compounds inhibit initiation of mammary tumors in the DMBA model by induction of GSH S-transferase activity [59]. The licorice-derived triterpene 18-β glycirrhizic acid has been the subject of recent work in preclinical and clinical trials sponsored by the National Cancer Institute. This compound has a number of anti-initiating and antipromotion effects in vitro and inhibits tumor development in rat and mouse chemical carcinogenesis models [73,143].

4.16. Polyphenols

The potential anticarcinogenic effects of plant-derived polyphenols are diverse. The best studied are green tea polyphenols, ellagic acid, and cucurmin.

Ellagic acid is a reactive epoxide scavenger [63], induces upregulation of antioxidant enzyme systems [62], and inhibits DNA methylation [144] and DNA topoisomerase [51]. Consumption of several components of green tea (tannic acid, phytic acid, γ-oryzanol, catechins, and catechol) have been evaluated in the rat DMBA model [140]. The greatest decrease in tumor numbers was induced by tannic acid, while the greatest decrease in tumor size and improvement in animal survival were associated with green tea catechins. The catechin epigallocatechin gallate inhibits growth of MCF-7 human breast tumor xenografts in nude mice when given parenterally [145] and inhibits mammary tumor cell proliferation in vitro [64,146], possibly by a tyrosine kinase-based mechanism [64]. A recent review by Stoner and Mukhtar [65] implicates several mechanisms by which tea polyphenols may be anticarcinogenic, including enhancement of antioxidant and phase II enzyme activities and gap junction intercellular communication; inhibition of lipid peroxidation, ornithine decarboxylase (ODC) and cyclooxygenase activities, and protein kinase C and cellular proliferation; and anti-inflammatory activity [65].

4.17. Seaweed polysaccharides

Polysaccharide molecules abundant in seaweed may have chemopreventive qualities [77]. In 1984, Teas et al. [147] demonstrated inhibition of DMBA-induced mammary tumorigenesis in rats by feeding them aqueous extracts of kelp (*Laminaria* spp). Seaweed polysaccharides have not been widely studied.

4.18. Caffeine

Epidemiologic data regarding coffee intake and breast cancer risk are inconclusive [148]. Evidence for a chemopreventive effect of caffeine on chemically induced mammary gland tumors in rodents is contradictory. Of nine rodent studies reviewed in 1994 by E1-Bayoumy [78], four showed a tumor-inhibiting effect, three showed enhanced tumorigenesis, and two had no effect or mixed results, depending on dose and time of administration. The lack of inhibition of the direct-acting carcinogen MNU in the mammary gland, compared to a chemopreventive effect seen in some studies with the procarcinogen DMBA, suggests that caffeine may alter carcinogen metabolism [78].

4.19. Studies of complex mixtures

Many studies have examined the effect of vegetable intake, or feeding of crude extracts, on chemical carcinogenesis in the mammary gland of rodents. Brussels sprouts, cauliflower, cabbage, broccoli, orange oil, rosemary oil, soybean isolates, coffee, and garlic are some of the test substances that have shown a chemopreventive effect (reviewed in [78]). The practical advantages of chemoprevention by such substances lie in the availability of vegetables and crude extracts and in their relative safety. Chemoprevention through the increase of fruit and vegetable intake also provides the potential advantage of multiple chemopreventive effects provided by differing compounds in the same plant product. The difficulty with studies lies more in the interpretation of the findings, given the wide variation in chemical composition between plants of different cultivars, different stage of maturity, or different growth conditions.

5. Prospective clinical trials

Strategies for the selection of putative chemopreventive agents for use in human trials have been the subject of several reviews [73,78,149,150]. Candidate compounds typically have been selected on the basis of epidemiologic observations and evidence of efficacy in in vitro and animal studies [73,150]. National Cancer Institute-supported phase III trials were reviewed by Kelloff et al. in 1994 [73]; trials relevant to breast and endometrial cancer prevention included beta carotene, vitamin E, glycirrhetinic acid, and vitamin D [73].

6. Summary

Although there is evidence that phytochemicals decrease the incidence of breast and endometrial cancer, many observations are only phenomenologic, and much work needs to be done to explore basic mechanisms and the strategic exploitation of their interactions. The multiplicity of phytochemical actions at different sites in the process of tumorigenesis may eventually lead to the development of a multiagent strategy designed to maximize the complementary effects of different agents.

A number of effects with possible relevance to cancer chemoprevention have been excluded from this review, including effects of phytochemicals on the immune response; the question of dietary restriction, which has a profound effect on tumorigenesis; the relatively low methionine levels in some phytochemicals such as soy, which may limit the synthesis of polyamines necessary for tumor growth [151]; and the fact that diets higher in plant products are usually lower in fat and result in leaner individuals with less potential for the synthesis of estradiol in adipose tissue. Also, many studies dealing solely with in vitro mutagenesis were excluded.

Acknowledgments

This work was supported in part by Grants USAMRID DAMD 17-91-4201, Department of the Army (JMC), and P01 RR08562, National Institutes of Health. The authors thank Karen Potvin Klein for editorial assistance.

References

1. Yu H, Harris RE, Gao YT, Gao R, Wynder EL. 1991. Comparative epidemiology of cancers of the colon, rectum, prostate and breast in Shanghai, China versus the United States. Int J Epidemiol 20:76–81.
2. Wynder EL, Fujita Y, Harris RE, Hirayama T, Hiyama T. 1991. Comparative epidemiology of cancer between the United States and Japan: a second look. Cancer 67:746–763.
3. Parkin DM, Muir CS, Whelan SL, Gao YT, Ferlay J, Powell J, eds. 1992. Cancer Incidence in Five Continents, vol. VI. Geneva: World Health Organization.
4. Ziegler RG, Hoover RN, Pike MC, Hildesheim A, Nomura AM, West DW, Wu-Williams AH, Kolonel LN, Horn-Ross PL, Rosenthal JF, Hyer MB. 1993. Migration patterns and breast cancer risk in Asian-American women. J Natl Cancer Inst 85:1819–1827.
5. Kato I, Tominaga S, Kuroishi T. 1987. Relationship between Westernization of dietary habits and mortality from breast and ovarian cancers in Japan. Jpn J Cancer Res 78:349–357.
6. Barbone F, Austin H, Partridge EE. 1993. Diet and endometrial cancer: a case–control study. Am J Epidemiol 137:393–403.
7. Kojima T, Tanaka T, Mori H. 1994. Chemoprevention of spontaneous endometrial cancer in female Donryu rats by dietary indole-3-carbinol. Cancer Res 54:1446–1449.
8. Howe GR, Hirohata T, Hislop TG, Iscovich JM, Yuan JM, Katsouyanni K, Lubin F, Marubini E, Modan B, Rohan T, Toniolo P, Shunzhang Y. 1990. Dietary factors and risk of breast cancer: combined analysis of 12 case–control studies. J Natl Cancer Inst 82:561–569.
9. Peto R, Doll R, Buckley JD, Sporn MB. 1981. Can dietary beta-carotene materially reduce human cancer rates? Nature 290:201–208.
10. Buring JE, Hennekens CH. 1995. Beta-carotene and cancer chemoprevention. J Cell Biochem Suppl 22:226–230.
11. Tallman MS, Wiernik PH. 1992. Retinoids in cancer treatment. J Clin Pharmacol 32:868–888.
12. Bollag W, Majewski S, Jablonska S. 1994. Cancer combination chemotherapy with retinoids: experimental rationale. Leukemia 8:1453–1457.
13. Khachik F, Beecher GR, Smith JC Jr. 1995. Lutein, lycopene, and their oxidative metabolites in chemoprevention of cancer. J Cell Biochem Suppl 22:236–246.
14. Block G. 1991. Vitamin C and cancer prevention: the epidemiologic evidence. Am J Clin Nutr 53:270S–282S.
15. Levi F, Franceschi S, Negri E, La Vecchia C. 1993. Dietary factors and the risk of endometrial cancer. Cancer 71:3575–3581.
16. Dorgan JF, Schatzkin A. 1991. Antioxidant micronutrients in cancer prevention. Hematol Oncol Clin North Am 5:43–68.
17. Wattenberg LW. 1985. Chemoprevention of cancer. Cancer Res 45:1–8.
18. Dimitrov NV, Pan RQ, Bauer J, Jones TI. 1994. Some aspects of vitamin E related to humans and breast cancer prevention. Adv Exp Med Biol 364:119–127.
19. Jennings E. 1995. Folic acid as a cancer-preventing agent. Med Hypoth 45:297–303.
20. Wainfan E, Poirier LA. 1992. Methyl groups in carcinogenesis: effects on DNA methylation and gene expression. Cancer Res 52 (7 Suppl):2071S–2077S.
21. Ip C, Lisk DJ. 1994. Enrichment of selenium in allium vegetables for cancer prevention. Carcinogenesis 15:1881–1885.
22. Weisburger JH, Reddy BS, Rose DP, Cohen LA, Kendall ME, Wynder EL. 1993. Protective mechanisms of dietary fibers in nutritional carcinogenesis. Basic Life Sci 61:45–63.
23. Shankar S, Lanza E. 1991. Dietary fiber and cancer prevention. Hematol Oncol Clin North Am 5:25–41.
24. Adlercreutz H, Höckerstedt K, Bannwart C, Bloigu S, Hämäläinen E, Fotsis T, Ollus A. 1987. Effect of dietary components, including lignans and phytoestrogens, on enterohepatic circulation and liver metabolism of estrogens and on sex hormone binding globulin (SHBG). J Steroid Biochem 27:1135–1144.

25. Rohan TE, Howe GR, Friedenreich CM, Jain M, Miller AB. 1993. Dietary fiber, vitamins A, C, and E, and risk of breast cancer: a cohort study. Cancer Causes Control 4:29–37.
26. Arts CJ, de Bie AT, van den Berg H, van't Veer P, Bunnik GS, Thijssen JH. 1991. Influence of wheat bran on NMU-induced mammary tumor development, plasma estrogen levels and estrogen excretion in female rats. J Steroid Biochem Mol Biol 39:193–202.
27. Baghurst PA, Rohan TE. 1994. High-fiber diets and reduced risk of breast cancer. Int J Cancer 56:173–176.
28. Kendall ME, Cohen LA. 1992. Effect of dietary fiber on mammary tumorigenesis, estrogen metabolism, and lipid excretion in female rats. In Vivo 6:239–245.
29. Steinmetz KA, Potter JD. 1991. Vegetables, fruit, and cancer. I. Epidemiology. Cancer Causes Control 2:325–357.
30. Steinmetz KA, Potter JD. 1991. Vegetables, fruit, and cancer. II. Mechanisms. Cancer Causes Control 2:427–442.
31. Bueding E, Ansher S, Dolan P. 1986. Anticarcinogenic and other protective effects of dithiolthiones. Basic Life Sci 39:483–489.
32. McDannell R, McLean AEM, Hanley AB, Heaney RK, Fenwick GR. 1988. Chemical and biological properties of indole glucosinolates (glucobrassicins): a review. Food Chem Toxicol 26:59–70.
33. Bradlow HL, Michnovicz JJ, Halper M, Miller DG, Wong GY, Osborne MP. 1994. Long-term responses of women to indole-3-carbinol or a high fiber diet. Cancer Epidemiol Biomarkers Prev 3:591–595.
34. Schutt HAJ, Dashwood RH. 1995. Inhibition of DNA adduct formation of 2-amino-1-methyl-6-phenylimidazo[4,5-*b*]pyridine (PhIP) by dietary indole-3-carbinol (I3C) in the mammary gland, colon, and liver of the female F-344 rat. Ann NY Acad Sci 768:210–214.
35. Dorant E, van den Brandt PA, Goldbohm RA. 1995. Allium vegetable consumption, garlic supplement intake, and female breast carcinoma incidence. Breast Cancer Res Treat 33: 163–170.
36. Talalay P, De Long MJ, Prochaska HJ. 1988. Identification of a common chemical signal regulating the induction of enzymes that protect against chemical carcinogenesis. Proc Natl Acad Sci USA 85:8261–8265.
37. Mäkelä S, Poutanen M, Lehtimäki J, Kostian ML, Santti R, Vihko R. 1995. Estrogen-specific 17beta-hydroxysteroid oxidoreductase type 1 (E.C. 1.1.1.62) as a possible target for the action of phytoestrogens. Proc Soc Exp Biol Med 208:51–59.
38. Sathyamoorthy N, Wang TTY, Phang JM. 1994. Stimulation of pS2 expression by diet-derived compounds. Cancer Res 54:957–961.
39. Edwards JM, Raffauf RF, Le Quesne PW. 1979. Antineoplastic activity and cytotoxicity of flavones, isoflavones, and flavanones. J Natl Prod 42:85–91.
40. Fiala ES, Reddy BS, Weisburger JH. 1985. Naturally occurring anticarcinogenic substances in foodstuffs. Annu Rev Nutr 5:295–321.
41. Das A, Wang JH, Lien EJ. 1994. Carcinogenicity, mutagenicity and cancer preventing activities of flavonoids: a structure-system-activity relationship (SSAR) analysis. Prog Drug Res 42:133–166.
42. Kennedy AR. 1995. The evidence for soybean products as cancer preventive agents. J Nutr 125 (Suppl 3):733S–743S.
43. Moy LY, Billings PC. 1994. A proteolytic activity in a human breast cancer cell line which is inhibited by the anticarcinogenic Bowman–Birk protease inhibitor. Cancer Lett 85:205–210.
44. Hughes CL. 1992. Plant sterols: are they mammalian reproductive hormones? Infertil Reprod Med Clin North Am 3:285–291.
45. Miksicek RJ. 1994. Interaction of naturally occurring nonsteroidal estrogens with expressed recombinant human estrogen receptor. J Steroid Biochem Mol Biol 49:153–160.
46. Messina MJ, Persky V, Setchell KDR, Barnes S. 1994. Soy intake and cancer risk: a review of the *in vitro* and *in vivo* data. Nutr Cancer 21:113–131.
47. Barnes S. 1995. Effect of genistein on *in vitro* and *in vivo* models of cancer. J Nutr 125 (Suppl 3):777S–783S.

48. Peterson TG, Barnes S. 1991. Genistein inhibition of the growth of human breast cancer cells: independence from estrogen receptors and the multi-drug resistance gene. Biochem Biophys Res Commun 179:661–667.
49. Akiyama T, Ishida J, Nakagawa S, Ogawara H, Watanabe S, Itoh N, Shibuya M, Fukami Y. 1987. Genistein, a specific inhibitor of tyrosine-specific protein kinases. J Biol Chem 262:5592–5595.
50. Okura A, Arakawa H, Oka H, Yoshimari T, Monden Y. 1988. Effect of genistein on topoisomerase activity and on the growth of [VAL12] Ha-*ras*-transformed NIH 3T3 cells. Biochem Biophys Res Commun 157:183–189.
51. Constantinou A, Stoner GD, Mehta R, Rao K, Runyan C, Moon R. 1995. The dietary anticancer agent ellagic acid is a potent inhibitor of DNA topoisomerases in vitro. Nutr Cancer 23:121–130.
52. Fotsis T, Pepper M, Adlercreutz H, Fleischmann G, Hase T, Montesano R, Schweigerer L. 1993. Genistein, a dietary-derived inhibitor of *in vitro* angiogenesis. Proc Natl Acad Sci USA 90:2690–2694.
53. Hoffman R. 1995. Potent inhibition of breast cancer cell lines by the isoflavonoid kievitone: comparison with genistein. Biochem Biophys Res Commun 211:600–606.
54. Adlercreutz H, Bannwart C, Wähälä K, Mäkelä T, Brunow G, Hase T, Arosemena PJ, Kellis JT Jr, Vickery LE. 1993. Inhibition of human aromatase by mammalian lignans and isoflavonoid phytoestrogens. J Steroid Biochem Mol Biol 44:147–153.
55. Rao AV, Sung MK. 1995. Saponins as anticarcinogens. J Nutr 125 (Suppl 3):717S–724S.
56. Shamsuddin AM. 1995. Inositol phosphates have novel anticancer function. J Nutr 125 (Suppl 3):725S–732S.
57. Thompson LU, Zhang L. 1991. Phytic acid and minerals: effect on early markers of risk for mammary and colon carcinogenesis. Carcinogenesis 12:2041–2045.
58. Elegbede JA, Maltzman TH, Elson CE, Gould MN. 1993. Effects of anticarcinogenic monoterpenes on phase II hepatic metabolizing enzymes. Carcinogenesis 14:1221–1223.
59. Wattenberg LW. 1983. Inhibition of neoplasia by minor dietary constituents. Cancer Res 43 (Suppl):2448S–2453S.
60. Haag JD, Lindstrom MJ, Gould MN. 1992. Limonene-induced regression of mammary carcinomas. Cancer Res 52:4021–4026.
61. Crowell PL, Gould MN. 1994. Chemoprevention and therapy of cancer by d-limonene, Crit Rev Oncogenesis 5:1–22.
62. Majid S, Khanduja KL, Gandhi RK, Kapur S, Sharma RR. 1991. Influence of ellagic acid on antioxidant defense system and lipid peroxidation in mice. Biochem Pharmacol 42:1441–1445.
63. Wood AW, Huang MT, Chang RL, Newmark HL, Lehr RE, Yagi H, Sayer JM, Jerina DM, Conney AH. 1982. Inhibition of the mutagenicity of bay-region diol epoxides of polycylic aromatic hydrocarbons by naturally occurring plant phenols: exceptional activity of ellagic acid. Proc Natl Acad Sci USA 79:5513–5517.
64. Komori A, Yatsunami J, Okabe S, Abe S, Hara K, Suganuma M, Kim SJ, Fujiki H. 1993. Anticarcinogenic activity of green tea polyphenols. Jpn J Clin Oncol 23:186–190.
65. Stoner GD, Mukhtar H. 1995. Polyphenols as cancer chemopreventive agents. J Cell Biochem Suppl 22:169–180.
66. Van't Veer P, Kolb CM, Verhoef P, Kok FJ, Schouten EG, Hermus RJJ, Sturmans F. 1990. Dietary fiber, beta-carotene and breast cancer: results from a case-control study. Int J Cancer 45:825–828.
67. Hunter DJ, Manson JE, Colditz GA, Stampfer MJ, Rosner B, Hennekens CH, Speizer FE, Willett WC. 1993. A prospective study of vitamins C, E, and A and the risk of breast cancer. N Engl J Med 329:234–240.
68. Levi F, La Vecchia C, Gulie C, Negri E. 1993. Dietary factors and breast cancer risk in Vaud, Switzerland. Nutr Cancer 19:327–335.
69. Potischman N, Swanson CA, Brinton LA, McAdams M, Barret RJ, Berman ML, Mortel R,

Twiggs LB, Wilbanks GD, Hoover RN. 1993. Dietary associations in a case–control study of endometrial cancer. Cancer Causes Control 4:239–250.
70. Shu XO, Zheng W, Potischman N, Brinton LA, Hatch MC, Gao YT, Fraumeni JF. 1993. A population-based case–control study of dietary factors and endometrial cancer in Shanghai, People's Republic of China. Am J Epidemiol 137:155–165.
71. Willett WC, Hunter DJ, Stampfer MJ, Colditz G, Manson JE, Spiegelman D, Rosner B, Hennekens CH, Speizer FE. 1994. Dietary fat and fiber in relation to risk of breast cancer. An 8-year follow-up. JAMA 268:2037–2044.
72. Negri E, La Vecchia C, Franceschi S, D'Avanzo B, Talamini R, Parpinel M, Ferraroni M, Filiberti R, Montella M, Falcini F, Conti E, Decarli A. 1996. Intake of selected micronutrients and the risk of breast cancer. Int J Cancer 65:140–144.
73. Kelloff GJ, Crowell JA, Boone CW, et al. Clinical development plans for cancer chemopreventive agents. J Cell Biochem Suppl 20:55–299.
74. Halter SA, Winnier AR, Arteaga CL. 1993. Pretreatment with vitamin A inhibits transforming growth factor alpha stimulation of human mammary carcinoma cells. J Cell Physiol 156:80–87.
75. Lee DC, Barlow KD, Gaido KW. 1996. The actions of 2,3,7,8-tetrachlorodibenzo-p-dioxin on transforming growth factor-$\beta 2$ promoter activity are localized to the TATA box binding region and controlled through a tyrosine kinase-dependent pathway. Toxicol Appl Pharmacol 137:90–99.
76. Swisshelm K, Ryan K, Lee X, Tsou HC, Peacocke M, Sager R. 1994. Down-regulation of retinoic acid receptor beta in mammary carcinoma cell lines and its up-regulation in senescing normal mammary epithelial cells. Cell Growth Differ 5:133–141.
77. Hocman G. 1989. Prevention of cancer: vegetables and plants. Comp Biochem Physiol 93B:201–212.
78. El-Bayoumy K. 1994. Evaluation of chemopreventive agents against breast cancer and proposed strategies for future clinical intervention trials. Cancinogenesis 15:2395–2420.
79. Adlercreutz H. 1988. Lignans and phytoestrogens: possible preventive role in cancer. Front Gastrointest Res 14:165–176.
80. Ingram DM, Roberts A, Nottage EM. 1992. Host factors and breast cancer growth characteristics. Eur J Cancer 28A:1153–1161.
81. Ingram D. 1994. Diet and subsequent survival in women with breast cancer. Br J Cancer 69:592–595.
82. Zheng W, Kushi LH, Potter JD, Sellers TA, Doyle TJ, Bostick RM, Folsom AR. 1995. Dietary intake of energy and animal foods and endometrial cancer incidence. The Iowa Women's Health Study. Am J Epidemiol 142:388–394.
83. Wattenberg LW. 1987. Inhibition of chemical carcinogenesis. J Natl Cancer Inst 60:11–18.
84. Clarke R, Dickson RB, Lippman ME. 1992. Hormonal aspects of breast cancer: growth factors, drugs, and stromal interactions. Crit Rev Oncol Hematol 12:1–23.
85. Nguyen B, Keane MM, Johnston PG. 1995. The biology of growth regulation in normal and neoplastic breast epithelium: from bench to clinic. Crit Rev Oncol Hematol 20:223–236.
86. Guidice LC. 1994. Growth factors and growth modulators in human uterine endometrium: their potential relevance to reproductive medicine. Fertil Steril 61:1–17.
87. Murphy LJ. 1994. Growth factors and steroid hormone action in endometrial cancer. J Steroid Biochem Mol Biol 48:419–423.
88. Jirtle RL, Haag JD, Ariazi EA, Gould MN. 1993. Increased mannose 6-phosphate/insulin-like growth factor II receptor and transforming growth factor beta 1 levels during monoterpene-induced regression of mammary tumors. Cancer Res 53:3849–3852.
89. Lamartiniere CA, Moore JB, Brown NM, Thompson R, Hardin MJ, Barnes S. 1995. Genistein supresses mammary cancer in rats. Carcinogenesis 16:2833–2840.
90. Whitten PL, Russell E, Naftolin F. 1992. Effects of a normal, human-concentration, phytoestrogen diet on rat uterine growth. Steroids 57:98–106.

91. Bryant-Greenwood GD, Schwabe C. 1994. Human relaxins: chemistry and biology. Endocr Rev 15:5–26.
92. Batzinger R, Bueding E, Reddy B, Weisburger J. 1978. Formation of a mutagenic drug metabolite by intestinal microoganisms. Cancer Res 38:608–612.
93. Marnett LJ. 1994. Generation of mutagens during arachidonic acid metabolism. Cancer Metastasis Rev 13:303–308.
94. De Flora S, Ramel C. 1988. Mechanisms of inhibitors of mutagenesis and carcinogenesis. Classification and overview. Mutat Res 202:285–306.
95. Thompson LU. 1994. Antioxidants and hormone-mediated health benefits of whole grains. Crit Rev Food Sci Nutr 34:473–497.
96. Yang CS, Smith TJ, Hong J-Y. 1994. Cytochrome P-450 enzymes as targets for chemoprevention against chemical carcinogenesis and toxicity: opportunities and limitations. Cancer Res 54 (Suppl 7):1982S–1986S.
97. Smith TJ, Yang CS. 1994. Effects of food phytochemicals on xenobiotic metabolism and tumorigenesis. In Huang M-T, Osawa T, Ho C-T, Rosen RT, eds. Food Phytochemicals for Cancer Prevention I. Fruits and Vegetables. Washington, D.C.: American Chemical Society, pp. 2–16.
98. Sipes IG, Gandolfi AJ, 1986. Biotransformation of toxicants. In Klaassen CD, Amdur MO, Doull J, eds. Casarett and Doull's Toxicology, 3rd ed. New York: Macmillan, pp. 64–98.
99. Rosenberg L. 1995. Nonsteroidal anti-inflammatory drugs and cancer. Prevent Med 24:107–109.
100. Kiguchi K, Glesne D, Chubb CH, Fujiki H, Huberman E. 1994. Differential induction of apoptosis in human breast tumor cells by okadaic acid and related inhibitors of protein phosphatases 1 and 2A. Cell Growth Differ 5:995–1004.
101. Lotan R. 1995. Retinoids and apoptosis: implications for cancer chemoprevention and therapy. J Natl Cancer Inst 87:1655–1657.
102. Li XS, Chen JC, Sheikh MS, Shao ZM, Fontana JA. 1994. Retinoic acid inhibition of insulin-like growth factor I stimulation of c-fos mRNA levels in a breast carcinoma cell line. Exp Cell Res 211:68–73.
103. Prasad KN, Edwards-Prasad J. 1990. Expressions of some molecular cancer risk factors and their modification by vitamins. J Am Coll Nutr 9:28–34.
104. Lamartiniere CA, Moore J, Holland M, Barnes S. 1995. Neonatal genistein chemoprevents mammary cancer. Proc Soc Exp Biol Med 208:120–123.
105. Russo J, Gusterson BA, Rogers AE, Russo IH, Wellings SR, van Zwieten MJ. 1990. Comparative study of human and rat mammary tumorigenesis. Lab Invest 62:244–278.
106. Constantinou A, Huberman E. 1995. Genistein as an inducer of tumor cell differentiation: possible mechanisms of action. Proc Soc Exp Biol Med 208:109–115.
107. Suh N, Luyengi L, Fong HH, Kinghorn AD, Pezzuto JM. 1995. Discovery of natural product chemopreventive agents utilizing HL-60 cell differentiation as a model. Anticancer Res 15:233–239.
108. Crowell PL, Kennan WS, Haag JD, Ahmad S, Vedejs E, Gould MN. 1992. Chemoprevention of mammary carcinogenesis by hydroxylated derivatives of d-limonene. Carcinogenesis 13:1261–1264.
109. Price KR, Fenwick GR. 1985. Naturally occurring estrogens in foods — a review. Food Addit Contam 2:73–106.
110. Markiewicz L, Garey J, Adlercreutz H, Gurpide E. 1993. *In vitro* bioassays of non-steroidal phytoestrogens. J Steroid Biochem Mol Biol 45:399–405.
111. Adlercreutz H, Mousavi Y, Clark J, Höckerstedt K, Hämäläinen E, Wähälä K, Mäkelä T, Hase T. 1992. Dietary phytoestrogens and cancer: in vitro and in vivo studies. J Steroid Biochem Mol Biol 41:331–337.
112. Adlercreutz H, Mousavi Y, Höckerstedt K. 1992. Diet and breast cancer. Acta Oncol 31:175–181.
113. Setchell KDR, Borriello SP, Hulme P, Kirk DN, Axelson M. 1984. Nonsteroidal estrogens of dietary origin: possible roles in hormone-dependent disease. Am J Clin Nutr 40:569–578.

114. Adlercreutz H, Honjo H, Higashi A, Fotsis T, Hämäläinen E, Hasegawa T, Okada H. 1991. Urinary excretion of lignans and isoflavonoid phytoestrogens in Japanese men and women consuming a traditional Japanese diet. Am J Clin Nutr 54:1093–1100.
115. Martin PM, Horwitz KB, Ryan DS, McGuire WL. 1978. Phytoestrogen interaction with estrogen receptors in human breast cancer cells. Endocrinology 103:1860–1867.
116. Mäkelä S, Davis VL, Tally WC, Korkman J, Salo L, Vihko R, Santii R, Korach K. 1994. Dietary estrogens act through estrogen receptor-mediated processes and show no antiestrogenicity in cultured breast cancer cells. Environ Health Perspect 102:572–578.
117. Bikfalvi A. 1995. Significance of angiogenesis in tumour progression and metastasis. Eur J Cancer 31A:1101–1104.
118. Dragsted LO, Strube M, Larsen JC. 1993. Cancer-protective factors in fruits and vegetables: biochemical and biological background. Pharmacol Toxicol 72 (Suppl 1):116–135.
119. Means AL, Gudas LJ. 1995. The roles of retinoids in vertebrate development. Annu Rev Biochem 64:201–233.
120. Sporn MB, Roberts AB. 1983. Role of retinoids in differentiation and carcinogenesis. Cancer Res 43:3034–3040.
121. Moon RC, Mehta RG, Detrisac CJ. 1992. Retinoids as chemopreventive agents for breast cancer. Cancer Detect Prevent 16:73–79.
122. Moon RC. 1994. Vitamin A, retinoids and breast cancer. Adv Exp Med Biol 364:101–107.
123. Turusov VS, Trukhanova LS, Parfenov YD. 1991. Modifying effect of ascorbic acid and sodium ascorbate on the promoting stage of uterine sarcomogenesis induced in CBA mice by 1,2-dimethylhydrazine and estradiol-dipropionate. Cancer Lett 56:29–35.
124. Ip C. 1982. Dietary vitamin E intake and mammary carcinogenesis in rats. Carcinogenesis 3:1453–1456.
125. Maucher A, von Angerer E. 1994. Antitumour activity of coumarin and 7-hydroxycoumarin against 7,12-dimethylbenz[a]anthracene-induced rat mammary carcinomas. J Cancer Res Clin Oncol 120:502–504.
126. Stoewsand GS. 1995. Bioactive organosulfur phytochemicals in Brassica oleracea vegetables — a review. Food Chem Toxicol 33:537–543.
127. Wattenberg LW, Loub WD. 1978. Inhibition of polycyclic aromatic hydrocarbon-induced neoplasia by naturally occurring indoles. Cancer Res 38:1410–1413.
128. Hecht SS. 1995. Chemoprevention by isothiocyanates. J Cell Biochem Suppl 22:195–209.
129. Bradlow HL, Michnovicz JJ, Telang NT, Osborne MP. 1991. Effects of dietary indole-3-carbinol on estradiol metabolism and spontaneous mammary tumors in mice. Carcinogenesis 12:1571–1574.
130. Zhang Y, Talalay P. 1994. Anticarcinogenic activities of organic isothiocyanates: chemistry and mechanisms. Cancer Res 54 (Suppl 7):1976S–1981S.
131. Dorant E, van den Brandt PA, Goldbohm RA, Hermus RJJ, Sturmans F. 1993. Garlic and its significance for the prevention of cancer in humans: a critical view. Br J Cancer 67:424–429.
132. Sundaram SG, Milner JA. 1993. Impact of organosulfur compounds in garlic on canine mammary tumor cells in culture. Cancer Lett 74:85–90.
133. Kennedy AR, Little JB. 1978. Protease inhibitors suppress radiation induced malignant transformation in vitro. Nature 276:825–826.
134. Umans RS, Weichselbaum RR, Johnson CM, Kenedy AR. 1984. Protease inhibitor antipain reduces nuclear binding of estrogen-receptor complex in MCF-7 breast tumor cells. Carcinogenesis 5:1355–1357.
135. Billings PC, St. Clair WH, Maki PA, Kennedy AR. 1992. Distribution of the Bowman Birk protease inhibitor in mice following oral administration. Cancer Lett 62:191–197.
136. Rao AV, Janezic SA. 1992. The role of dietary phytosterols in colon carcinogenesis. Nutr Cancer 18:43–52.
137. Folman Y, Pope GS. 1966. The interaction in the immature mouse of potent oestrogens with coumestrol, genistein and other utero-vaginotrophic compounds of low potency. J Endocrinol 34:215–225.

138. Barnes S, Peterson TG. 1995. Biochemical targets of the isoflavone genistein in tumor cell lines. Proc Soc Exp Biol Med 208:103–108.
139. Wei H, Bowen R, Cai Q, Barnes S, Wang Y. 1995. Antioxidant and antipromotional effects of the soybean isoflavone genistein. Proc Soc Exp Biol Med 208:124–130.
140. Price KR, Johnson IT, Genwick GR. 1987. The chemistry and biological significance of saponins in foods and feedstuffs. Crit Rev Food Sci Nutr 26:27–135.
141. Hirose M, Hoshiya T, Akagi K, Futakuchi M, Ito N. 1994. Inhibition of mammary gland carcinogenesis by green tea catechins and other naturally occurring antioxidants in female Sprague–Dawley rats pretreated with 7,12-dimethylbenz[a]anthracene. Cancer Lett 83: 149–156.
142. Elson CE, Maltzman TH, Boston JL, Tanner MA, Gould MN. 1988. Anti-carcinogenic activity of d-limonene during the initiation and promotion/progression stages of DMBA-induced mammary carcinogenesis. Carcinogenesis 9:331–332.
143. Gould MN. 1995. Prevention and therapy of mammary cancer by monoterpenes. J Cell Biochem Suppl 22:139–144.
144. Steele VE, Moon RC, Lubet RA, Grubbs CJ, Reddy BS, Wargovich M, McCormick DL, Pereira MA, Crowell JA, Bagheri D, Sigman CC, Boone CW, Kelloff GJ. 1994. Preclinical efficacy evaluation of potential chemopreventive agents in animal carcinogenesis models: methods and results from the NCI chemoprevention drug development program. J Cell Biochem Suppl 20:32–54.
145. Dixit R, Gold B. 1986. Inhibition of n-methyl-n-nitrosourea induced mutagenicity and DNA methylation by ellagic acid. Proc Natl Acad Sci USA 83:8039–8043.
146. Liao S, Umekita Y, Guo J, Kokontis JM, Hiipakka RA. 1995. Growth inhibition and regression of human prostate and breast tumors in athymic mice by tea epigallocatechin gallate. Cancer Lett 96:239–243.
147. Araki R, Inoue S, Osborne MP, Telang NT. 1995. Chemoprevention of mammary pre-neoplasia. *In vitro* effects of a green tea polyphenol. Ann NY Acad Sci 768:215–222.
148. Teas J, Harbison ML, Gelman RS. 1984. Dietary seaweed (*Laminaria*) and mammary carcinogenesis in rats. Cancer Res 44:2758–2761.
149. Lamarine RJ. 1994. Selected health and behavioral effects related to the use of caffeine. J Commun Health 19:449–466.
150. Lippman SM, Benner SE, Hong WK. 1993. Chemoprevention. Strategies for the control of cancer. Cancer 72:984–990.
151. Szarka CE, Grana G, Engstrom PF. 1994. Chemoprevention of cancer. Curr Probl Cancer 8:6–79.
152. Hawrylewicz EJ, Zapata JJ, Blair WH. 1995. Soy and experimental cancer: animal studies. J Nutr 125 (Suppl 3):698S–708S.

8. Hormonal strategies for the prevention of breast cancer

Mark R. Olsen and Richard R. Love

1. Introduction

The first successful systemic therapy for breast cancer was described by Beatson exactly one century ago [1]. By translating his observations of the ovarian control of mammary epithelial proliferation in lactating sheep to the epithelial proliferation seen in human cancer, he reasoned that oophorectomy might play a role in controlling the growth of breast cancer. The first oophorectomy in an attempt to suppress breast cancer was carried out on June 15, 1895, and the patient had and excellent response. Subsequently, oophorectomy has become a standard therapy for advanced breast cancer in premenopausal women. Over the intervening years, various hormonal manipulations have been developed to treat earlier stages of breast carcinoma. Favorable results from these interventions, in combination with a growing understanding of the biology of breast carcinoma, have fostered the hope that hormonal manipulations may prevent breast cancers.

In devising hormonal strategies for the prevention of early breast cancer, biological models of mammary carcinogenesis are critical. These offer our present picture of both the development of breast cancers and the likely mechanism(s) by which proposed prevention interventions might operate. Clearly, current models of normal and malignant breast biology are incomplete but do offer a beginning picture of critical growth stimulatory and inhibitory events at a molecular level. With a working model, the addressing of several important intervention issues follows more logically. For example, does the intervention attempt to 'prevent' disease from its inception, or does it prevent the appearance of clinical disease by suppressing preclinical but recognizable tissue abnormalities? Second, can one define a population for which the intervention is suited and then identify and enroll that population in a specific trial? Third, do the benefits of the prevention strategy outweigh the costs?

In this chapter, several hormonal strategies for the prevention of breast cancer will be discussed. Each will be approached with regard to the rationale for its use and the likely point at which each intervention might act in a multistep model for mammary carcinogenesis. Prevention strategies will also be considered from the standpoint of benefits and risks. Finally, potential future hormonal prevention strategies will be suggested.

2. Carcinogenesis and models of breast cancer development

Carcinogenesis is thought to be a multistep process. The first of these steps, initiation, is the process by which DNA is damaged, and is generally felt to be an irreversible process. This step is followed by a promotion stage, which involves stimulation of cell division, typically by hormonal or other mitogenic agents. Finally, a small clone of transformed cells undergoes progression, the process of development into a frank neoplastic lesion.

A large number of initiators (chemical, radiation, and biologic) in breast cancer have been described, and in general these share the property of genotoxicity. In humans, a role for tumor viruses in the initiation of breast cancer has not been described. Radiation exposure is, however, a well-known risk factor, presumably mediated by the generation of mutations ultimately leading to tumors [2–4]. The evidence that chemical carcinogens initiate breast cancer is more limited. There is evidence that cigarette smoking may act as an initiator, and while this evidence is not strong, the available data cannot be ignored [5]. Finally, the role of genetic susceptibility in breast carcinoma is becoming increasingly clear with the description of the BRCA-1 and -2 genes [6–8]. Neoplasms directly attributable to these inherited genetic changes likely represent approximately 5%–10% of all breast cancers. The role of these defects in the development of breast carcinomas remains to be discovered, but emerging evidence suggests that the BRCA 1 gene may be responsible for producing an extracellular protein that is functionally behaving as a tumor suppressor [9]. Genetic susceptibility is also reflected by increased rates of breast carcinomas in families with ataxia–telangiectasia. The gene for this disorder is associated with increased sensitivity to ionizing radiation. Swift and associates [10] have demonstrated an increased risk for breast carcinoma in heterozygotes for this gene. Heterozygotes for this disorder may constitute up to 1.4% of the American population, and it is estimated that 9%–18% of all persons with breast cancer in the United States carry this mutation [10]. Table 1 depicts the stages at which major risk factors for breast carcinogenesis appear to have their major impact.

A promotional stage of tumorigenesis in breast cancer is most understood at present and appears to offer the greatest potential for hormonal prevention of breast cancer. As stated above, promotion may be defined as a reversible process in which an initiated cell or cells are stimulated to undergo mitoses, resulting in a population of transformed cells. For mammary carcinogenesis, broadly, two major physiologic models have been described. The first is essentially a differentiation model. The identification of age of first full-term pregnancy as the single most powerful physiologic predictive factor for breast tumor development ([11]; summarized in figure 1) prompted laboratory inves-

Table 1. Major risks for mammary cancer

Stage: Initiation	⟶ Promotion	⟵⟶ Progression
Genetic susceptibility Cigarette smoking Irradiation Chemical carcinogens??	Years of ovulation Age at full-term pregnancy	

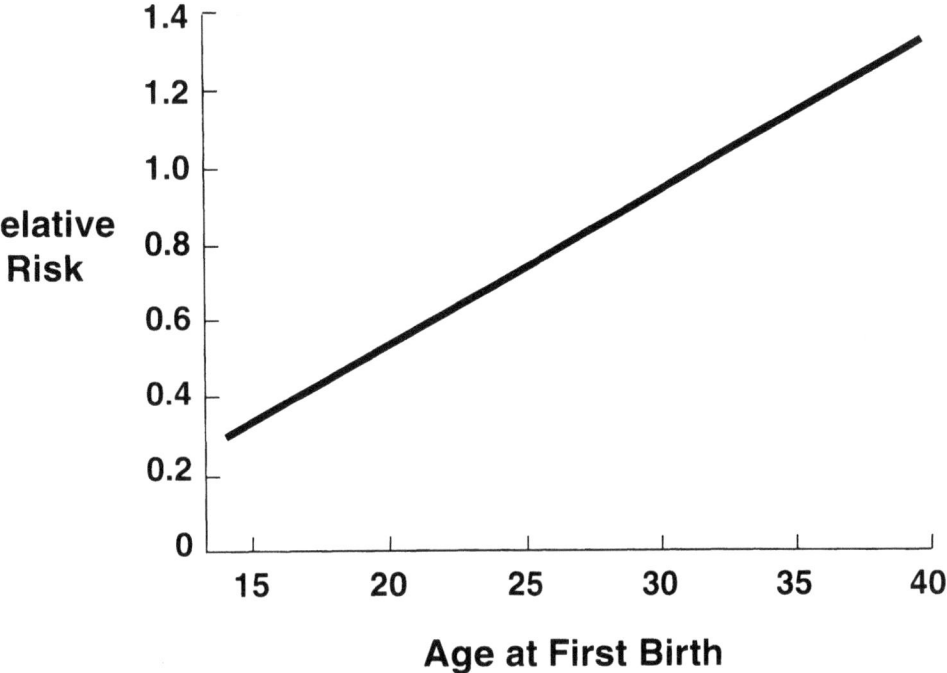

Figure 1. Age at first birth in 4323 cases and 12,699 controls and relative risk of breast cancer. (Adapted from MacMahon et al. [11].)

tigations into the hormonal modulation of mammary carcinogenesis. The subsequent identification of lactation as a protective factor further underpins the model that has evolved. The 7,12-dimethylbenz(a)anthracene (DMBA)-induced rat mammary cancer model has been well studied with regard to mammary gland development and the effects of hormonal manipulations on the subsequent development of breast tumors. The relatively high susceptibility of the mammary gland in the virgin animal to the carcinogenic effects of DMBA has been shown to depend on the presence of undifferentiated terminal end buds [12,13]. The epithelium of these terminal end buds has high proliferative capacity and is highly sensitive to initiation by DMBA. Once initiated. epithelial cells undergo hormone-driven proliferation during the estrous cycle, with development of frank carcinomas. The hormonal stimulation during each estrous cycle does induce the differentiation of terminal end buds into alveolar buds and subsequently lobules, which have markedly reduced susceptibility to the initiating effects of DMBA, but this process proceeds in a progressive fashion, leaving significant amounts of mammary epithelium in a state of high susceptibility to carcinogenesis [14]. If, however, the rat completes a full-term pregnancy, the mammary gland is able to undergo complete differentiation and from that point on is almost completely refractory to carcinogenic effects of DMBA [14–16]. In humans, the lobular structure of the breast appears similar, specifically, the degree of lobular differentiation (classified by numbers of alveoli per lobule) has been found to be directly related to parity. As in the rat, however, the human mammary gland exhibits a significant degree of heterogeneity with regard to lobular differentiation [17].

Further work from the DMBA-induced rat mammary cancer model has demonstrated that interruption of pregnancy halts the differentiation process of the terminal end buds. If this interruption occurs at the beginning of the second half of gestation, the terminal end buds are found to be in a hormonally primed state for differentiation into alveolar buds [14]. At this point in the differentiation process, the epithelial cells are no less susceptible to carcinogenesis than in virgin rats.

Pregnant or lactating rats appear to have intermediate sensitivity to the carcinogenic effects of DMBA [18,19]. These lines of evidence suggested that placental hormones produced during pregnancy are affecting mammary gland development. Attempts at dissecting the mechanism by which the placental hormones influence mammary epithelium development have generally involved exogenous administration of placental hormones. Varying effects on the susequent development of mammary tumors have been observed. Human chorionic gonadotropin is able to reduce the incidence of mammary carcinomas in a dose-dependent fashion when administered to animals prior to DMBA treatment. While mammary hyperplasia is observed during administration of the hormone, it would appear that partial differentiation and mammary gland involution commences upon cessation of treatment. Placental lactogen, on the other hand, has been shown to stimulate the production of terminal end buds without enhancing the differentiation process. Thus, DMBA treatment following placental lactogen administration results in a significant increase in the number of carcinomas observed [20]. It would appear that completion of the lobular differentiation process and mammary gland involution is required for acquisition of resistance to DMBA-induced carcinogenesis.

The application of this differentiation model of mammary carcinogenesis to human hormonal prevention strategies generally involves schemes to produce as complete differentiation of the mammary gland as possible at as early an age as is practical. The goal of these strategies is to bring about a gland that is resistant to carcinogenesis due to near or total terminal differentiation.

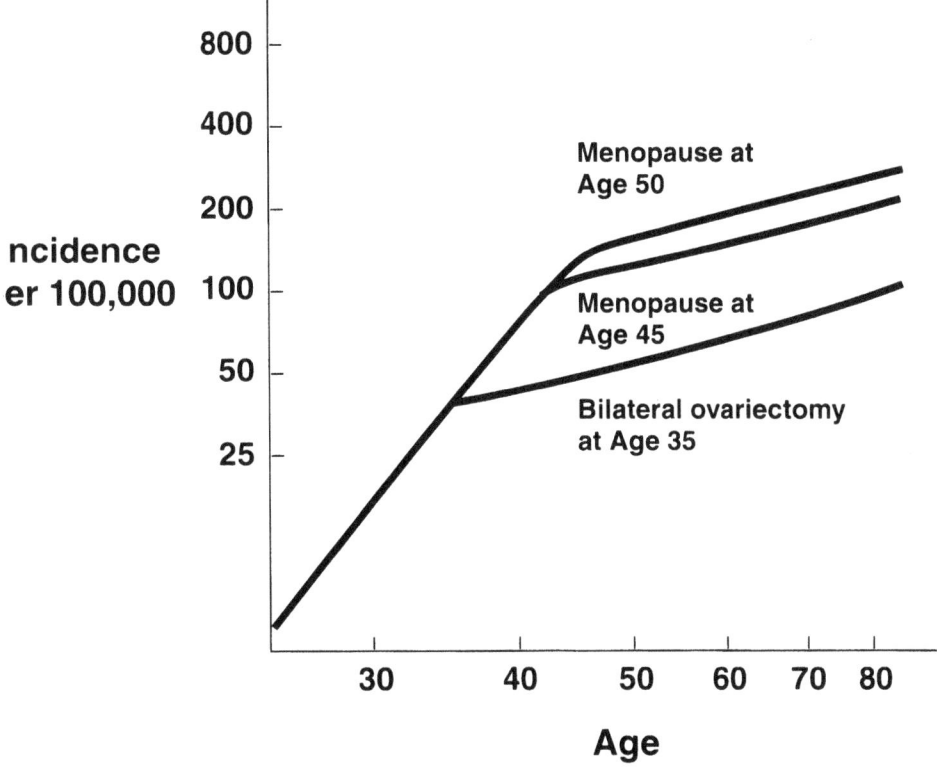

Figure 2. Age-incidence of breast cancer. Age-incidence curves of breast cancer for (working from top curve down) women with natural menopause at age 50 and at age 45, and with a bilateral ovariectomy at age 35, respectively (with no HRT given to any group). (Adapted from Pike et al. [34].)

A second major model for mammary carcinogenesis can be viewed as a duration of ovulation or estrogen–progesterone cycle, hormone-exposure model. Epidemiologic evidence has clearly identified early age at menarche, anovulatory cycles (as a consequence of lactation, for example), the immediate postpregnancy years, higher estradiol levels as in Western vs. Asian women, and late age at menopause as risk factors for breast cancer [21]. Pike has emphasized the consistency of the epidemiologic data and the major impact these factors have on age incidence of breast cancer (figure 2). Each of these factors contributes to increased numbers of regular ovulatory cycles and/ or more hormone exposure to the breast, with the associated increases and decreases in estrogen and progesterone. The sex steroid changes are considered to drive epithelial proliferation in the promotion stage for already initiated cells. During the menstrual cycle, normal breast tissue undergoes cyclical cell proliferation and loss. In the follicular phase, cell division remains at a relatively low rate. During the luteal phase, however, progesterone drives epithelial proliferation at a rate 2–3 times greater than the follicular phase rates [22–24]. If fertilization does not occur, progesterone levels decline and epithelial cell division rates fall. This change is followed by apoptosis of the lobular cells [25]. With successful fertilization, lobular cell division rates increase substantially. This proliferation continues until the beginning of the second half of pregnancy, when the lobules undergo differentiation. Rates of cell division decline significantly at this point [26]. The hormonal role in mammary carcinogenesis appears to involve synergistic estrogen and progestin actions. In this model, estrogen 'primes' breast epithelial cells such that they are more susceptible both to the proliferative effects of progestin and to the initiating effects of carcinogens [24]. Other data complicate the acceptance of this simplified analysis. The hypothesis that progestin-driven epithelial proliferation increases risk for subsequent development of breast cancers is based on the definition of tumor promotion requiring cell division. While progestin-driven proliferation of estrogen-primed normal breast tissue is well described, growth-inhibitory effects of progestins for hormone-responsive breast cancer cells are also known [27,28]. The time point at which hormonal responsiveness to progestins changes along the continuum from a normal breast epithelial cell to an initiated, promoted, and frankly malignant cell is not known, and the biologic basis for this alteration in hormone growth sensitivity is not well understood. The importance of estrogen priming in the differentiation pathway has been described and may account for conflicting observations regarding the effects of progestins [29]. Hypotheses related to altered steroid receptor activity or associations at key enhancer sites as well as altered profiles of autocrine or paracrine transforming growth factors have been suggested to explain this change. In contrast to the idea that progesterone increases risk for tumor development, it is thought that progestins actually decrease the risk of benign breast disease and that progestins are generally breast protective [30–33]. An argument against a significant role for progestin in the generation of breast tumors is the finding that progestins decrease the rate of cell division in the presence of estradiol, an effect that has been termed *antiestrogenic* [28].

These apparently contrasting findings may be equally valid and may arise from our incomplete understanding of the subtleties involved in the sequential exposure of normal breast epithelial cells to both estrogens and progestins as well as the peptide growth factors generated by exposure of the cells to sex steroids. For these reasons, there is considerable interest in assessing the benefits and potential risks of modulation of ovarian activity (i.e., steroid hormone levels), as well as in defining the types and doses of hormone replacement therapies in healthy postmenopausal women to minimize the risk for breast cancer and achieve optimal benefits for cardiovascular and skeletal organ systems. As noted in the introduction to this chapter, the initial attempts at modulation of breast tumor growth involved reducing the levels of endogenous sex steroids by oophorectomy [1]. Current models of breast carcinoma progression are characterized by essentially three major steps. An initial, hormone-dependent stage is characterized by the requirement of initiated breast epithelial cells for sex-steroid growth stimulation both to fix mutations and for the development of a clone of malignant cells. In a second stage, an established focus of carcinoma is able to survive in the absence of sex steroids, but growth remains hormone responsive. Finally, selection pressures will often produce a hormone-independent clone of tumor cells that is able to proliferate in the absence of sex steroids.

Reducing sex-steroid exposure is a well-established method for treating patients with breast tumors. Several techniques are currently availabley, including ovarian ablation by surgery, radiation, or chemical means (gonadotropin-releasing hormone agonists or as a side effect of systemic chemotherapy). These and other methods for altering sex-steroid exposure will be discussed later.

While both these biological (the differentiation and hormone-exposure) models of hormonal action on the mammary gland and mammary carcinogenesis provide considerable explanation of the means by which the hormonal environment may alter a woman's risk for breast cancer, significant gaps remain in our understanding of the process at the molecular level. While hormonal effects have been sufficiently characterized to attempt a series of interventions at the clinical level, it is likely that the cascade of events generated by our interventions is far more complex than our current level of understanding is able to recognize. Clearly, it is of importance to continue to investigate the mechanisms underlying the biology of hormonal manipulations in order to devise improved strategies.

The remainder of this chapter is devoted to specific hormonal intervention strategies for the prevention of early breast carcinoma. These strategies will be considered from the point of view of the aforementioned models of mammary carcinogenesis. Further consideration will be given to potential suitable target populations for the prevention strategy as well as to the inherent risks, benefits, and side effects of each. For a given intervention, a key issue involves attempting to determine whether the risk–benefit profile would allow widespread use versus more limited application in selected, defined patient subgroups.

3. Prevention strategies based on induction of mammary gland differentiation — pseudopregnancy

While early first full-term pregnancy (and probably lactation) are well-described protective factors for breast carcinoma development due to the induction of mammary epithelial differentiation, general application of this information is possible for only some women. However, given the strength of the association between early full-term pregnancy and breast cancer risk (figure 1), a potential prevention strategy might seek to mimic as closely as possible the endocrine state of pregnancy, with a goal of the induction of complete mammary gland lobular development. It is likely that a re-creation of the conditions leading up to and including the midpoint of the pregnancy would be required to bring about complete epithelial differentiation. It is not entirely clear what the requirements are for hormones other than estrogens and progestins, e.g., insulin, prolactin, chorionic gonadotropin, and placental lactogen. In experimental models, the role of chorionic gonadotropin is to stimulate mammary epithelial proliferation, with involution and partial differentiation occurring upon withdrawal of the hormone. The overall effect is protective. Placental lactogen appears only to stimulate proliferation, resulting in enhanced susceptibility to the carcinogenic effects of DMBA [20]. In experimental animals, estrogen and progestin alone in sufficient doses are able to induce full mammary development [35]. In humans, the timing and optimal combination of differentiation-inducing hormones are not yet known. While the suggested risk reduction following full mammary maturation is large, the risks of a course of high-dose sex steroids of uncertain duration may be significant. One concern is for increased occcurrence of thromboembolic disease. In addition, the suggestion that certain oral contraceptives used in young women increase the risk of breast cancer [36] shows the pitfalls inherent in generalizing a potentially favorable hormonal treatment without a clear understanding of the temporal and compositional requirements of the intervention.

4. Prevention strategies exhibiting differentiating as well as hormone-modulating activity

4.1. Retinoids

Retinoids exhibit several properties that may allow them to act as prevention agents for breast carcinoma: they have inhibitory effects on cellular proliferation, induce differentiation, and have some cytostatic activity. An inhibitory effect on terminal end-bud proliferation and ductal branching was demonstrated in Sprague–Dawley rats treated with the vitamin A derivative fenretinide [37]. Fenretinide reduced the incidence of mammary cancers in rats treated with nitrosomethyl urea (NMU), with a dose-dependent effect on the latency period for tumor development [38]. In vitro growth inhibition by fenretinide of a human breast tumor cell line has also been demonstrated [39].

In human studies, fenretinide is well tolerated, but a major side effect is loss of night vision [40]. This problem can be avoided by incorporating a three-day drug 'holiday' each month [41]. Two prevention trials testing fenretinide are under way. In a large Italian study, patients with T1–2, N0 breast cancer are being randomized to placebo vs. fenretinide 200 mg po qd. The endpoint of this study is the incidence of contralateral breast cancer [42]. (A second non-breast trial is examining prevention of oral leukoplakia [43]).

The molecular mechanism of action of fenretinide is not known. The demonstration that fenretinide is able to antagonize IGF-I and IGF-II as well as estradiol-stimulated growth of MCF-7 cells [44], taken in combination with the findings that fenretinide administration in humans reduces circulating levels of IGF-I [42,45] and raises c-AMP levels in rats [46], suggests that fenretinide is able to bring about growth inhibition by interfering with growth-stimulatory pathways as well as possible enhancing growth-inhibitory pathways. A further potential action of fenretinide is modulation of binding of the retinoic acid receptor with receptor-associated proteins, affecting the transcriptional specificities of the receptor complex [47].

4.2. Retinoids in combination with antiestrogens

In a series of experiments in a NMU-treated rat model, Ratko et al. demonstrated that the chemopreventive actions of fenretinide were potentiated by tamoxifen [48]. Findings included a reduction in the number of tumors per rat, an increase in the latency period, and improved survival compared to that seen in rats treated with fenretinide alone. In a phase I/II human trial, tamoxifen at 20 mg/day in combination with fenretinide up to 700 mg/day resulted in several responses in a population of previously untreated patients with hormone receptor-positive metastatic disease [49,50]. This promising result has led to a phase III double-blind, prospective, randomized comparison of adjuvant tamoxifen vs. tamoxifen and fenretinide in 1500 postmenopausal patients with receptor-positive, axillary lymph node-positive disease (Intergroup trial INT-0151).

Mechanistically, the synergistic effects of tamoxifen and fenretinide may be partially explained by reduction in IGF levels and responsiveness [45]. Further, alterations in the interactions of steroid hormone receptors with their specific receptor-associated proteins are likely to be brought about by binding of the hormone analogues tamoxifen and fenretinide. Alterations of these interactions are likely to result in modification of transcriptional control of hormonally responsive genes [47]. For example, inhibition of transcription of the IGF and/or TGF-α genes may result. For tamoxifen, another possibility is that alterations in the microenvironment of receptor-interacting proteins might result in the loss of negative transcriptional control of certain target genes such as TGF-β. As the molecular mechanisms of hormone action in breast carcinomas are elucidated, it is likely that additional hormone analogues and combinations of drugs will be developed for evaluation in the prevention setting.

5. Prevention strategies based on control of sex-steroid exposure

5.1. Antiestrogens

A number of estrogen antagonists have been synthesized, the most well known and widely used being the triphenylethylene derivative tamoxifen. This drug was discovered and developed in 1962 by Dr. Arthur L. Walpole, then at ICI as head of the fertility control program. Initially intended for use as an oral contraceptive based on studies in rats [51], the drug was found to induce ovulation in humans [52]. As the role of estrogen receptors in hormone-dependent breast cancer was elucidated, Walpole encouraged clinical testing of tamoxifen [53]. The use of tamoxifen in breast cancer developed from in vitro work that suggested that the compound had tumoricidal activity [54]. Subsequently, Jordan demonstrated that tamoxifen administration to DMBA-treated rats could not only delay the onset of mammary carcinomas but also prevent appearance of the majority of tumors if given continuously [55,56].

Tamoxifen and its metabolites exhibit a complex pharmacology [57]. Depending on the tissue and species, it may behave as a pure antiestrogen, a partial agonist, and even as a pure estrogen agonist. The parent compound exhibits approximately 1/100th of the binding affinity to the estrogen receptor, as does estradiol. The active metabolite of tamoxifen, 4-hydroxytamoxifen, exhibits binding affinity equal to or slightly greater than estradiol. This compound represents on the order of 2% of the concentration of the parent drug in serum from patients receiving 20 mg of tamoxifen BID [58].

In humans, tamoxifen has been demonstrated to function as an antagonist in patients with primary (estrogen receptor (ER)-positive) breast cancers while showing agonist activity in bone, liver, and vaginal epithelial tissues in postmenopausal women [59]. Relatively little is known with regard to the effect of tamoxifen on normal breast tissue. The published body of data is insufficient to allow definitive conclusions regarding effects in premenopausal women as well as multiyear treatment effects in postmenopausal women [60]. This situation is of major relevance to prevention studies, particularly those in premenopausal subjects.

A favorable impact of tamoxifen on the natural history of early-stage breast cancer is supported by several lines of evidence. First, the demonstrated efficacy of tamoxifen in treating metastatic breast carcinoma suggested a role in the suppression of micrometastatic disease; indeed, the use of tamoxifen as adjuvant hormonal therapy in patients with axillary node-positive disease as well as in those with node-negative, hormone-receptor positive disease is associated with improved disease-free and overall survival [61]. Of interest is the finding that short duration of treatment with tamoxifen (1–2 years) is associated with decreases in recurrence rates and improved survival 10 and 15 years later, an observation that suggests that tamoxifen is cytocidal in addition to being cytostatic in its activity. The suggestion that axillary node-negative patients do not derive additional benefit from 10 years of adjuvant treatment with tamoxifen as opposed to five years may be interpreted to support this hypothesis [62]. This latter finding, however, from the NSABP B14 trial, has yet to be examined in detail.

Various hypotheses have been offered to explain the actions of tamoxifen on mammary carcinomas: arrest at G1; induction of apoptosis or possibly

Table 2. Major biochemical effects of tamoxifen on breast cancer cells

1. Competitive binding to estrogen receptor
2. G1 blockade
3. Increased production of TGF-beta
4. Inhibition of TGF-alpha production
5. Decreased IGF_1
6. Increased sex hormone-binding globulin

differentiation into quasi-normal epithelial cells; and binding to the estrogen receptor with induction of altered receptor activation via a series of conformational changes that may be antagonistic or agonistic in different tissues and/or species and that result in changes in production of several growth-influencing proteins [63–65]. The major biochemical effects of tamoxifen on breast cancer cells are summarized in table 2. While the molecular basis for these differential activities is not clearly understood, an emerging body of evidence suggests that the specific microenvironment of receptor-associated chromatin proteins at specific gene enhancer sites may play a central role in determining the estrogenic or antiestrogenic properties of a particular ER ligand [47]. Tamoxifen has been convincingly demonstrated to modulate growth factor levels in breast tumor cells lines as well as in patients with breast cancer [66,67]. This property may be very important in explaining the success of tamoxifen in preventing the progression of small foci of breast carcinoma. It is well known that breast tumors are a heterogeneous mix of cells that are under constant selection pressures. If one performs immunocytochemistry with antibodies to the estrogen receptor, a typical result is that the tumor cells stain for ER to widely varying degrees. One can conclude that when estrogen receptor content is assayed in breast tumor specimens by hormone-binding techniques, the receptor values reported are in fact an average not only of a spectrum of ER-containing tumor cells but also of receptor-negative tumor cells and very likely (receptor-containing) adjacent normal breast tissue. Several conclusions may be drawn from these facts. First, measurements of the ER content in tumors is, at best, a gross oversimplification of the actual situation in the tumor with regard to expression of the estrogen receptor. Second, while the decision to pursue hormonal therapy is based on the average ER value for the assayed specimen, it is not possible to say at present whether a tumor that has a modest but homogeneous distribution of ER throughout will respond better, worse, or the same as a tumor with highly heterogeneous receptor distribution. One could argue that a subfraction of tumor cells that were highly receptor positive might secrete large amounts of inhibitory growth factors, resulting in overall inhibition of tumor growth. This issue requires further investigation in order to gain an understanding of exactly how to integrate immunohistochemistry data with current techniques of hormone receptor assay to arrive at more accurate prognostic information. For example, the specific quantity and distribution of steroid hormone receptors in a breast tumor biopsy specimen might allow the clinician to select a particular type of hormonal treatment from the array of specifically tailored therapies. The third conclusion that one may be tempted to draw from the finding that breast tumors are heterogeneous with regard to steroid hormone receptor content is that receptor-negative cells are those that will eventually progress to hormone independence and result in clinical failure of the hormonal treatment being used. This possibility is certainly open to debate, however, and an equally convincing argument can be made that, in fact, the loss of hormonal responsiveness is secondary to the loss of a functional estrogen receptor system in a receptor-positive cell, which then is able to escape suppression to develop into refractory disease. This possibility might also be seen as a decrease in local production of TGF-β. Additionally, more direct alterations of tumor responsiveness to transforming growth factors could be expected to result in a loss of growth suppression by tamoxifen.

These factors must be taken into account when considering both the likely mechanisms by which hormonal prevention strategies operate and the most likely reasons for their failure. First, hormonal prevention strategies based on the use of hormone antagonists or suppression of endogenous sex steroids do not prevent mammary cancers from developing but rather act to suppress tumors at a preclinical level. It is only through induction of mammary epithelial differentiation that carcinomas are likely to be prevented at a cellular level. Additionally, the failure of hormonal strategies that actually suppress preclinical disease is not a failure to prevent, per se, but rather the act of natural selection of a clone of malignant cells that is able to circumvent the growth-suppressive actions of the treatment. These concepts are important when one considers the target populations for intervention (those without disease but with risks sufficient to warrant a preventive intervention versus those patients likely to have preclinical disease requiring suppressive treatment), especially since the most efficacious treatments for each group may be quite different. For example, a prevention strategy based on treating patients with a course of high-dose sex steroids to induce mammary gland differentiation would have the potential to stimulate the growth of preclinical carcinomas in another, less suitable target population. As with all prevention strategies, identification of suitable target populations presents significant challenges.

The primary biological rationale for the use of tamoxifen as a preventive agent for early breast cancer stems primarily from the DMBA–rat experiments referred to earlier [52,53]. An important finding from these and other experiments is that the duration of treatment with tamoxifen has a significant impact on the development and numbers of mammary tumors. The experimental evidence for tamoxifen as a preventive agent is given additional support by human clinical data demonstrating a reduction in incidence of second primary breast cancers in women with stage I and II tumors who received adjuvant tamoxifen. A meta-analysis of these trials has revealed an overall odds reduction of 39% for second primary breast cancers (from 2.4% to 1.6%)

[61]. Significant observations in support of this broad conclusion are available in specific trials. The Stockholm trial [69] demonstrated a 40% reduction in the rate of contralateral breast cancer in postmenopausal women treated with tamoxifen at 40 mg per day (equal efficacy with 2 or 5 years of treatment) compared to controls. The NSABP B14 trial with premenopausal and postmenopausal subjects demonstrated a 50% reduction in contralateral breast tumors in women with hormone receptor-positive, node-negative breast cancer treated with 20 mg tamoxifen daily for five or more years [70]. While both tamoxifen dose and duration of use have varied among these trials, the consistent result is compelling.

At present, three large-scale prevention trials with tamoxifen are under way. In a British trial, participants are randomized to receive tamoxifen 20 mg qd versus placebo for three years. Eligibility criteria include age over 40 years and the single risk factor of strong family history (defined as a first-degree relative with bilateral breast cancer or breast cancer at less than 40 years of age) [71,72]. An accrual goal of 2000 patients was reached by June 1993. The American NSABP P1 trial has different eligibility requirements, including age greater than 60 with or without risk factors or ages 35–59 with a predicted risk for the development of breast cancer equivalent to a 60-year-old woman based on the Gail model [73,74]. Any woman 35 years or older with lobular carcinoma in situ (LCIS) treated by biopsy alone is eligible. Treatment of five years is planned with an accrual goal of 13,000 patients. A third trial is being conducted by the National Cancer Institute (NCI) of Milan, Italy. Here, subjects must be age 45 or greater and must have been hysterectomized. Participants will be randomized to receive tamoxifen 20 mg daily versus placebo. The accrual goal is 20,000 women.

As can be readily noted from the brief descriptions of these trials, significant differences exist in study populations. Essentially, these reflect differing views regarding the risk–benefit profile of tamoxifen as applied to the breast cancer risk profiles for different target populations. While the epidemiologic risks for breast cancer are fairly well characterized, major logistical hurdles exist in the identification and enrollment of individual high-risk patients in these trials. Ultimately, decisions must be made regarding the number and type of risk factors required for subjects to enroll in prevention trials, balancing the greater numbers of eligible subjects with relatively lower risk and the fewer subjects at the highest risk [75].

In addition to the protective effects of tamoxifen demonstrated by the reduction of breast cancer recurrences, several other potential benefits of this therapy have been described. Tamoxifen has been shown to preserve bone mineral density in postmenopausal women [76]; whether this effect will result in decreased fracture rates over the long term remains to be seen. In addition, tamoxifen has favorable effects on coagulation proteins and lipid profiles again best described in postmenopausal women [77]. The long-term benefits of tamoxifen therapy on these parameters is currently under investigation. One can argue that the agonist properties of tamoxifen in the osseous and hepatic tissues are of significant benefit both to the postmenopausal patient and to the patient who is premenopausal at diagnosis but subsequently undergoes ovarian ablation (see below). Of note, however, is that these potentially clinically important effects have not been well studied in premenopausal women; indeed, where they have been investigated, some findings have been untoward. For example, in premenopausal women, Powles and colleagues have found decreased bone mineral density with tamoxifen treatment [78].

Unfortunately, long-term use of tamoxifen is also associated with several toxicities. These are well described elsewhere [59,79-81] but primarily involve constitutional side effects (hot flushes), increased risk for thromboembolism, possible ocular toxicity, and increased risk for endometrial cancer (on the order of 1%-2% over five years). Major side effects of tamoxifen are summarized in table 3.

Potential participants in a prevention trial must consider the relative risks and benefits to them as individuals. For tamoxifen, the current prevention trials attempt to select for patients at high risk for breast cancer based on a profile of risk factors balanced against the risks and benefits of the drug (table 3). As data from these studies are examined, it will be necessary to consider the risk-benefit profiles for patients with regard to the length of treatment planned and the cumulative exposure to the drug. As noted above, there is a significant lack of information regarding the long-term effects of tamoxifen in premenopausal women (with induced and relatively high levels of competing estrogens). Data on contralateral breast cancer occurrences from the NSABP B14 adjuvant trial suggest that the use of tamoxifen in premenopausal women is beneficial, but this trial selected the subset of women with hormone receptor-positive primary tumors [61]. The efficacy of tamoxifen as a long-term preventive agent in the estrogen-rich environment of the premenopausal breast has been presumed to be minimal, although recent data suggest that in the adjuvant setting significant benefit may be derived, at least with regard to disease-free survival [82]. Given that the growth of normal breast tissue, as well as initiated breast cancer cells, is stimulated by estrogen, careful consideration must be given to the risks associated with a treatment that results in elevation of the levels of endogenous estrogens [83].

Table 3. Major side effects of tamoxifen

1. Constitutional side effects (hot flushes)
2. Reduction in second primary breast cancers
3. Preservation of bone mineral density (postmenopausal subjects only)
4. Favorable changes on serum lipoproteins
5. Increased risk of endometrial cancer
6. Reduction in ovarian cancer (?; postmenopausal subjects)
7. Increase in thrombophlebitis (?)
8. Increase in cholelithiasis (?)
9. Ocular toxicity (?)

A potential means of avoiding the concerns regarding endogenous estrogen stimulation by tamoxifen is to induce menopause in the patient at the time that tamoxifen prevention is initiated. This approach is described more fully later in this chapter, but ovarian ablation carries the distinct advantage that the competitive effects of endogenous estrogens are obviated, allowing unopposed antiestrogen activity.

An alternative approach involves the use of newer antiestrogens. When long-term use of these 'pure' antiestrogens is contemplated, a significant issue is the absence of estrogen agonist effects with these agents.

5.2. Antiprogestins

As discussed, the normal mammary gland undergoes cyclic epithelial proliferation. Following estrogen-dependent priming of the cells during the follicular phase, progesterone drives cell division during the luteal phase at several times the rate seen in the follicular phase. If fertilization does not occur, progesteronel levels fall and the epithelium involutes. Given the role of progesterone as a potent stimulator of breast epithelial proliferation, antiprogestins should be considered as hormonal-preventive agents for breast carcinomas. The most thoroughly studied antiprogestin to date is RU486; in humans, this investigation has occurred primarily in its role as an abortifacient. Inhibitory effects on breast cell proliferation have been demonstrated both in vitro and in vivo (rodent models). It is thought that at least a portion of the antiproliferative effects of RU486 is due to enhanced production of the inhibitory growth factor TGF-β [84], and possibly modulation of P53 [85] as well as decreased expression of growth factor receptors [86]. In at least one report, however, RU486 has been demonstrated to exhibit weakly estrogenic properties [87]. The authors made use of a reporter gene under ERE (estrogen response element) control to demonstrate that RU486 was able to stimulate transcription of the reporter gene, the progesterone receptor and induce MCF-7 cell proliferation as well as to decreasel levels of TGF-β2 and TGF-β3 mRNA. These actions were able to be blocked by the addition of the antiestrogens monohydroxytamoxifen or ICI 164,384. While the translation of conclusions from work in rodent systems and tissue culture to humans is difficult, this work points to the need to further elucidate the potential estrogenic as well as antiprogestogenic actions of RU486. These findings raise the possibility that RU486 would need to be utilized in combination with an antiestrogen to negate its weakly estrogenic properties. Additionally, the significant antiglucocorticoid activities of RU486 present challenges with long-term use.

5.3. Modulation of ovarian function

Modulation of ovarian function as a prevention strategy follows logically from the duration of ovulation model: sex steroids act as tumor promoters by driving epithelial proliferation. While antiestrogen/antiprogestin therapies may be viewed as indirect modulators of ovarian function by interfering with ovarian hormones, more direct methods for suppressing the influence of the ovarian hormones deserve attention. Surgical or radiation oophorectomy as such a direct strategy is appealing as a single, permanent treatment with minimal morbidity (figure 2). The permanence of this intervention is disadvantageous in younger women who might wish to become pregnant in the future. In such women, reversible chemical suppression of ovarian function with luteinizing hormone-releasing hormone (LHRH) agonists might be more acceptable. Ovarian ablation by adjuvant cytotoxic chemotherapy has been argued to be responsible for a significant portion of the survival benefit derived from this treatment. The challenges in applying this concept in the healthy-woman prevention setting concern the spectrum of associated toxicities.

The suppression of ovarian function by goserelin (a widely evaluated LHRH agonist) appears to produce response rates similar to those following surgical or radiotherapeutic oophorectomy in premenopausal women with estrogen receptor-positive metastatic breast carcinoma [88]. Thus, from the standpoint of efficacy, one can argue that there is little to choose between the two techniques. Cost issues are, however, a first hurdle. Given the likely time span that such an individual would need in order to receive gonadotropin-releasing hormone agonist (GnRHA) therapy, the $350–450 cost per month, contrasted with surgical oophorectomy at a one-time cost of approximately $1600 in physician fees (as well as hospital charges) and radiotherapeutic ovarian ablation at $1000–2000, makes the reversible chemotherapeutic approach less attractive.

Another factor to be taken into account when attempting to minimize exposure to endogenous estrogen is that circulating estrogen is not reduced to negligible levels by ovarian ablation. The peripheral aromatization of adrenal steroids continues to represent a source of estrogen that can stimulate the growth of hormone-dependent or hormone-responsive breast carcinomas. Several strategies are available to minimize the role of peripheral aromatization of adrenal steroids in stimulating tumor growth. The first of these is the use of aromatase inhibitors such as aminoglutethimide or arimidex. While best known from their use in the metastatic setting, the aromatase inhibitors have a potential role in the development of preventive therapies that seek to control levels of circulating estrogens. Aromatase inhibitors might be useful in some type of combination regimen involving suppression of ovarian function, inhibition of peripheral aromatization, and potentially the direct blockade of estrogen action at the receptor level with antiestrogens.

An attempt to answer the question of the importance of ovarian ablation in conjunction with tamoxifen in premenopausal patients with established stage I ER-positive tumors is currently being addressed in an adjuvant phase III trial (figure 3).

Using the approach of estrogen blockade by ovarian ablation and/or

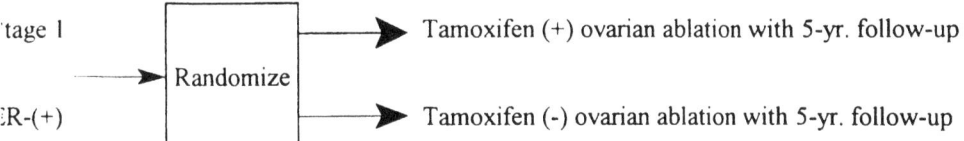

Figure 3. Scheme for tamoxifen ± ovarian ablation for stage I ER-positive patients.

aromatase inhibition, potentially in combination with antiestrogens, has the potential not only for preventing tumors in high-risk patients but also for halting progression of hormone-dependent and hormone-responsive early breast tumors. However, the potential side effects of what is essentially early and complete menopause are barriers. For young women, the long-term expected increased risks of coronary artery disease and osteoporosis are not insignificant. There risks may be reduced in part by the use of agonist/antagonist antiestrogens such as tamoxifen. The overall risk–benefit ratio will depend significantly on the risk profile of an individual subject.

5.4. An 'ideal' combination oral contraceptive

An alternative to *complete* estrogen blockade is precise control of the levels of sex steroids. One such strategy is based on the suppression of ovarian function with a GnRH agonist (monthly leuprolide acetate), with replacement estrogen (conjugated estrogens at 0.625 mg po on 6 of 7 days), and progestogen (medroxyprogesterone acetate 10 mg po for 13 days every fourth 28-day cycle) given to replace needed hormones [24,89,90]. The proponents hypothesize that the use of GnRHA alone should result in rates of breast cancer equal to those in oophorectomized women (see figure 2). The addition of supplemental sex steroids may have a weak promoting effect on breast cancer development (above that which follows ovarian ablation or suppression alone) equivalent to that associated with postmenopausal estrogen replacement therapy. The authors estimate that using such an ideal contraceptive regimen over any 10-year period between first full-term pregnancy and age 40 is likely to reduce lifetime breast cancer risk by more than 50%.

This regimen, modified with the addition of low-dose androgens, has been demonstrated to preserve bone mineral density. This androgen may also have the added benefit of compensating for some loss of libido reported by users of GnRHA. Likely consequent to the addition of exogenous estrogen and progesterone, a rise in HDL cholesterol was observed, suggesting that at least a portion of the increased cardiovascular risk due to ovarian suppression may be negated. Early results demonstrate a mammographic reduction in breast parenchymal density, which suggests that significant suppression of breast proliferation is being achieved [91]. Whether an actual reduction in breast cancer risk is observed in the treated cohort, as well as whether other clinical endpoints associated with ovarian suppression such as bone fracture or major changes in bone density and cardiovascular disease will occur at reduced frequencies, remains to be demonstrated.

6. Future directions

This chapter has described a number of strategies that hold promise for the preventive treatment of breast cancer. It is also clear that significant gaps exist in our understanding both of this disease and of the physiology of the normal mammary gland at the molecular level. These gaps include both the complex hormonal interactions in the normal mammary gland and the as yet undefined molecular events along the continuum from normal breast to malignant epithelium. Futher, many if not all of the currently proposed prevention treatments have pleomorphic effects on multiple target tissues. The development of better-targeted, model-based approaches will be required if broad application to large populations is to be accomplished.

A major focus of breast cancer prevention research involves completion of the current series of prevention trials, an effort that will stretch into the next century. Given the length of time required for follow-up of young patients, trials involving premenopausal women can be envisioned to require decades to develop comprehensive data on risks and benefits. Such trials will therefore require major commitments from subject-participants, funding agencies, and investigators. In fact, several generations of investigators may ultimately become involved with large-scale prevention trials.

A second major effort regarding prevention relates to the continued search for active agents or combinations of agents. Implicit in this search is the desire to uncover treatments that are not only more efficacious regarding breast cancers but also possess improved side effect profiles. For example, an ideal antiestrogen might exhibit pure antiestrogen properties in breast tissue while providing protective effects in bone and vascular systems. To pursue drug development in this arena, new discoveries in the field of steroid hormone-receptor biology will be necessary in order to better refine biological models for control of mammary growth and differentiation. Implicit in this endeavor is the need to continually question the current dogma for hormone action, tumorigenesis, and prevention strategies. Current models of steroid action have begun to account for the observations that the receptors for these hormones have multiple interactions distinct from the ligand and DNA. An emerging body of evidence suggests that these proteins are involved in interactions at chromatin sites with transcription factors and protein kinases [92] and possibly small molecules (such as polyamines) as well. Knowledge of the spectrum of interacting proteins and the specific interactions at a molecular level will enable investigators to consider the development of rationally designed compounds that alter the interactions of steroid hormone receptors at their chromatin enhancer sites. Preliminary work has resulted in the ability to identify unique peptides cleaved from model proteins known to interact with and alter the hormone-binding ability of the estrogen receptor (M.R. Olsen and G.C. Mueller, unpublished). The development of such approaches will allow construction of peptide mimetic drugs that are able to alter specifically the activities of estrogen receptors at target genes. At least a portion of the agonist–antagonist actions of compounds such as tamoxifen may be due to the influence of the particular spectrum of receptor-associated proteins in various target tissues. The development of specific peptide-mimetic agents may allow minimization of unwanted antiestrogenic side effects (primarily with regard to bone mineral density and atherosclerosis) while providing the required breast cancer protective activity.

Finally, the combination of antiestrogens with agents such as retinoids, currently being investigated in the adjuvant setting, may eventually become useful in the prevention arena, especially as the results of the Italian retinoid trial become known.

7. Conclusion

A number of hormonal strategies exist or are under development that hold promise for the treatment of early breast cancers. In order for these treatments to find widespread use, several key issues must be addressed. These include the profile of risks and benefits for each form of therapy and the suitability for use in particular target populations being considered for intervention. More broadly, the ability to identify and recruit suitable patients from the general population for hormonal prevention efforts presents a considerable challenge. Additional issues to be considered include questions of cost–benefit in an era of increasing fiscal constraints as well as the ability to carry out the required long-term investigations required to rigorously assess the efficacy of proposed interventional strategies.

References

1. Beatson GT. 1896. On the treatment of inoperable cases of carcinoma of the mamma: suggestions for a new method of treatment with illustrative cases. Lancet 2:104–107.
2. Tokunaga M, Land CE, Yamamoto T, et al. 1984. Breast cancer among atomic bomb survivors. In Boice JD Jr, Fraumeni JF Jr, eds. Radiation Carcinogenesis: Epidemiology and Biological Significance. New York: Raven Press, pp. 45–55.
3. Tokunaga M, Land CE, Yamamoto T, et al. 1987. Incidence of female breast cancer among atomic bomb survivors, Hiroshima and Nagasaki, 1950–1980. Radiat Res 112:243–272.
4. Committee on the Biological Effects of Ionizing Radiations. 1990. Health Effects of Exposure to Low Levels of Ionizing Radiation: BEIR V. Washington, DC: National Academy Press, pp. 253–267.
5. Hirayama T. 1988. Health effects of active and passive smoking. In Aoki M, Hisamian S, Taminoga S, eds. Smoking and Health 1987. Amsterdam: Elsevier, pp. 75–86.

6. Ford D, Easton DF. 1995. The genetics of breast and ovarian cancer. Br J Cancer 72:805–812.
7. Miki Y, Swensen J, Shattuck-Eidens D, et al. 1993. A strong candidate for the breast and ovarian cancer susceptibility gene BRCA1. Science 266:66–71.
8. Wooster R, Neuhausen SL, Mangion J, et al. 1994. Localization of a breast cancer susceptibility gene, BRCA2, to chromosome 13q12–13. Science 265:2088–2090.
9. Jensen RA, Thompson ME, Jetton TL, et al. 1996. BRCA1 is secreted and exhibits properties of a granin. Nat Genet 12:303–308.
10. Swift M, Morrell D, Massey RB, et al. 1991. Incidence of cancer in 161 families affected by ataxia–telangiectasia. N Engl J Med 325:1831–1836.
11. MacMahon B, Cole P, Lin TM, et al. 1970. Age at first birth and breast cancer risk. Bull WHO 43:209–221.
12. Russo J, Russo IH. 1978. DNA labeling index and structure of the rat mammary gland as determinants of its susceptibility to carcinogenesis. J Natl Cancer Inst 61:1451–1459.
13. Russo J, Russo IH. 1980. Influence of differentiation and cell kinetics on the susceptibility of the rat mammary gland to carcinogenesis. Cancer Res 40 (8, pt 1): 2677–2687.
14. Russo J, Russo IH. 1980. Susceptibility of the mammary gland to carcinogensis. II. Pregnancy interruption as a risk factor in tumor incidence. Am J Pathol 100:497–512.
15. McCormick GM, Moon RC. 1965. Effect of pregnancy and lactation on growth of mammary tumors induced by 7,12-dimethylbenz(a)anthracene (DMBA). Br J Cancer 19:160–166.
16. Ciocca DR, Parente A, Russo J. 1982. Endocrinologic milieu and susceptibility of the rat mammary gland to carcinogenesis. Am J Pathol 109:47–56.
17. Russo J, Russo IH. 1987. Development of the human mammary gland. In Neville MC, Daniel C, eds. The Mammary Gland Development, Regulation and Function. New York: Plenum, pp. 67–93.
18. Dao TL, Bock FG, Greiner MJ. 1960. Mammary carcinogenesis by 3-methylcholanthrene II. Inhibitory effect of pregnancy and lactation on tumor induction. J Natl Cancer Inst 25:991–1003.
19. Huggins C, Grand LC, Brillantes F. 1959. Critical significance of breast structure in the induction of mammary cancer in the rat. Proc Natl Acad Sci USA 45:1294–1300.
20. Russo J. 1983. Basis of cellular autonomy in susceptibility to carcinogenesis. Toxicol Pathol 11:149–166.
21. MacMahon B. 1993. General Motors Cancer Research Prizewinners Laureates Lectures. Charles S. Mott Prize. Reproduction and cancer of the breast. Cancer 71:3185–3188.
22. Longacre TA, Bartow SA. 1986. A correlative morph0logic study of human breast and endometrium in the menstrual cycle. Am J Surg Pathol 10:382–393.
23. Potten CS, Watson RJ, Williams GT, et al. 1988. The effect of age and menstrual cycle upon proliferative activity of the normal human breast. Br J Cancer 58:163–170.
24. Spicer DV, Krecker EA, Pike MC. 1995. The endocrine prevention of breast cancer. Cancer Invest 13(5):495–504.
25. Anderson TJ, Ferguson DJP, Raab GM. 1982. Cell turnover in the 'resting' human breast: influence of parity, contraceptive pill, age and laterality. Br J Cancer 46:376–382.
26. Dawson EK. 1935. A histological study of the normal mamma in relation to tumour growth: II The mature gland in pregnancy and lactation. Edin Med J 42:569–598.
27. Gompel A, Malet C, Spritzer P, et al. 1986. Progestin effect on cell proliferation and 17 beta-hydroxysteroid dehydrogenase activity in normal human breast cells in culture. J Clin Endocrinol Metab 63:1174–1180.
28. Vignon F, Bardon S, Chalbos D, Rochefort H. 1983. Antiestrogenic effect of R5020, a synthetic progestin, in human breast cancer cells in culture. J Clin Endocrinol Metab 56:1124–1130.
29. Murphy LC, Dotzlaw H. 1989. Endogenous growth factor expression in T47D, human breast cancer cells, associated with reduced sensitivity to antiproliferative effects of progestins and antiestrogens. Cancer Res 49:599–604.
30. Cowan LD, Gordis L, Tonascia JA, et al. 1981. Breast cancer incidence in women with a history of progesterone deficiency. Am J Epidemiol 144:209–217.

31. Gonzalez ER. 1983. Chronic anovulation may increase postmenopausal breast cancer risk. JAMA 249:445–446.
32. Pike MC, Henderson BE, Krailo MD, et al. 1983. Breast cancer and oral contraceptives: reply to critics. Lancet 2:1414.
33. Royal College of General Practitioners. 1977. Effect on hypertension and benign breast disease of progestagen component in combined oral contraceptives. Lancet 1:624–626.
34. Pike MC, Ross RK, Lobo RA, et al. 1989. LHRH agonists and the prevention of breast and ovarian cancer. Br J Cancer 60:142–148.
35. Key TJA, Pike MC. 1988. The role of oestrogens and progestagens in the epidemiology and prevention of breast cancer. Eur J Cancer Clin Oncol 24:29–43.
36. Drife JO. 1991. Avoiding hormone-related risk factors. In Stoll BA, ed. Approaches to Breast Cancer Prevention. Dordrecht: Kluwer, pp. 61–72.
37. Radcliffe JD, Moon RC. 1975. Effect of N-(4-hydroxyphenyl)retinamide on food intake, growth, and mammary gland development in rats (41736). Proc Soc Exp Biol Med 174:270–275.
38. Moon RC, Thompson HJ, Becci PJ, et al. 1979. N-(4-hydroxyphenyl) retinamide, a new retinoid for prevention of breast cancer in the rat. Cancer Res 39:1339–1346.
39. Bhatnagar R, Abou-Issa H, Curley RW Jr, et al. 1991. Growth suppression of human breast carcinoma cells in culture by N-(4-hydroxyphenyl)retinamide and its glucuronide and through synergism with glucarate. Biochem Pharmacol 41:1471–1477.
40. Rotmensz N, DePalo G, Formelli F, et al. 1991. Long-term tolerability of fenretinide (4-HPR) in breast cancer patients. Eur J Cancer 27:1127–1131.
41. Formelli F, Carsana R, Costa A, et al. 1989. Plasma retinol level reduction by the synthetic retinoid fenretinide: a one year follow-up study of breast cancer patients. Cancer Res 49:6149–6152.
42. Veronesi U, DePalo G, Costa A, et al. 1992. Chemoprevention of breast cancer with retinoids. Monogr Natl Cancer Inst 12:93–97.
43. Chiesa F, Tradati N, Marazza M, et al. 1992. Prevention of local relapses and new localisations of oral leukoplakias with the synthetic retinoid fenretinide (4-HPR). Preliminary results. Eur J Cancer B Oral Oncol 28B:97–102.
44. Gupta MK, Posch A, Budd T, et al. (Cleveland Clinic). 1992. Inhibition of IGF-I- and IGE-II-induced growth of human breast cancer cells (MCF-7) by N-(4-hydroxyphenyl) retinamide. Proc Annu Meet Am Assoc Cancer Res 33(275):A1643.
45. Torrisi R, Pansa F, Orengo M, et al. 1993. The synthetic retinoid fenretinide lowers plasma insulin-like growth factor I levels in breast cancer patients. Cancer Res 53:4769–4771.
46. Abou-Issa H, Wilcox KA, Webb TE. 1992. Signal transduction system may mediate the growth-inhibitory effects of retinoids and calcium glucarate in the rat mammary tumor model. Proc Annu Meet Am Assoc Cancer Res 33(90):A541.
47. Halachmi S, Marden E, Martin G, et al. 1994. Estrogen receptor-associated proteins: possible mediators of hormone-induced transcription. Science 264:1455–1458.
48. Ratko TA, Detrisac CJ, Dinger NM, et al. 1989. Chemopreventive efficacy of combined retinoid and tamoxifen treatment following surgical excision of a primary mammary cancer in female rats. Cancer Res 49:4472–4476.
49. Cobleigh MA, Dowlatshahi K, Deutsch TA, et al. 1993. Phase I/II trial of tamoxifen with or without fenretinide, an analogue of vitamin A, in women with metastatic breast cancer. J Clin Oncol 11:474–477.
50. Cobleigh MA, Lincoln S, Mullane M, Benson AB, Minn F. 1993. Phase I/II trial of tamoxifen (tam) + fenretinide (4HPR) in Stage IV, receptor-positive, previously-untreated breast cancer. Breast Cancer Res Treat 21:51.
51. Harper MJK, Walpole AL. 1967. Mode of action of ICI 46,474 in preventing implantation in rats. J Endocrinol 37:83–92.
52. Williamson JG, Ellis JD. 1973. The induction of ovulation by tamoxifen. J Obstet Gynecol Br Common 80:844–847.
53. Jordan VC. 1994. The development of tamoxifen for breast cancer therapy. In Jordan VC, ed.

Long-Term Tamoxifen Treatment for Breast Cancer. Madison: University of Wisconsin, pp. 3–26.

54. Lippman ME, Bolan G. 1975. Oestrogen-responsive human breast cancer in long term tissue culture. Nature 256:592–593.
55. Jordan VC. 1978. Use of the DMBA-induced rat mammary carcinoma system for the evaluation of tamoxifen as a potential adjuvant therapy. Rev Endocr Rel Cancer (October supplement):49–55.
56. Jordan VC, Dix CJ, Allen KE. 1979. The effectiveness of long-term treatment in a laboratory model for adjuvant hormone therapy of breast cancer. In Salmon SE, Jones SE, eds. Adjuvant Therapy of Cancer, vol. 2. New York: Grune and Stratton, pp. 19–26.
57. Jordan VC, Murphy CS. 1990. Endocrine pharmacology of antiestrogens as antitumor agents. Endocr Rev 11:578–610.
58. Daniel P, Gaskell SJ, Bishhop H, Nicholson RI. 1979. Determination of tamoxifen and an hydroxylated metabolite in plasma from patients with advanced breast cancer using gas chromatography–mass spectrometry. J Endocrinol 83:401–408.
59. Love RR. 1994. Multisystem biological and symptomatic toxicity of tamoxifen in postmenopausal women. In Jordan VC, ed. Long-Term Tamoxifen Treatment for Breast Cancer. Madison: University of Wisconsin, pp. 57–81.
60. Walker KJ, Price-Thomas JM, Candlish W, et al. 1991. Influence of the antioestrogen tamoxifen on normal breast tissue. Br J Cancer 64:764–768.
61. Early Breast Cancer Trialists' Collaborative Group. 1992. Systemic treatment of early breast cancer by hormonal, cytotoxic or immune therapy. 133 randomized trials involving 31,000 recurrences and 24,000 deaths among 75,000 women. Lancet 339:1–15, 71–85.
62. National Cancer Institute. 1995. Adjuvant Therapy of Breast Cancer—Tamoxifen Update. Bethesda, MD: NCI, pp. 1–7.
63. Johnston SR, MacLennan KA, Sacks NP, Salter J, Smith IE, Dowsett M. 1994. Modulation of Bcl-2 and Ki-67 expression in oestrogen receptor-positive human breast cancer by tamoxifen. Eur J Cancer 30A:1663–1669.
64. Perry RR, Kang Y, Greaves BR. 1995. Relationship between tamoxifen-induced transforming growth factor beta 1 expression, cytostasis and apoptosis in human breast cancer cells. Br J Cancer 72:1441–1446.
65. Colletta AA, Benson JR, Baum M. 1994. Alternative mechanisms of action of anti-oestrogens. Breast Cancer Res Treat 31:5–9.
66. Kopp A, Jonat W, Schmahl M, et al. 1995. Transforming growth factor beta 2 (TGF-beta 2) levels in plasma of patients with metastatic breast cancer treated with tamoxifen. Cancer Res 55:4512–4515.
67. Noguchi S, Motomura K, Inaji H, Imaoka S, Koyama H. 1993. Down-regulation of transforming growth factor-alpha by tamoxifen in human breast cancer. Cancer 72:131–136.
68. Jordan VC. 1993. Growth factor regulation by tamoxifen is demonstrated in patients with breast cancer. Cancer 72:1–2.
69. Fornander T, Rutqvist LE, Cedermark B, et al. 1989. Adjuvant tamoxifen in early breast cancer: occurrence of new primary cancers. Lancet 1:117–120.
70. Fisher B, Costantino J, Redmond C, et al. 1989. A randomized clinical trial evaluating tamoxifen in the treatment of patients with node-negative breast cancer who have estrogen-receptor-positive tumors. N Engl J Med 320:479–484.
71. Powles TJ, Hardy JR, Ashley SE, et al. 1989. A pilot trial to evaluate the acute toxicity and feasibility of tamoxifen for prevention of breast cancer. Br J Cancer 60:126–131.
72. Powles TJ, Jones AL, Ashley SE, et al. 1994. The Royal Marsden Hospital pilot tamoxifen chemoprevention trial. Breast Cancer Res Treat 31:73–82.
73. Gail MH, Brinton LA, Byar DP, et al. 1989. Projecting individualized probabilities of developing breast cancer for white females who are being examined annually. J Natl Cancer Inst 81:1879–1886.
74. Bondy ML, Lustbader ED, Halabi S, et al. 1994. Validation of a breast cancer risk assessment model in women with a positive family history. J Natl Cancer Inst 86:620–625.

75. Vogel VG, Love RR. 1991. High risk groups and cost strategies. In Stoll BA, ed. Approaches to Breast Cancer Prevention. Dordrecht: Kluwer, pp. 207–220.
76. Love RR, Barden HS, Mazess RB, et al. 1994. Effect of tamoxifen on lumbar spine bone mineral density in postmenopausal women after 5 years. Arch Intern Med 154:2585–2588.
77. Love RR, Wiebe DA, Feyzi JM, et al. 1994. Effects of tamoxifen on cardiovascular risk factors in postmenopausal women after 5 years of treatment. J Natl Cancer Inst 86:1534–1539.
78. Powles TJ, Hickish T, Kanis JA, et al. 1996. Effect of tamoxifen on bone mineral density measured by dual-energy x-ray absorptiometry in healthy premenopausal and postmenopausal women. J Clin Oncol 14:78–84.
79. Fisher B, Costantino JP, Redmond CK, et al. 1994. Endometrial cancer in tamoxifen-treated breast cancer patients: findings from the National Surgical Adjuvant Breast and Bowel Project (NSABP) B-14. J Natl Cancer Inst 86:527–537.
80. Rutqvist LE, Johansson H, Signomklao T, et al. 1995. Adjuvant tamoxifen therapy for early stage breast cancer and second primary malignancies. Stockholm Breast Cancer Study Group. J Natl Cancer Inst 87:645–651.
81. Nayfield SG, Gorin MB. 1996. Tamoxifen-associated eye disease — a review. J Clin Oncol 14: 1018–1026.
82. Jaiyesimi IA, Buzdar AU, Decker DA, Hortobagyi GN. 1995. Use of tamoxifen for breast cancer: twenty-eight years later. J Clin Oncol 13:513–529.
83. Jordan VC, Fritz NF, Langan-Fahey S, et al. 1991. Alteration of endocrine parameters in premenopausal women with breast cancer during long-term adjuvant therapy with tamoxifen as the single agent. J Natl Cancer Inst 83:1488–1491.
84. Dickens TA, Colletta AA. 1993. The pharmacological manipulation of members of the transforming growth factor beta family in the chemoprevention of breast cancer. Bioessays 15(1):71–74.
85. Hurd C, Khattree N, Alban P, et al. 1995. Hormonal regulation of the p53 tumor suppressor protein in T47D human breast carcinoma cell line. J Biol Chem 270:28507–28510.
86. Sapi E, Flick MB, Gilmore-Hebert M, et al. 1995. Transcriptional regulation of the c-fms (CSF-1R) proto-oncogene in human breast carcinoma cells by glucocorticoids. Oncogene 10(3):529–542.
87. Jeng MH, Langan-Fahey SM, Jordan VC. 1993. Estrogenic actions of RU486 in hormone-responsive MCF-7 human breast cancer cells. Endocrinology 132(6):2622–2630.
88. Boccardo F, Rubagotti A, Perrotta A, et al. 1994. Ovarian ablation versus goserelin with or without tamoxifen in pre-perimenopausal patients with advanced breast cancer: results of a multicentric Italian study. Ann Oncol 5:337–342.
89. Spicer DV, Shoupe D, Pike MC. 1991. GnRH agonists as contraceptive agents: predicted significantly reduced risk of breast cancer. Contraception 44:289–310.
90. Spicer DV, Pike MC, Pike A, et al. 1993. Pilot trial of a gonadotropin hormone agonist with replacement hormones as a prototype contraceptive to prevent breast cancer. Contraception 47:427–444.
91. Spicer DV, Ursin G, Parisky YR, et al. 1994. Changes in mammographic densities induced by a hormonal contraceptive designed to reduce breast cancer risk. J Natl Cancer Inst 86: 431–436.
92. Traynor A. 1995. Recent advances in hormonal therapy for cancer. Curr Opin Oncol 7: 572–581.

9. Ovarian ablation as adjuvant therapy for early-stage breast cancer

Kathleen I. Pritchard

1. Background and rationale

Ovarian ablation was first used by Beatson [1] before the turn of the century and proved useful in shrinking tumors in women with widespread metastatic disease. It was Schinzinger, however, who first suggested, around the same time, that oophorectomy be done before or at the time of mastectomy in order to 'involute' the breast, thus 'containing tumour cells' [2]. The subsequent development of methods for radiation ovarian ablation led others to suggest that radiation castration following radical mastectomy might prevent or postpone the development of metastatic disease [3]. A series of small trials of adjuvant ovarian ablation were subsequently carried out, but the small size of the studies, poor study design, lack of sophisticated methodology for analysis, and the apparently minimal effects seen in these trials led to a loss of interest in this modality, which was exacerbated by the promising early results of adjuvant chemotherapy in the mid 1970s [4–6].

By the early 1980s, however, it was apparent that combination chemotherapy as well was limited in its effects [7]. It was becoming clear that chemotherapy, at least as given at that time, provided little improvement in postmenopausal women and that even in the premenopausal population, it was not a panacea. In turn, the more widespread availability of measurements of estrogen receptors (ERs) and progesterone receptors (PRs) and the development of several new hormonal agents [7–9] encouraged a reexamination of adjuvant endocrine therapy. It became obvious, early in its use, that adjuvant tamoxifen, particularly in postmenopausal patients, had an effect not dissimilar from that of adjuvant combination chemotherapy in premenopausal women. With this conceptual shift to the use of adjuvant endocrine therapy in postmenopausal women, there was renewed interest in the role of ovarian ablation in the premenopausal population. The development, in 1984, of the Early Breast Cancer Trialists Collaborative Group (EBCTG), a consortium of investigators interested in examining adjuvant hormonal and chemotherapy trials with the meta-analysis or overview technique, led to the application of modern analysis methodology to the available trials of ovarian ablation and to the observation that ovarian ablation had a substantial effect when given as adjuvant therapy in premenopausal women [10–12].

In women with metastatic breast cancer, ablative or additive endocrine therapies produce response rates of 30% in unselected patients [13–15], around 50% in women with ER-positive (+ve) tumors [16,17] and as high as 80% in women with ER+ve, PR+ve tumors [16,17]. In contrast, fewer than 5%–10% of ER negative (−ve) or ER−ve, PR−ve tumors will respond to hormonal manipulations [16,17]. Response rates are proportional to the levels of hormone receptor measured [17,18]. Receptor levels measured in primary tumors correspond quite closely to levels measured in recurrent disease, at least in the absence of intervening hormonal therapy [19]. Thus the receptor status of the primary tumor probably corresponds quite closely to that of any occult metastases left after primary surgery, and so it would seem likely that adjuvant endocrine therapy of any type would prove most effective in women with high ER and PR levels at the time of primary surgery.

2. Trials of adjuvant ovarian ablation versus no other systemic therapy

Following the proposal of adjuvant oophorectomy by Schinzinger [2], there have been over 20 trials of various types of ovarian ablation, with or without the addition of prednisone, which has been hypothesized to further reduce estrogen levels in the body by turning off adrenal activity. Many of these trials, however, were done in an era in which randomized clinical trial methodology was not widely accepted. In addition, virtually all these trials were done before the widespread availability of ER or PR measurements, so appropriate subgroup entry criteria, stratification, or analyses could not be done.

The first trials of ovarian ablation consisted mainly of series of patients from single institutions, often with historical nonmatched, nonrandomized controls [20–27]. Interpretation of the results of these trials was hampered by the lack of the modern statistical methodology for life table analysis which is currently widely used and allows efficient comparisons of disease-free and overall survival [28]. Furthermore, at the time these trials were carried out, information was seldom present on such now well-appreciated prognostic factors as nodal status [29]. In spite of the problems with these early studies, however, most of them suggested some advantage in favor of ovarian ablation. A little later, several studies were carried out using surgical or radiation castration, with matched but nonrandomized control groups [30–34]. Some of these studies also suggested a degree of benefit for patients who received ovarian ablation [32,34], although others found neither benefit nor detriment [30,31,33].

Currently of course, randomized controlled trials are considered the best methodology for the evaluation of any therapy, since randomization minimizes the possibility of bias. As this methodology came into more common usage, several prospective randomized trials of ovarian ablation were carried out (see table 1) [35–43] [44,45].

Table 1. Randomized trials of ovarian ablation versus no systemic therapy

Trial	Ovarian treatment	Accrual period	Randomized <50 yrs	Randomized >50 yrs	Data available	Published [ref]
Paterson (Christie)	450 rads	1948–50	178	11	Yes	Yes [35,36]
Nissen-Meyer (Norweigen)	1000 rads	1957–63	151	195	Yes	Yes [37–39]
Nevinny (Boston)	Surgery	1961–[b]		143	No	Yes [45]
Ravdin (NSABP)	Surgery	1961–67	184	0	Yes	Yes [40]
Bryant & Weir (Saskatchewan)	Surgery	1964–74	255	124	Yes	Yes [44]
Meakin & Hayward (Princess Margaret Hospital, Toronto)	2000 rads[a]	1965–72	349	430	Yes	Yes [41–43]
Ontario Cancer Research and Treatment Foundation	1500 rads	1968–77	9	323	Yes	Yes [48]
CRFB Cancer Agency	900/1400 rads	1971–76	1	51	Yes	Yes [49]
Bradford RI	Surgery	1974–85	42	9	Yes	No
Subtotal: (except Nevinny)		1948–85	1169	1143	Yes	

[a] Stratum 1: control vs 2000 rads.
[b] Although 143 patients were randomized, no individual patient data are available on accrual period, age distribution, or outcome.
Abbreviations: NSABP, National Surgical Adjuvant Breast Project; RI, Radiotherapy Institute; CFRB, Centre Regionale Francois Baclesse; yrs, years of age.

In the first of these, conducted at the Christie Hospital in Manchester, England, from 1948 to 1955, patients who received irradiation to the ovaries had significantly fewer recurrences, both local and distant, and showed improved survival at three years of follow-up for all patients [35]. Updates of the same study showed reduction in both local and distant metastases at five and seven years of follow-up and marginally improved survival at five ($p < 0.07$) but not at seven years ($p = 0.14$). Survival at 10 years of follow-up was almost significantly improved ($p = 0.07$) but at 15 years showed only a trend toward improvement [36]. Interpretation of this study is complicated by several factors. First, there has been considerable confusion about the methodology of the randomization used in the trial and hence the degree of protection from bias it provided. It is now understood that during the first years of the trial, randomizations were done by birthdate, but in a blinded fashion so that the proposed allocation could not be known to the participating physician before his/her patient was actually randomized. This method probably provided appropriate randomization with protection from bias. Some of the patients who entered later in the study, however, were randomized by birthdate in an open fashion, so protection from bias was probably not present, at least to the same degree. Because of this, some patients from this study have not been included in the most recent Early Breast Cancer Trialists Collaborative Group (EBCTCG) or Oxford Overview analysis, while those randomized in the first part of the trial in what is believed to be a blinded fashion are included in the analysis [46]. Furthermore, 13% of the women castrated by irradiation in this study resumed menses at some later date [36].

Somewhat later, Nissen-Meyer published results of a small study of stage I premenopausal and stage I and II postmenopausal women randomized to receive either irradiation ovarian castration or no further therapy following treatment of their primary tumor. Peculiarly, these data showed a significant improvement in both overall survival and disease-free survival in postmenopausal women, but only disease-free interval was improved ($p = 0.05$) in the premenopausal group, while significant effects on overall survival in these younger women were not seen [37,38]. The results of this trial have been recently updated [39].

In 1967, a group from Boston published a randomized study of surgical ovarian ablation in pre- and peri- (up to five years post) menopausal women. Once again, the relapse rate was lower and survival higher in the castrated group, but by this analysis, statistical significance was not reached. Only 63 of 159 patients had been followed for a minimum of five years at the time of this report, and survival analysis examined only those 34 patients who had died, thus tending to minimize any survival benefit [45]. The National Surgical Adjuvant Breast Project (NSABP) study of 136 women who received surgical oophorectomy compared to 257 who received placebo or no further therapy showed no significant difference in relapse rate (56% vs. 66%) or in survival (71% vs. 76%) at five years of follow-up [40]. Unfortunately, a number of logistic difficulties have prevented further follow-up, analysis, and independent publication of these data.

Meakin and Hayward randomized 705 patients to receive radiation castration (R), R plus prednisone 7.5 mg for five years (P), or no further therapy (C) after primary treatment for breast cancer [41]. In several publications over the years, they have reported a consistently statistically significant improvement in recurrence-free rate and in overall survival in favor of R + P in premenopausal women over 45 (premenopausal women under 45 were randomized only between C and R). There has also been a trend toward improved survival and reduced relapse rate in premenopausal women over and under 45 who received ovarian irradiation alone (R) [41–43]. As mentioned earlier, prednisone was initially added to these regimens in the belief that it would further reduce estrogen levels by eliminating adrenal production of the precursor hormones that lead to estrogen production in the body. It is still not clearly understood how prednisone works in this setting, but it has been documented that prednisone produces a small objective response rate when given alone in a small proportion of women with metastatic disease [47]. In any case, the addition of prednisone in this randomized study appears to have provided some benefit and was repeated in other regimens of this type.

Bryant and Weir, from the Saskatchewan Cancer Foundation, studied 177 patients randomized to receive surgical ovarian ablation in comparison to 182 controls. These women were either menstruating or showed evidence of ovarian activity based on vaginal cornification indices. Both relapse-free rate ($p < 0.05$) and overall survival ($p < 0.05$) were significantly improved in the castrated group. This effect was most apparent in those women under 50 with 1–3 positive lymph nodes, although women with stage I disease showed a marginal benefit in survival as well ($p = 0.051$). Subsequent analyses from the Saskatchewan Group have shown improved relapse-free and overall survival rates for both stage I and II patients, and although these updated data have been included in the past and recent overviews [10,11,46], they have not as yet been separately published. (personal communication, Dr. A. Bryant and Mrs. J. Krushen).

In addition to these studies, all of which have been published at least once as individual reports, there are three further trials of ovarian or surgical ablation that have now been discovered and examined as a result of the EBCTG or Oxford Overview process. These include an Ontario Cancer Treatment and Research Foundation (OCTRF) study of 332 women randomized to receive or not receive radiation castration [48]; the Centre Regionale Francois Baclesse (CRFB) Caen trial, in which 52 patients were randomized to receive or not receive ovarian ablation with 900 or 1400 rads [49]; and the Bradford Radiation Institute trial, in which 51 patients were randomized to receive or not receive surgical ovarian ablation (personal communication, Richard Gray, Oxford). These trials are all included in the previous [10,11] and most recent [46] Oxford Overview analyses. Many of the above described studies of ovarian ablation have not been published as individual studies in their updated forms, the exceptions being the Meakin and Hayward and Nissen-Meyer studies, which have been updated and published at relatively regular intervals. All of the above studies, however, with the exception of the Nevinny trial, have provided updated information to the Oxford Overview process, and so their most recently available results are included in that analysis [46].

3. Trials of ovarian albation plus chemotherapy versus the same chemotherapy used alone

In addition to the studies of ovarian ablation versus no further systemic therapy, there are at least five trials in which women were randomized to receive ovarian ablation by either surgery or radiation in addition to systemic therapy versus the same systemic therapy used alone (see table 2). These trials in general began somewhat later, and as a result, only two of them have been published in individual form [50,51], although three others have provided updated information to the Oxford Overview process. Ragaz and colleagues

Table 2. Randomized trials of ovarian ablation plus chemotherapy versus chemotherapy alone

Trial	Ovarian treatment	Common systemic therapy	Accrual period	Randomized <50yrs	Randomized >50yrs	Data available	Published [ref]
Bradford RI	Surgery	M + TT	1974–85	38	5	Yes	No
Toronto–Edmonton Study Group	1500 rads +P	CMF[a] (some ± TT)	1978–88	241	56	Yes[b]	No
Ragaz BCCA Vancouver	1600 rads +P	CMF	1979–85	111	23	Yes[b]	Yes [50]
IBCSG/ Ludwig II	Surgery	CMF + P	1978–81	281	75	Yes[b]	Yes [51]
SWOG 7827 B	Surgery	CMFVP	1979–89	262	52	Yes[b]	No
Subtotal:			1974–89	933	211		

[a] First patients were cross-randomized to receive or not receive immunotherapy with oral BCG (Bacillus Calmette-Guerin).
[b] Estrogen receptors available only in these trials.
Abbreviations: RI, Radiotherapy Institute; IBCSG, International Breast Cancer Study Group; BCCA, British Columbia Cancer Agency; SWOG, South West Oncology Group; IT, immunotherapy; C, cyclophosphamide; M, methotrexate; F, 5-fluorouracil; V, vincristine; P, prednisone; TT, thiotepa; yrs, years of age.

from Vancouver randomized 134 women receiving CMF chemotherapy to receive or not receive ovarian ablation given with 1600 rads, plus 7.5 mg of prednisone given for five years. There was also a cross-randomization to receive or not receive postoperative regional radiotherapy. This trial shows no difference in the number of events (recurrence or death) for either therapy [50]. The International Breast Cancer Study Group (IBCSG) (formerly Ludwig Group) randomized 356 premenopausal women with four or more positive axillary nodes who were receiving CMF chemotherapy plus prednisone to receive or not receive surgical ovarian ablation. This trial has reported no advantage for the overall group at a median of 48 months of follow-up [51] and subsequently of 13 years of follow-up [52] from the addition of ovarian ablation in these women. A high incidence of amenorrhea (89%) was seen in the group receiving CMFP alone, suggesting that surgical oophorectomy might therefore be rendered superfluous. An analysis of the ER+ve subset in this IBCSG/Ludwig Trial, however, has shown a trend closely approaching statistically significant improvement in disease-free and overall survival for the group receiving ovarian ablation [52]. Thus, it may be true that in the receptor-positive and therefore more highly hormonally responsive women in this trial, ovarian ablation does add some benefit to CMFP chemotherapy. This possibility remains to be confirmed, however, in a prospective randomized study of this particular group of patients.

In addition to these published studies, three small trials involving 43

Table 3. Randomized trials of medical ovarian ablation

Trial	Ovarian treatment	Coomon systemic therapy	Accrual period	Randomized <50 yrs	Randomized >50 yrs	Data available	Published [ref]
CRC under 50's	Goserelin (Zoladex)	±Tam	1987–SR	972	0	No	No
FNCLCC France	Triptorelen or Goserelin (Zoladex)	FAC or FEC	1989–SR	746	120	No	No
SE Sweden	Goserelin (Zoladex)	±Tam	1989–SR	191	0	No	No
ECOG EST 5188	Goserelin (Zoladex)	FAC ± Tam	1989–94	1382	155	No	No
Subtotal:			1987–	3291	275		

Abbreviations: F, 5-fluorouracil; A, Adriamycin (doxorubicin); SR, Still randomizing patients; FNCLCC, ••; SE, Southeast; ECOG, Eastern Cooperative Oncology Group; EST, ••; C, Cyclophosphamide; E, Epirubicin; ± = randomization; V, vincristine; yrs, years of age; CRC, Cancer Research Campaign; Tam, tamoxifen.

(Bradford RI), 297 (Toronto-Edmonton Breast Cancer Study Group), and 314 (SWOG 7827B) women have been undertaken but not as yet analyszed and published. These studies have provided data to the EBCTCG or Oxford Overview Group, however, and their results are included in that analysis [46].

4. Trials of medical ovarian ablation or suppression

At the time of the 1995 Oxford Overview update [46], four trials in which premenopausal women were randomized to receive or not receive medically induced ovarian suppression were registered (see table 3). There were no data available for the 1995 Overview analysis from any of these trials, and no results have as yet been published. These studies include a Cancer Research Campaign (CRC) trial in which women under 50 are randomized to receive or not receive therapy with goserelin (Zoladex) with a cross-randomization to receive or not receive tamoxifen. Nine hundred and seventy-two women, many of whom were receiving or had received various types of adjuvant chemotherapy, have been randomized as part of this study, which began in 1987 and is still ongoing. The second trial is the Fédération Nationale d'Centres d'Lutte Contre Le Cancer of France (FNCLCC) trial in which women, in addition to receiving chemotherapy with FAC (5-FU, Adriamycin, and Cyclophosphamide), were randomized to receive or not receive triptorelen or goserelin (Zoladex). Nine hundred and ninety-six women have been randomized to this study, which began in 1989. Randomization is still ongoing. A third study, the Southeast Sweden trial, has cross-randomized 191 women since 1989 to receive or not receive goserelin and also to receive or not receive tamoxifen.

Randomization is still ongoing. The Eastern Cooperative Oncology Group (ECOG) completed a fourth study, their EST 5188 trial, in 1994. In that study, 1535 premenopausal women receiving FAC chemotherapy were randomized to receive or not receive tamoxifen and were also cross-randomized to receive or not receive goserelin (Zoladex). No results are as yet available.

5. Early breast cancer Trialists' collaborative group (EBCTCG) or oxford overview of ovarian ablation in early breast cancer: the 1995 update

In 1995, the Early Breast Cancer Trialists' Collaborative Group based in Oxford sought information on each patient in any randomized trial of ovarian ablation or suppression versus control that had begun before 1990, for the purpose of an updated overview or meta-analysis. Data were available for 12 of the 13 known studies assessing ovarian ablation by radiation or surgery, but not for any of the four known studies assessing ovarian suppression by drugs, all of which began after 1980. Because menopausal status was not consistently defined across these trials, the 1995 Oxford Overview main analysis has been carried out in women under 50, as was done in past years [10,11]. While the Overview attempted to analyze results according to estrogen receptors, these measurements were only available in the later trials, namely, those of ovarian ablation plus chemotherapy versus the same chemotherapy alone.

5.1. Effects in women under 50

The 1995 Overview analysis [46] reports the results from 2102 women aged less than 50 when randomized. At the time of the 1995 analysis, there had been 1130 deaths and an additional 153 recurrences in these women. The analysis shows that 15-year recurrence-free survival was highly significantly improved among those allocated to ovarian ablation (45.0% vs. 39.0%; difference = 6% ± standard deviation [SD] = 2.3; $p = 0.0007$; see figure 1). Overall survival was also significantly improved (52.4% vs. 46.1%; difference = 6.3 ± SD = 2.3; $p = 0.001$; see figure 2). The numbers of events in the study, although large, are too small for really reliable subgroup analyses.

Attempts to analyze the results in node-negative versus node-positive women in the Overview are heavily confounded by the fact that almost all the node-negative women were entered into trials of ovarian ablation versus no therapy, whereas almost all the node-positive women were entered into trials of chemotherapy plus ovarian ablation versus the same chemotherapy given alone. Thus, the relative effectiveness of ovarian ablation with respect to nodal status could only be assessed in the overview in ovarian ablation trials in which chemotherapy was not given. In the trials of ovarian ablation alone versus no other systemic therapy, proportional risk reductions for node-positive and for node-negative women appeared similar, while the absolute risk reduction was nonsignificantly greater for node-positive women. For both recurrence and survival, there was a significant improvement within both node-negative ($p = 0.01$ for recurrence; $p = 0.01$ for survival) and node-positive ($p = 0.0002$ for recurrence; $p = 0.0007$ for survival) subgroups of women receiving ovarian ablation (see figures 3 and 4).

Estrogen-receptor measurements on the primary tumor were available for 4 of 5 trials in which women were randomized to receive chemotherapy plus ovarian ablation versus the same chemotherapy used alone. Among the 194 women with ER-poor primary tumors, there was no apparent benefit to the addition of ovarian ablation in terms of recurrence-free or overall survival. Among the 550 women with ER+ve primary tumors, however, the addition of ovarian ablation appeared beneficial both for recurrence-free survival (odds reduction = 13%, ±SD = 11; nonsignificant [NS]) and for overall survival (odds reduction 17%, ±SD = 13; NS), but these differences were not statistically significant.

Analyses were done to examine the degree of benefit provided by ovarian ablation added to cytotoxic chemotherapy, in comparison to its benefit when given in the absence of cytotoxic chemotherapy. The proportional improvement in annual odds of recurrence in women in the absence of chemotherapy was 25% ± SD = 7; $p = 0.0005$, while the proportional improvement in annual odds of recurrence in the presence of chemotherapy was only 10% ± SD = 9; $p > 0.1$, NS (see figure 5). Similarly, the proportional improvement in annual odds of death was 24% ± SD = 7; $p = 0.0006$ in the absence of chemotherapy, but only 8% ± SD = 10; $p > 0.1$; NS in the presence of chemotherapy (see figure 6). Because of the small numbers of deaths, however, it is difficult to tell whether these differences are actually reliable.

5.2. Effects in women over 50

In the 1995 Overview analysis, data were available on 1354 women aged 50 or over who were randomized to receive or not receive ovarian ablation. Most of these would have been perimenopausal or postmenopausal. There was only a small and nonsignificant improvement in survival and in recurrence-free survival in this subset. By year 15 after randomization, there were 3.1 (±SD = 2.6; NS) fewer recurrences or deaths per 100 women allocated to ovarian ablation. There were 32% alive without recurrence in the ovarian ablation group versus 28.9% in the controls (NS) and 36.9% alive overall in the ovarian ablation group versus 34.5% of controls (NS).

5.3. Late effects and effects on non-breast cancer deaths

The late effects of ovarian ablation can be clearly examined in this Overview analysis. Most of the patients in these trials were randomized before 1970, and for most survivors there is follow-up information going beyond 1990. Thus, there is a large amount of information beyond year 15. Even during this later time period, the annual death rates for all women in the Overview remain

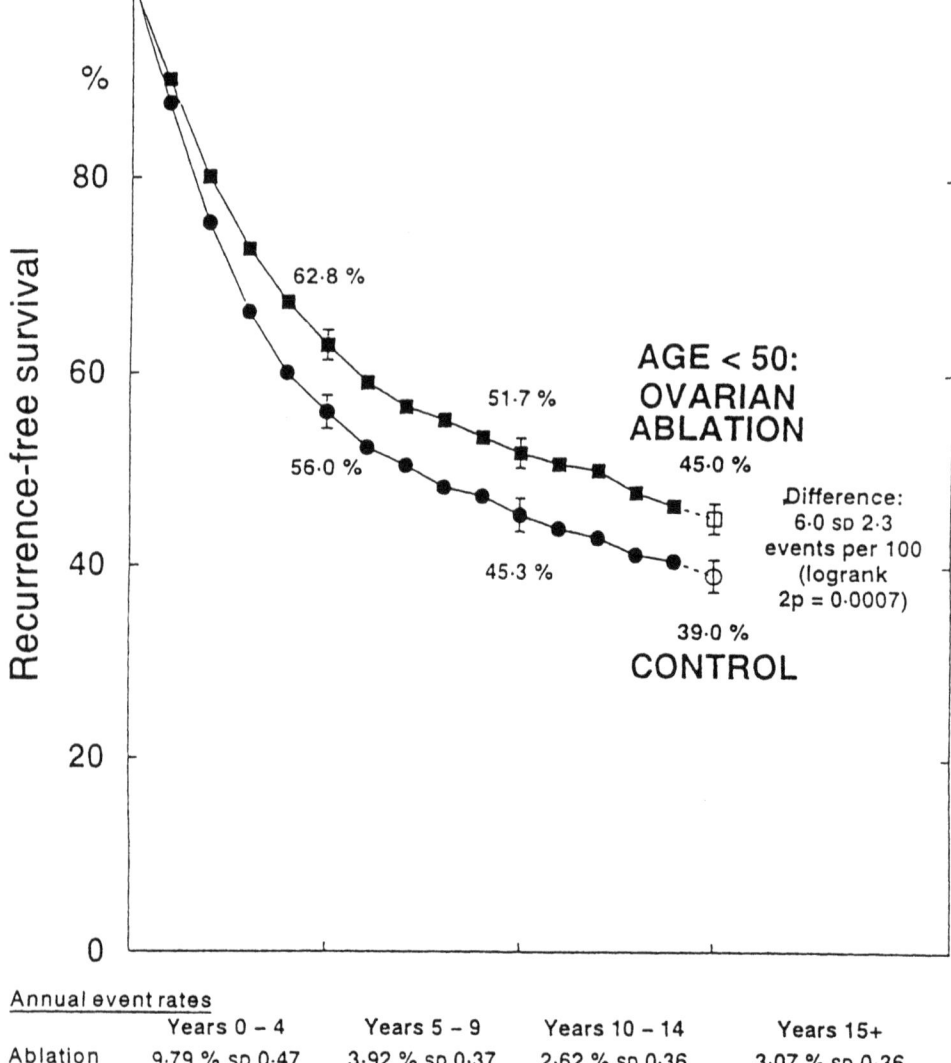

Figures 1 and 2. **Absolute effects of ovarian ablation in all trials combined among women aged under 50 at entry.** Recurrence-free survival (figure 1) and overall survival (figure 2) for 2102 women aged under 50 when randomized between ovarian ablation (squares) and control (circles). Bars indicate standard deviations (SD).

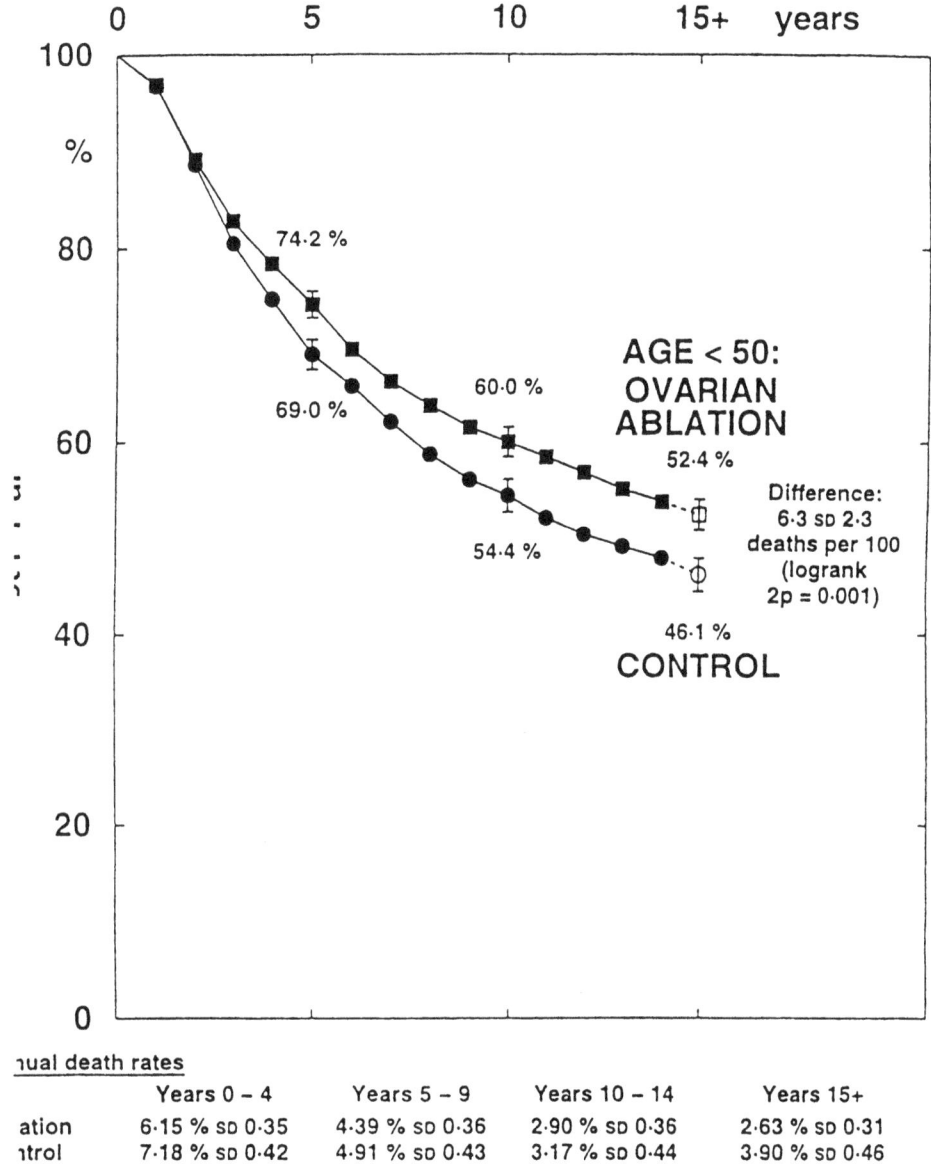

ual death rates	Years 0 – 4	Years 5 – 9	Years 10 – 14	Years 15+
ation	6·15 % SD 0·35	4·39 % SD 0·36	2·90 % SD 0·36	2·63 % SD 0·31
itrol	7·18 % SD 0·42	4·91 % SD 0·43	3·17 % SD 0·44	3·90 % SD 0·46

Figure 2

lower among those who were originally allocated to ovarian ablation (2.6% ± SD = 0.3) than among the controls (3.9% ± SD = 0.5). Thus, the effects of ovarian ablation appear to persist long after the women received this maneuver.

The Overview also attempted to study information on cause-specific mor-

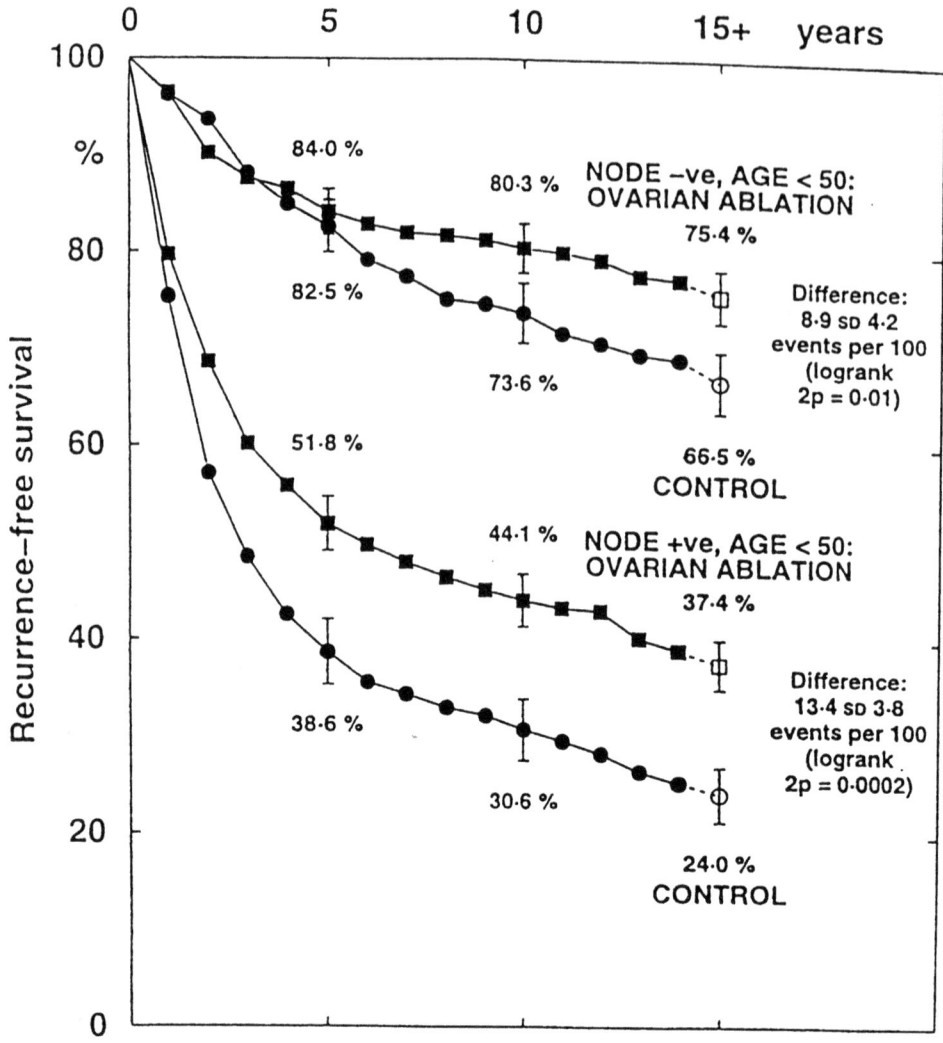

Figures 3 and 4. **Absolute effects of ovarian ablation in the absence of routine chemotherapy in all trials combined among women aged under 50 at entry.** Recurrence-free survival (figure 3) and overall survival (figure 4) for 473 node-negative and 696 node-positive women who were aged under 50 when randomized between ovarian ablation (squares) and control (circles) in the trials, or parts of trials, where cytotoxic therapy was not routinely used. Among node-negative women, in years 0–4 there were 28 deaths out of 1170 person-years in the ablation group versus 25 of 1037 in the controls (annual death rates: 2.4% SD 0.5 versus 2.4% SD 0.5); in years 5–9, there were 15 of 1030 versus 21 of 884 (1.5% SD 0.4 versus 2.4% SD 0.5); in years 10–14, there were 12 of 931 versus 15 of 779 (1.3% SD 0.4 versus 1.9% SD 0.5); and in years 15+ there were 33 of 1580 versus 43 of 1309 (2.1% SD 0.4 versus 3.3% SD 0.5). Among node-positive women, the corresponding values are years 0–4, 166 of 1620 versus 134 of 997 (10.3% SD 0.8 versus 13.4% SD 1.2); years 5–9, 55 of 1077 versus 37 of 577 (5.1% SD 0.7 versus 6.4% SD 1.1); years 10–14, 29 of 870 versus 23 of 426 (3.3% SD 0.6 versus 5.4% SD 1.1); and years 15+, 40 of 1151 versus 28 of 491 (3.5% SD 0.6 versus 5.7% SD 1.1). Format as in figure 1.

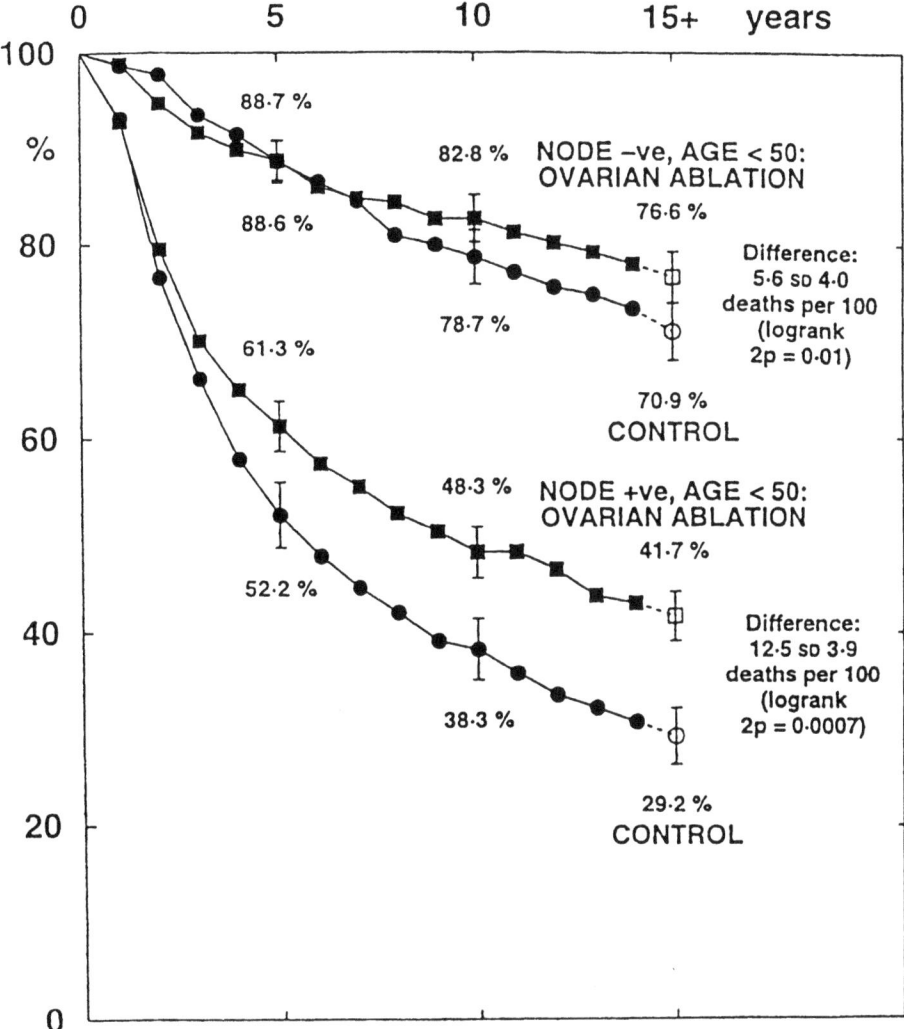

Figure 4

tality. Among women under 50 who died without any record of distant recurrence of their breast cancer, 116 were classified as having died of non-breast cancer causes. Taking into account the fact that those allocated ovarian ablation survived longer and were therefore at more prolonged risk of death from other causes, there was then no significant difference between the treatment groups in vascular deaths (22 of 922 in the ovarian ablation group vs. 20 of 824 in the controls) in trials for which data were provided. Similarly, there was no difference in non-breast cancer, nonvascular deaths (44 of 929 vs. 30 of 824), or in all non-breast cancer deaths.

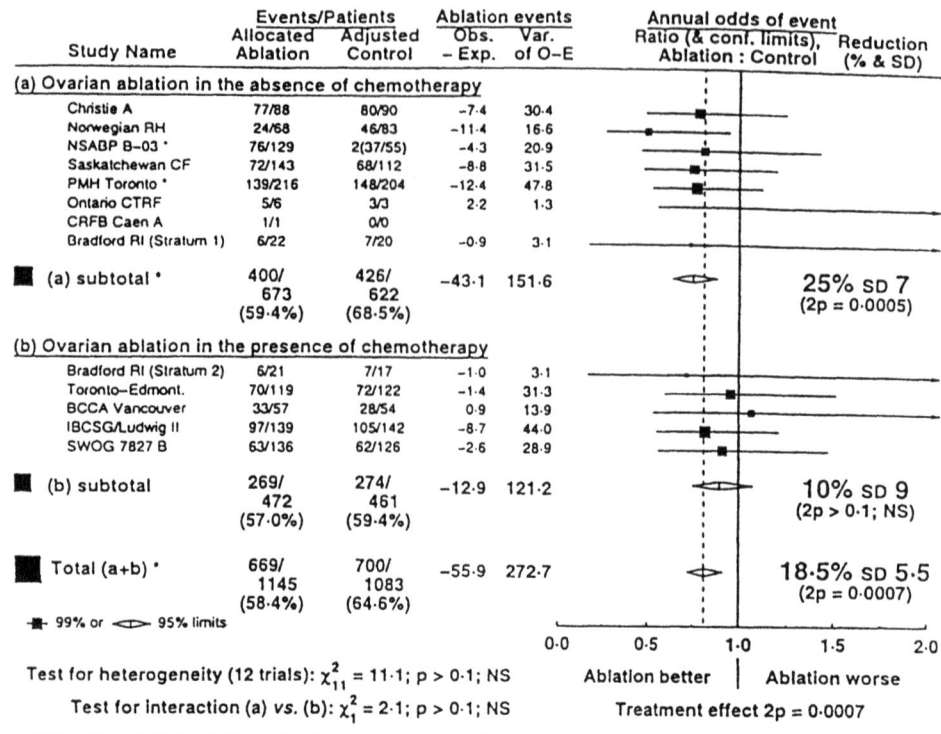

Figures 5 and 6. Proportional effects of ovarian ablation in each trial and overall, with subdivisions by absence or presence of chemotherapy, among women aged under 50 at entry. Recurrence-free survival (figure 5) and overall survival (figure 6) for women aged under 50 when randomized, with subtotals for strata in the absence and in the presence of routine cytotoxic chemotherapy. Each trial, or part of a trial, is described by a single line of information, showing the numbers of events and patients and summary logrank statistics. For each of these strata, the ratio of the annual event rate in the ovarian ablation group to that in the control group (the odds ratio) is plotted as a solid square, with the 99% confidence interval shown. For the subtotals and total, the 95% confidence interval is represented by a diamond. The solid vertical line indicates an odds ratio of 1.0 (i.e., no difference between ovarian ablation and control), whereas the broken vertical line indicates the 'typical odds ratio' in the total of all these trial results. For balance, control patients in the 2:1 randomizations (i.e., NSABP and part of PMH) are counted twice in the adjusted control totals but not in the statistical calculations.

5.4. Second breast primaries

An attempt was made to look at the incidence of contralateral breast cancer, but there was not enough information to examine this issue. Only 30 contralateral breast cancers were recorded as the first event among 712 women allocated to ovarian ablation, compared to 32 of 679 women in the control arm in trials for which data were provided.

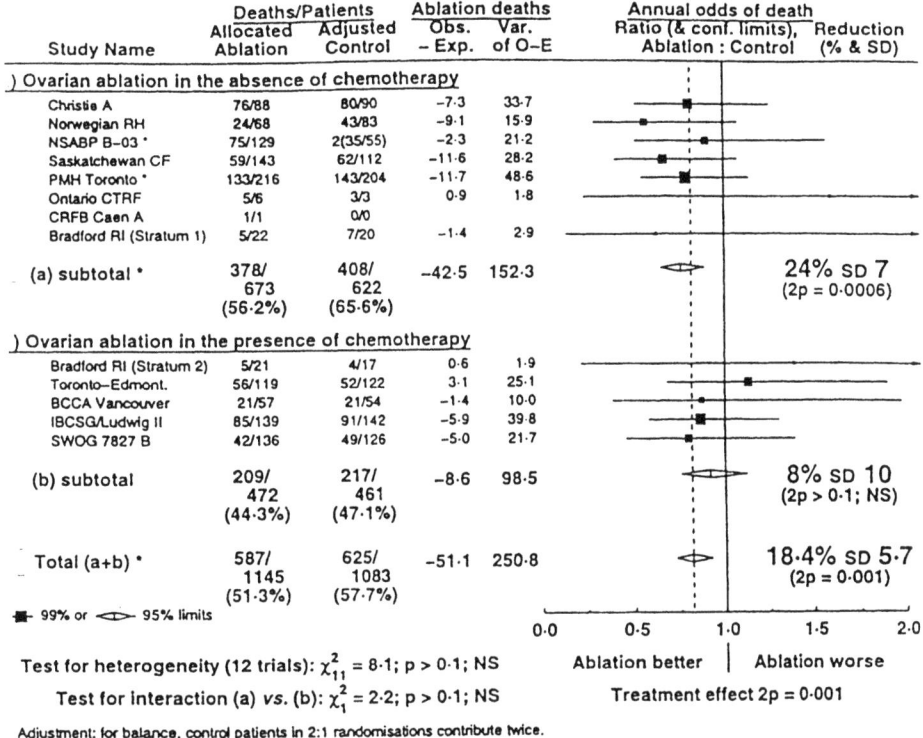

Figure 6

5.5. 1995 overview: summary

In summary, the Overview confirms suggestions from individual trials that ovarian ablation in premenopausal women provides a small but statistically significant benefit in terms of recurrence-free and overall survival. This benefit appears similar for node-positive and node-negative women. There appears to be some degree of benefit both in the presence and in the absence of chemotherapy. The degree of benefit appears larger when ovarian ablation is given in the absence rather than in the presence of chemotherapy, but this appearance is not confirmed by formal statistical testing (test of heterogeneity = NS). From the few trials for which estrogen receptor measurements are available, the effect of ovarian ablation appears significant in those women with estrogen receptor in their tumors and not significant in those without it. The numbers available to examine this issue are very small, however. Similarly, it is difficult to draw firm conclusions regarding non-breast cancer deaths, or regarding the incidence of second primary breast cancers. There is no obvious difference in the incidence of noncancer deaths in those randomized to ovarian ablation, however.

6. Relationship between response to chemotherapy and amenorrhea in randomized trials in premenopausal women

The results outlined above, particularly those of the Oxford Overview, suggest that ovarian ablation may not be as effective when it is added to chemotherapy as it is when given alone. An obvious explanation of this outcome could involve the degree of ovarian suppression provided by chemotherapy. A number of investigators have attempted to examine this issue, with conflicting results. Unfortunately, many trials of chemotherapy do not provide information concerning the proportion of women who become amenorrheic, or if they do, do not provide long-term follow up on how many of these women remain permanently amenorrheic and how many resume normal menstrual function. Furthermore, it is not clear how closely amenorrhea mirrors a complete lack of ovarian function. It is possible that some ovarian function may persist even in the absence of regular menses, but this possibility has not been well studied. The incidence of amenorrhea has been reported from several trials of cytotoxic chemotherapy in premenopausal women and ranges from 40% to 90% [51,53–58]. Several investigators have attempted to examine whether chemotherapy acts through ovarian ablation in their trials, by attempting to correlate the effectiveness of chemotherapy with amneorrhea in women within each randomized trial. Three investigators have found that women who develop amenorrhea have a longer disease-free and/or overall survival [53–55], but three others have not found this relationship [56–58]. These conflicting data suggests that while more investigation is required, part of the explanation for the better effects of cytotoxic chemotherapy in younger or premenopausal women may be that a medical castration is achieved in many of these women [53–55]. Clearly, however, this effect does not explain the entire action of cytotoxic chemotherapy in this setting [56–58]. Thus, it is probable that the results of the Oxford Overview, in which ovarian ablation does not appear to add as much benefit in women who are also receiving cytotoxic chemotherapy, may relate to the fact that the cytotoxic chemotherapy is already achieving castration in even the non-ovarian ablation control group in these trials.

7. Comparability of ovarian ablation to chemotherapy

Very few studies exist comparing chemotherapy directly to ovarian ablation. One small study by the Scottish Cancer Trials Breast Group [59] compared adjuvant ovarian ablation to CMF (cyclophosphamide, methotrexate, and 5-FU) in premenopausal women with pathological stage II breast cancer. In this group, ovarian ablation was comparable in its effects to CMF in terms of both disease-free and overall survival for the entire group of women randomized. When the patients were divided into ER+ve and ER−ve groups, however, it seemed that ovarian ablation produced a substantially better effect in women with ER+ve tumors, while chemotherapy produced a substantially better effect in women with ER−ve disease. It is worth noting that the CMF given in this study was not particularly dose intensive and that more aggressive or intensive types of chemotherapy, such as the classic Bonnadonna regimen [5] given in full doses or the newly reported CEF (cyclophosphamide, epirubicin, and 5-FU) regimen, which appears superior to classic Bonnadonna CMF [60], may provide more substantial effects and thus presumably be superior to ovarian ablation used alone. This sort of indirect conclusion is somewhat unsatisfactory, however, and it is to be hoped that more direct comparisons of ovarian ablation and chemotherapy will be carried out in the future in order to further delineate their relative roles in premenopausal women.

8. Equivalence of ovarian medical suppression and surgical or radiation ovarian ablation

Although a number of the newer trials outlined above are now substituting medical ovarian ablation for radiation or surgical ablation, the equivalence of this treatment or indeed the equivalence of ovarian ablation by surgery and by radiation is unclear.

Ovarian irradiation has been assumed to produce an effect similar to that of surgical oophorectomy. Considerable data, however, suggest that, following ovarian irradiation, depending on the dose, dose schedule, and age of the patient, ovarian function may not be totally destroyed. For example, in the study of Nissen-Meyer and others, 13% of the women castrated by irradiation resumed menses at some later date [38]. Similarly, Meakin and others found that 3.3% of women receiving 2000 rads to the ovaries in five fractions resumed menstruation over subsequent years. An even higher percent of those under 45 at the time of therapy resumed menstruation (7%) [41]. Thus, ovarian irradiation may not produce the complete and permanent ablation that is presumably achieved by surgery. In spite of this, there seems no obvious difference between the results of ovarian ablation and surgical ablation in the various trials or in the Oxford Overview analysis.

Similarly, medical ablation with drugs such as Zoladex is in some ways assumed to be equivalent to surgical oophorectomy. In ongoing adjuvant trials, however, the LHRH analogues are given for periods of time that range from 2 to 5 years. In none are they given permanently. Depending on the age of the patients involved, five years of an LHRH analogue may take the patients through the time when they would normally reach a physiologic menopause in any case. In younger women, however, the discontinuation of the LHRH analogue would usually lead to resumed ovarian function, since the endocrine effects of these analogues are reversible, with the return of menses usually occurring within 1–2 months after discontinuation of therapy [61]. The importance of the length and completeness of ovarian ablation in this setting has not been studied and remains to be established. However, the LHRH agonist, goserelin (Zoladex), has been shown to suppress ovarian function and to produce clinical responses, in premenopausal and perimenopausal women with advanced breast cancer, that are comparable to those previously reported for other hormonal therapies [62–65]. One large randomized study [65a] has shown Zoladex to be equivalent to ovarian ablation in the metastatic setting. Thus, it seems likely that an LHRH analogue produces the same effects as surgical or radiation ovarian ablation on all body systems and on any remaining breast cancer cells, at least while it is being given. Presumably, however, the length of the ovarian suppression will affect its efficacy as adjuvant therapy, perhaps in a similar way to the effects demonstrated with varying lengths of tamoxifen [66,67]. The relative importance of length of treatment in this setting has been poorly studied to date and remains to be clarified in future trials.

9. Effects of ovarian ablation on other body systems

It is well recognized that premature ovarian ablation can have deleterious effects on the cardiovascular and skeletal systems [68,69]. Whether this finding assumes a major role in terms of competing risks of death in comparison to the risk of dying from breast cancer has not been clearly established, however, Certainly the most updated information from the Oxford Overview does not suggest any strong trend toward increased cardiac or non-breast cancer deaths in the women randomized to receive ovarian ablation. The difficulty of establishing cause of death, particularly in a meta-analysis setting in which information is obtained retrospectively from multiple centers, may obscure a relatively small or even moderately large effect on deaths from other causes, however. Alternatively, the competing risk of death from breast cancer may be so high that it greatly outweighs any effect on deaths from other causes. In particular, deaths related to reduced osteoporosis will not be as frequent as those from breast cancer, nor will they occur until the patients have had 20–30 years of follow-up after ovarian ablation. Cardiac deaths, being both more common and occurring at younger ages, may be of greater concern, but to date this has not been demonstrated in any individual study nor in the Overview Analysis. Further data concerning these long-term risks of death remain to be accumulated.

10. Conclusions and future directions

It seems clear that ovarian ablation has a small but significant effect on disease-free and overall survival in premenopausal women, particularly those with positive estrogen receptors. This effect appears significant and fairly similar in both node-positive and node-negative women, although it appears to have a greater absolute effect in those with positive nodes. The effect appears more dramatic when ovarian ablation is used alone than when it is given in the presence of cytotoxic chemotherapy. The indirect comparisons of treatment effects in different circumstances (that is, node negative versus node positive, or ovarian ablation in the presence versus in the absence of chemotherapy), however, are to be interpreted with more caution than the results obtained from direct comparisons within each randomized trial and from the summaries of those direct comparisons obtained in the Overview. Much additional follow-up information will be available on each of these individual trials over the next 5–10 years and for the next cycle of the Overview, which will occur in the year 2000. For example, one Chinese trial of ovarian ablation that began in 1991 has already randomized more than 3000 premenopausal women. In addition, there are over 3000 women in the recent trials of ovarian suppression with LHRH agonists. As well, a large study comparing tamoxifen plus ovarian ablation as adjuvant therapy versus tamoxifen plus ovarian ablation at the time of recurrence is now taking place in Vietnam (personal communication, Dr. Richard Love, Madison, WI). These trials will add considerable additional information to that which is already available.

It would still be useful, however, to undertake further large randomized trials assessing the additional effects of ovarian ablation in the presence of cytotoxic chemotherapy as well as the additional effects of cytotoxic chemotherapy in the presence of ovarian ablation, and to further assess the effects of both or either of these modalities in the presence of prolonged tamoxifen therapy. Such trials could be designed as three-way comparisons of ovarian ablation versus cytotoxic chemotherapy versus both, which would add data in each of the areas one might wish to further examine. Until further information becomes available, however, it would seem that there is enough information to conclude that ovarian ablation is useful in premenopausal women with positive estrogen receptors, producing effects comparable to those of CMF-type chemotherapy in that setting. Although there is a far larger body of data establishing the role of CMF or comparable types of chemotherapy in the premenopausal setting, certainly enough data exist to suggest that ovarian ablation might be used as an alternative in ER+ve women for whom chemotherapy is either unacceptable or unsuitable for whatever reasons. In the meantime, one must await further data before recommending ovarian ablation as a routine alternative to chemotherapy in any group of premenopausal women and before recommending it for routine addition to chemotherapy in that setting.

References

1. Beatson GT. 1896. On the treatment of inoperable cases of carcinoma of the mamma: suggestions for a new method of treatment with illustrative cases. Lancet 2:104–107.
2. Schinzinger A. 1889. Ueber carcinoma mammae. Verh Dtsch Ges Chir 18:28–29.
3. Taylor GW. 1934. Artificial menopause in carcinoma of the breast. N Engl J Med 211:1138–1140.

4. Fisher B, Carbone P, Economou SG, Frelick R, Glass A, Lerner H, Redmond C, Zelen M, Band P, Katrych DL, Wolmark N, Fisher ER. 1975. L-phenylalanine mustard (L-PAM) in the management of primary breast cancer: a report of early findings. N Engl J Med 292:117–122.
5. Bonadonna G, Brusamolino E, Valagussa P, Rossi A, Brugnatelli L, Brambilla C, De Lena M, Tancini G, Bajetta E, Musumeci R, Veronesi U. 1976. Combination chemotherapy as an adjuvant treatment in operable breast cancer. N Engl J Med 294:405–410.
6. Holland JF. 1976. Major advance in breast cancer therapy. N Engl J Med 294:440–441.
7. Legha SS, Carter SK. 1976. Antiestrogens in the treatment of breast cancer. Cancer Treat Rev 3:205–216.
8. Legha SS, Davis HLJ, Muggia FM. 1978. Hormonal therapy of breast cancer: new approaches and concepts. Ann Intern Med 88:69–77.
9. Santen RJ, Samojik E, Lipton A, Harvey H, Ruby EB, Wells SA, Kendall J. 1977. Kinetic, hormonal and clinical studies with aminoglutethimide in breast cancer. Cancer 39:2948–2958.
10. Early Breast Cancer Trialists' Collaborative Group. 1990. Treatment of Early Breast Cancer. 1: Worldwide Evidence 1985–1990. A Systematic Overview of All Available Randomized Trials of Adjuvant Endocrine and Cytotoxic Therapy. Oxford: Oxford University Press.
11. Early Breast Cancer Trialists' Collaborative Group. 1992. Systemic treatment of early breast cancer by hormonal, cytotoxic, or immune therapy. Lancet 339:71–85.
12. Pritchard KI. 1992. Ovarian ablation as adjuvant therapy for premenopausal women with early breast cancer: phoenix arisen? (Editorial.) Lancet 339:95–96.
13. Kennedy BJ, Fortuny IE. 1964. Therapeutic castration in the treatment of advanced breast cancer. Cancer 17:1197–1202.
14. Stoll BA. 1969. Hormonal Management in Breast Cancer. London: Pitman, p. 3.
15. Welbourn RB, Burn JI. 1972. Treatment of advanced mammary cancer. N Engl J Med 287:398–400.
16. Osborne CK, Yochmowitz MG, Knight WA, McGuire WL. 1980. The value of estrogen and progesterone receptors in the treatment of breast cancer. Cancer 46:2884–2888.
17. Bloom ND, Tobin EH, Schreibman B, Degenshein GA. 1980. The role of progesterone receptors in the management of advanced breast cancer. Cancer 45:2972–2977.
18. Leclercq G, Heuson JC. 1977. Therapeutic significance of sex-steroid hormone receptors in the treatment of breast cancer. Eur J Cancer 13:1205–1215.
19. Allegra JC, Barlock A, Huff KK, Lippman ME. 1980. Changes in multiple or sequential estrogen receptor determinations in breast cancer. Cancer 45:792–794.
20. Horsley JS. 1944. Bilateral oophorectomy with radical operation for cancer of the breast. Surgery 15:590–601.
21. Adair FE, Treves N, Farrow JH, Scharnagel IM. 1945. Clinical effects of surgical and x-ray castration in mammary cancer. JAMA 128:161–167.
22. Horsley GW. 1951. Carcinoma of the breast: radical mastectomy, oophorectomy and hormone therapy. Virginia Med Monthly 78:226–231.
23. Horsley GW. 1947. Treatment of cancer of the breast in premenopausal patients with radical amputation and bilateral oophorectomy. Ann Surg 125:703–711.
24. Siegert A. 1952. Kastration and mamma-ca. Strahlentherapie 87:62–64.
25. Smith GV, Smith OW. 1953. Carcinoma of the breast. Results, evaluation of x-irradiation, and relation of age and surgical castration to length of survival. Surg Gynecol Obstet 97:508–516.
26. Rosenberg MF, Uhlmann EM. 1959. Prophylactic castration in carcinoma of the breast. Arch Surg 78:376–379.
27. Treves N. 1957. An evaluation of prophylactic castration in the treatment of mammary carcinoma. Cancer 10:393–407.
28. Mantel N. 1966. Evaluation of survival data and two new rank order statistics arising in its consideration. Cancer Chemother Rep 50:163–170.
29. Fisher B, Slack NH. 1970. Number of lymph nodes examined and the prognosis of breast carcinoma. Surg Gynecol Obstet 131:79–88.
30. McWhirter R. 1956. Some factors influencing prognosis in breast cancer. J Fac Radiol Lond 8:220–234.

31. Huck P. 1952. Artificial menopause as an adjunct to radical treatment of breast cancer. NZ Med J 51:364–367.
32. Kennedy BJ, Mielke PW, Fortuny IE. 1964. Therapeutic castration versus prophylactic castration in breast cancer. Surg Gynecol Obstet 118:524–540.
33. Alrich EM, Liddle HV, Morton CB. 1957. Carcinoma of the breast: results of surgical treatment: some anatomic and endocrine consideration. Ann Surg 145:779–806.
34. Rennaes S. 1960. Prophylactic ovarian irradiation. Acta Chir Scand 266:85–90.
35. Paterson R, Russell MH. 1959. Clinical trials in malignant disease. Part II — Breast cancer: value of irradiation of the ovaries. J Faculty Radiologists 10:130–133.
36. Cole MP. 1975. A clinical trial of an artificial menopause in carcinoma of the breast. In Namer M, Lalanne CM, eds. Hormones and Breast Cancer. Paris: INSERM, pp. 143–150.
37. Nissen-Meyer R. 1967. The role of prophylactic castration in the therapy of human mammary cancer. Eur J Cancer 3:395–403.
38. Nissen-Meyer R. 1975. Ovarian suppression and its supplement by additive hormonal treatment. In Namer M, Lalanne CM, eds. Hormones and Breast Cancer. Paris: INSERM, pp. 151–158.
39. Nissen-Meyer R. 1991. Primary breast cancer: the effects of primary ovarian ablation. Ann Oncol 2:343–346.
40. Ravdin RG, Lewison EF, Slack NH, Gardner B, State D, Fisher B. 1970. Results of a clinical trial concerning the worth of prophylactic oophorectomy for breast carcinoma. Surg Gynecol Obstet 131:1055–1064.
41. Meakin JW, Allt WEC, Beale FA, et al. 1979. Ovarian irradiation and prednisone therapy following surgery and radiotherapy for carcinoma of the breast. Can Med Assoc J 19:1221–1238.
42. Meakin JW, Allt WEC, Beale FA, et al. 1983. Ovarian irradiation and prednisone following surgery and radiotherapy for carcinoma of the breast. Breast Cancer Res Treat 3:45–48.
43. Meakin JW, Hayward JL, Panzarella T, et al. 1996. Ovarian irradiation and prednisone therapy following surgery and radiotherapy for carcinoma of the breast. Breast Cancer Res Treat 37:11–19.
44. Bryant AJS, Weir JA. 1981. Prophylactic oophorectomy in operable instances of carcinoma of the breast. Surg Gynecol Obstet 153:660–664.
45. Nevinny HB, Nevinny D, Roscoff CB, Hall TC, Muench H. 1969. Prophylactic oophorectomy in breast cancer therapy. Am J Surg 117:531–536.
46. Early Breast Cancer Trialists' Collaborative Group. In press. Ovarian ablation in early breast cancer: an overview of the randomized trials. Lancet.
47. Stuart-Harris RC, Smith IE. 1984. Aminoglutethimide in the treatment of advanced breast cancer. Cancer Treat Rev 2:189–204.
48. Clarke EA, Fetterly JC, Ryan NC. 1990. The Ontario Cancer Treatment and Research Foundation clinical trial on the comparative effect of ovarian irradiation in carcinoma of the breast in the postmenopausal patient. In Early Breast Cancer Trialists' Collaborative Group, ed. Treatment of Early Breast Cancer 1: Worldwide Evidence 1985–1990. A Systematic Overview of All Available Randomized Trials of Adjuvant Endocrine and Cytoxic Therapy. Oxford: Oxford University Press, p. 106.
49. Delozier T, Juret P, Couette JE, Mace-Lesech J. 1990. Ovarian irradiation in postmenopausal women with breast cancer and positive axillary nodes. In Early Breast Cancer Trialists' Collaborative Group, ed. Treatment of Early Breast Cancer. 1: Worldwide Evidence 1985–1990. A Systematic Overview of All Available Randomized Trials of Adjuvant Endocrine and Cytoxic Therapy. Oxford: Oxford University Press, p. 114.
50. Ragaz J, Jackson S, Nilson K, Plenderleith IH, Knowling M, Basco V, Ng V. 1988. Randomized study of locoregional radiotherapy and ovarian ablation in premenopausal patients with breast cancer treated with adjuvant chemotherapy (abstract). Proc Am Soc Clin Oncol 7:12.
51. Ludwig Breast Cancer Study Group. 1985. Chemotherapy with or without oophorectomy in high risk premenopausal patients with operable breast cancer. J Clin Oncol 13:1059–1067.
52. Castiglione-Gertsch M, Johnsen C, Goldhirsch A. 1994. The International (Ludwig) Breast Cancer Study Group Trials I–IV: 15 years follow up. Ann Oncol 5:717–724.

53. Howell A, George WD, Crowther D, Bush H, Howat JM, Sellwood RA, Rubens RD, Hayward JL, Bulbrook RD, Fentiman IS. 1984. Controlled trial of adjuvant chemotherapy with cyclophosphamide, methotrexate and fluorouracil for breast cancer. Lancet 2:307–311.
54. Pourquier H. 1981. The results of adjuvant chemotherapy are predominantly caused by the hormonal changes such therapy induces. In Van Scoy-Moscher MB, ed. Medical Oncology. Controversies in Cancer Treatment. Boston: Hall, pp. 83–89.
55. Ludwig Breast Cancer Study Group. 1985. Adjuvant combination chemotherapy with or without prednisone in premenopausal breast cancer patients with metastases in 1 to 3 axillary lymph nodes: a randomized trial. Cancer Res 45: 4454–4459.
56. Bonadonna G, Valagussa P, DePalo G. 1981. The results of adjuvant chemotherapy are predominantly caused by the hormonal changes such therapy induces. In Van Scoy-Moscher MB, ed. Medical Oncology. Controversies in Cancer Treatment. Boston: Hall, pp. 100–109.
57. Fisher B, Sherman B, Rockette H, Redmond C, Margolese R, Fisher ER. 1979. L-phenylalanine mustard (L-PAM) in the management of premenopausal patients with primary breast cancer: lack of association of disease-free survival with depression of ovarian function. Cancer 44:847–857.
58. Rubens RD, Knight RK, Fentiman IS, Hayward JL, Bulbrook RD, Chaudary M, Howell A, Bush H, Crowther D, Sellwood RA, George WD, Howat JM. 1983. Controlled trial of adjuvant chemotherapy with melphalan for breast cancer. Lancet 1:839–843.
59. Scottish Cancer Trials Breast Group. 1993. Adjuvant ovarian ablation versus CMF chemotherapy in premenopausal women with pathological stage II breast carcinoma: the Scottish trial. Lancet 341:1293–1298.
60. Levine M, Bramwell V, Bowman D, et al. 1995. A clinical trial of intensive CEF versus CMF in premenopausal women with node positive breast cancer (abstract). Proc 31st Annu Meeting Am Soc Clin Oncol 14:103.
61. West CP, Baird DT. 1987. Suppression of ovarian activity by Zoladex depot (ICI 118 630), a long acting luteinizing hormone releasing hormone agonist analogue. Clin Endocrinol 26:213–220.
62. Kaufmann M, Jonat W, Kleeberg UR. 1989. Goserelin, a depot gonadotropin-releasing hormone agonist in the treatment of premenopausal patients with metastatic breast cancer. J Clin Oncol 7:1113–1119.
63. Kaufmann M, Jonat W, Schachner-Wunschmann E. 1991. The depot GnRH analogue goserelin in the treatment of premenopausal patients with metastatic breast cancer — a 5 year experience and further endocrine therapies. Onkologie 14:22–30.
64. Blamey RW, Jonat W, Kaufmann M. 1992. Goserelin depot in the treatment of premenopausal advanced breast cancer. Eur J Cancer 28A:810–814.
65a. Taylor CW, Green S, Dalton WS, Martino S, Ingle JN, Robert NJ, Rector DJ, Osborne CK, 1995. Participating investigators of the Southwest Oncology Group, North Central Cancer Treatment Group and Eastern Cooperative Oncology Group. A multicentered randomized trial of Zoladex versus surgical oophorectomy in premenopausal patients with receptor positive metastatic breast cancer. Breast Cancer Res. Treat 37:31.
65. Blamey RW, Jonat W, Kaufmann M. 1993. Survival data relation to the use of goserelin depot in the treatment of premenopausal advanced breast cancer. Eur J Cancer 29A:1498.
66. Gallen M, Alonso MC, Ojeda B, et al. 1994. Randomized multicentre trial comparing two different time-span of adjuvant tamoxifen therapy (ATT) in women with operable node positive breast cancer (abstract). Proc Am Soc Clin Oncol 13:76.
67. Swedish Breast Cancer Cooperative Group. 1996. Randomized trial of 2 versus 5 years of adjuvant tamoxifen in postmenopausal early-stage breast cancer (abstract). Proc Am Soc Clin Oncol 15:126.
68. Colditz GA, Willett WC, Stampfer MJ. 1987. Menopause and the risk of coronary heart disease in women. N Engl J Med 316:1105–1110.
69. Knoweldon J, Buhr AJ, Dunbar O. 1964. Incidence of fractures in persons over 35 years of age: a report to the M.R.C. working party on fractures in the elderly. Br J Prev Soc Med 18:130–141.

10. The duration of adjuvant tamoxifen therapy

Malcolm M. Bilimoria and V. Craig Jordan

1. Introduction

Ever since the first clinical trials demonstrated a disease-free and overall survival benefit from tamoxifen use in breast cancer patients, the optimal duration of tamoxifen use has remained controversial. Despite the numerous clinical trials over the last 10 years, this question remains. Previously, we have noted that results from several large clinical trials are needed to determine whether five years of therapy or longer is the best therapeutic regimen [1]. We concluded that the proven length of therapy would depend largely on the amount and degree of tamoxifen resistance within the heterogeneous clinical sample.

The National Cancer Institute has recently issued a clinical alert concerning the duration of tamoxifen use. Using unpublished data from the National Surgical Adjuvant Breast Program (NSABP) study B14 and the Scottish Trial, they concluded that for node-negative, estrogen receptor- (ER-) positive women, the optimal duration of tamoxifen therapy is five years. Their overall conclusion is that for node-negative women, the benefits after five years of treatment are not significantly improved by longer treatment. Indeed, there is a stated concern that iatrogenic side effects may offset the advantages of tamoxifen. This chapter will highlight the possible mechanisms that can account for some women receiving optimal benefit from just five years while others may benefit from longer therapy. In addition, we will take a closer look at the NSABP B14 trial and the Scottish Trial and finally describe the newer trials recently launched to answer the question of whether five years or longer is needed to achieve the maximal benefit from tamoxifen.

2. Clinical studies

Tamoxifen is the first-line endocrine therapy for early-stage breast cancer, largely due to this agent's proven efficacy in clinical trials. The treatment strategies employed, however, are the result of concepts developed in the laboratory and translated through clinical trials into general practice. During the mid-1970s, the concept of adjuvant therapy was being tested in node-positive breast cancer patients, with the goal of prolonging survival. One year of therapy was initially selected because this was the average duration of response observed in the treatment of metastatic disease [2–5]. In contrast, laboratory studies demonstrated that short-term therapy was not an appropriate strategy to control the appearance of carcinogen-induced rat mammary tumors [6]. Long-term treatment, for 25% of the animal's life span, with clinically equivalent per-kilogram doses (250 µg/kg) of tamoxifen, however, almost completely prevented tumor occurrence [7–9]. Thus, the concept of long-term therapy with a competitive inhibitor of estrogen action became a reasonable rationale to test in clinical trials.

The Nolvadex Adjuvant Trial Organization (NATO) was the first to demonstrate a survival advantage for breast cancer patients receiving two years of adjuvant tamoxifen [10]. Clinical trials since that time have largely investigated tamoxifen in axillary node-positive disease; however, a few trials have either studied node-negative patients versus controls or have reanalyzed their data by focusing on only the smaller proportion of node-negative patients. Tamoxifen therapy in early-stage breast cancer appears to increase the disease-free survival, but the effects on overall survival are more difficult to discern from individual clinical trials. Some trials demonstrate a clear increase in overall survival while others do not [11–13].

In hopes of clearing up much of the confusion involving breast cancer therapy, the Early Breast Cancer Trialist's Collaborative Group performed an overview analysis of 133 randomized clinical trials involving over 75,000 women, 30,000 of whom were enrolled in clinical trials studying tamoxifen therapy. The analysis confirmed that adjuvant tamoxifen therapy has proven efficacy in early-stage breast cancer [14]. For node-negative women taking tamoxifen for an average of two years, the 10-year analysis found a 5.1% reduction in recurrence-free survival and a 3.5% reduction in mortality. Of note is that even though the average duration of therapy was only two years, there was a statistically significant increase in recurrence-free survival and overall survival when these were measured at both the 5- and 10-year mark.

Indirectly, the analysis demonstrates that both node-positive and node-negative patients who had taken longer courses of tamoxifen (>two years) had decreased annual odds of recurrence and mortality when compared to those that were treated with shorter courses of tamoxifen (<two years). Patients averaging greater than two years of tamoxifen therapy had a 38% reduction in annual odds of recurrence and a 24% reduction in annual odds of death compared to 16% and 11% reductions, respectively, for patients on less than two years of tamoxifen. Clearly, the overview analysis shows that tamoxifen in early-stage breast cancer increases disease-free and overall survival, with an increase in benefit noted if the duration of therapy is greater than two years.

Since the overview analysis, the ideal duration of tamoxifen therapy has remained controversial because there are no firm clinical trials data available to answer this important question. Nevertheless, the National Cancer Institute recently released a clinicians' alert after analysis of the NSABP B14 trial found no increased benefit for lymph node-negative, ER-positive women randomized to 10 years of tamoxifen versus women who took the drug for only five years. They recommended that clinicians could stop tamoxifen therapy after five years for this subgroup of breast cancer patients because no significant benefits could be detected after a short-term follow-up.

3. Drug resistance to tamoxifen

While the majority of women with node-negative, ER-positive breast cancer will be cured of their disease, it is clear that approximately one third will have a recurrence of disease within 10 years [14]. Since the recurrences are often observed as late as 10 years after the diagnosis of breast cancer, trials studying 10 years of tamoxifen use make sense intuitively. An important determinant of whether long-term (10 years to indefinite therapy) tamoxifen therapy will prove useful depends on drug resistance.

There is virtually no clinical information about the change from tamoxifen-sensitive to -resistant or -stimulated growth. We will therefore consider numerous laboratory studies to formulate possible clinical situations that could occur during long-term adjuvant tamoxifen treatment. Laboratory studies demonstrate that short-term (one-month) tamoxifen treatment will only delay the appearance of mammary tumors and will not control tumorigenesis in the majority of rats [8]. Similar observations are seen when MCF-7 cells are implanted into athymic mice that are treated with long-term tamoxifen [15]. If tamoxifen is stopped, estrogen will reactivate the tumor. The conclusion from these laboratory studies using homogenous tumors is that 'longer is better' for the control of hormone-responsive disease and that tamoxifen should not be stopped prematurely [16]. Clinically, this finding may represent the premenopausal woman who, after a short course (1–2 years) of tamoxifen therapy, has regrowth of breast cancer metastases as a result of high circulating estrogen levels.

Alternatively, continuous tamoxifen given to athymic mice transplanted with MCF-7 cells can result in tamoxifen-stimulated growth of the tumor [17,18]. The tumors in this instance remain ER positive and, therefore, will grow in response to estradiol or tamoxifen. This growth can occur clinically in some breast cancer patients who often respond to a second-line endocrine therapy. A pure antiestrogen is being developed and is showing promise as an endocrine therapy for women who fail long-term tamoxifen therapy [19,20].

Yet another model has been noted when MCF-7 tumors have been serially transplanted for several years into tamoxifen-treated athymic mice. Tumors in this model may regress when tamoxifen is stopped and physiologic doses of estrogen are administered [21]. Clearly, this tumoricidal effect of estrogen

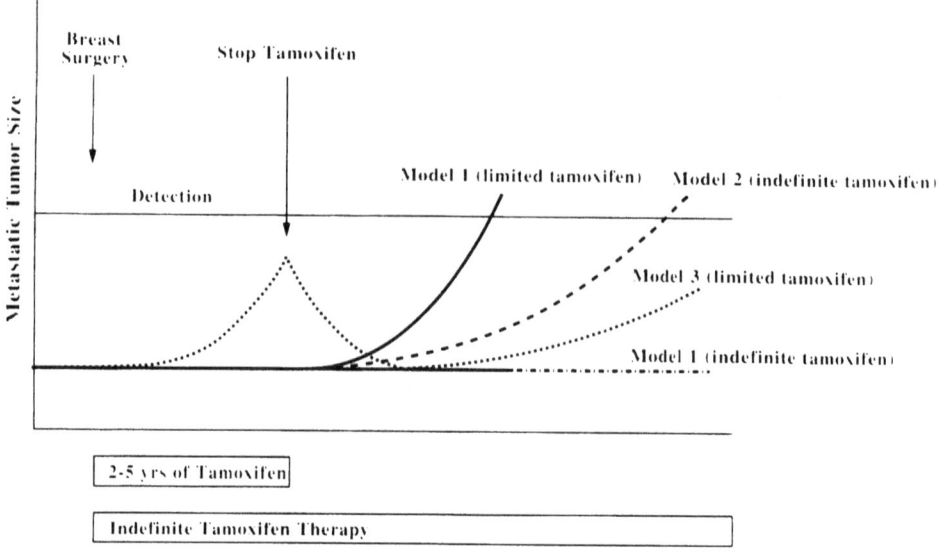

Figure 1. Graph demonstrating possible growth patterns of metastatic breast cancer during and after tamoxifen therapy. Model 1 (—) shows regrowth of the metastasis following cessation of 2–5 years of tamoxifen. However, if continuous tamoxifen therapy is used, the tumoristatic action of the drug may control tumor recurrence (model 1-··-). In contrast, continuous tamoxifen therapy might eventually result in the development of tamoxifen-stimulated tumors (model 2----). Alternatively, model 3 (···) depends on tamoxifen-stimulated tumors developing early with subsequent tumor supersensitivity to the women's own estrogen that causes tumor regression. The tumor eventually develops clones of cells that are estrogen dependent. (From Bilimoria et al. 1996. Cancer J Sc Am 2:140–150, with permission.)

could be responsible for the long-term survival advantages seen when even short-term tamoxifen therapy is used [14]. Stopping tamoxifen before tamoxifen-dependent cancer cells were detected would result in rapid regression of a sensitized micrometastasis once the women's estrogen is free to act.

Each laboratory model (figure 1) is an example of what might occur clinically. Only prospective randomized trials, similar to NSABP B14, can demonstrate the true effect of tamoxifen resistance clinically. A closer examination of the available trials, however, make generalizations based on current data unwise.

4. A closer look at NSABP B14

In 1981, the NSABP initiated protocol B14 to determine the efficacy of tamoxifen in women with early-stage breast cancer. The trial has 2892 node-negative, ER-positive breast cancer patients randomized to receive either tamoxifen (20 mg/day) for five years or placebo [13] (figure 2). The updated

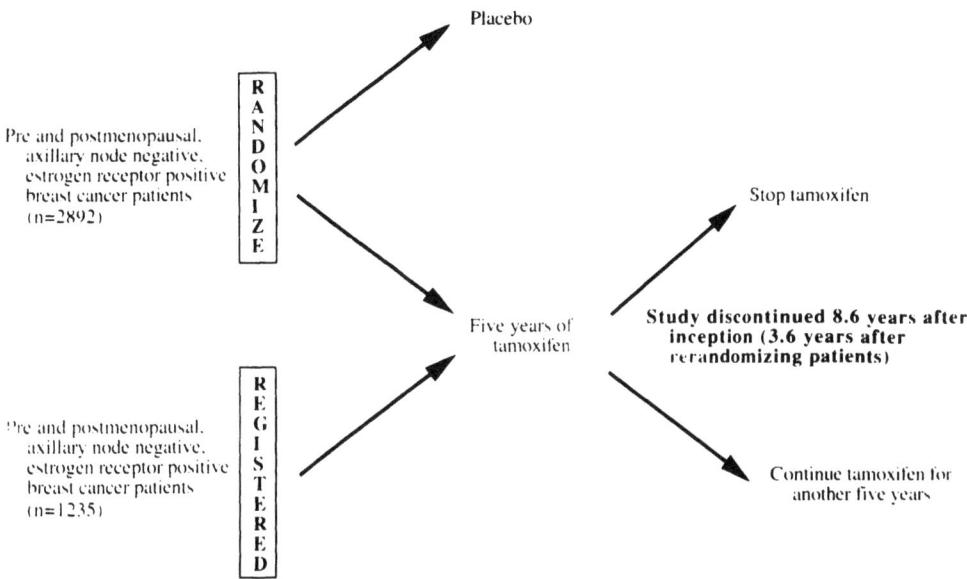

Figure 2. Study protocol of the National Surgical Adjuvant Breast Project trial B14.

10-year disease-free survival was 68% for the tamoxifen-treated group and 57% for the placebo-controlled group ($p < 0.0001$). A concomitant increase in overall survival was also noted for the tamoxifen-treated group, namely, 78% vs. 75% ($p = 0.0370$). Similar to the finding of the overview analysis, it was clearly demonstrated that the beneficial effects of tamoxifen seem to be evident long after the therapy has stopped. In this trial, women who had stopped the therapy five years earlier continued to have clear benefits with respect to disease-free and overall survival.

Of the women who had taken tamoxifen for five years and remained disease free, a second randomization to receive either placebo or an additional five years of tamoxifen therapy was initiated. In order to increase the number of tamoxifen-treated patients in this second randomization, 1235 patients who fulfilled the same eligibility criteria were registered into the study. However, only 1166 women (from both the randomized and registered group) were randomized to either continue tamoxifen for five more years ($n = 591$) or to stop therapy ($n = 575$). Less than four years after this rerandomization, preliminary data from this study revealed that the actuarial disease-free survival for the five years of tamoxifen followed by placebo group was 92% vs. 86% for the group randomized to take a longer duration of tamoxifen. Overall, the actuarial survival was noted to be 96% in the five years tamoxifen followed by placebo group vs. 94% in the group randomized to take tamoxifen for 10 years.

It must be noted that after rerandomization, the intended trial was never completed. Therefore, in essence, the trial compared tamoxifen for five years vs. tamoxifen for 8.6 years with analysis occurring 8.6 years after the study began. As the results from NSABP B14, as well as the overview analysis, have illustrated, the beneficial effects of tamoxifen are known to remain many years after tamoxifen therapy has been discontinued, so it will be extremely important to follow these patients to discover whether the responses change after 10 years of tamoxifen-free life. Clearly, it will be virtually impossible to compare the groups for cardiovascular risks, since they are very similar with regard to duration of therapy.

Also of concern is that there is no separate analysis of premenopausal or postmenopausal women in the study. It is important to appreciate that postmenopausal patients stand to benefit much more from tamoxifen's bone-preserving and cardioprotective effects when they consider long-term (10-year) tamoxifen use. Unfortunately, no data exist on this subgroup of patients, and there is no way to predict what the disease-free or overall survival effects would be if these data were analyzed 5 and 10 years after a full 10 years of tamoxifen.

Another important distinction that was not analyzed in the study was tumor size. It is clear that for node-negative patients, tumor size is an important determinant of disease-free and overall survival [22]. Most importantly, however, there is no analysis of response to tamoxifen with respect to tumor size. Since clinicians in general must deal with the individual patient and make decisions on a case-by-case basis, information with respect to tumor size and response to five years or longer of tamoxifen therapy will now be unavailable. Regrettably, there are too few patients in the current database to make any definitive conclusions about all stages of breast cancer.

Since the analysis of NSABP B14 showed no statistical difference in actuarial disease-free survival between 5 and 8.6 years of tamoxifen, the primary concern becomes a fear of endometrial cancer in postmenopausal patients alone. A closer look at the incidence of second primary cancers in the two groups showed no significant differences between 5 and 8.6 years of treatment, but the results do add to the perceptions regarding the concern about endometrial cancer. The group of patients receiving tamoxifen for 3.6 years longer than the other group had three times the rate of endometrial cancer (six diagnosed tumors) when compared to the five-year tamoxifen group (two diagnosed tumors) — despite the fact that large reviews of tamoxifen-associated endometrial cancer have shown that longer durations of therapy are not associated with an increased risk of endometrial cancer when compared to shorter durations of tamoxifen [23]. Still others have noted that the risk of endometrial cancer remains steady for at least five years after tamoxifen is discontinued [24]. One therefore has to question why there are three times more cases of endometrial cancer in the women taking tamoxifen for 8.6 years if the risk of developing endometrial cancer remains elevated in the women who stopped at five years. Overall, the difficulty in making a definitive conclusion is that the database is too small for vigorous analysis. The information from the NSABP is also incomplete because the numbers of postmenopausal women at risk are not stated. Despite the current concerns and uncertainty, it is reassuring to note the fact that tens of thousands of node-positive and node-negative patients have been maintained on tamoxifen, often for more than a decade, without serious side effects or aggressive recurrent disease.

5. Scottish trial

In addition to the NSABP B14 trial, the NCI clinical alert has cited unpublished data from the Scottish Tamoxifen Trial as additional evidence for their recommendation to stop tamoxifen at five years. The Scottish Tamoxifen Trial, which began in 1978, randomized 1312 breast cancer patients to receive either five years of tamoxifen or no treatment until relapse [12] (figure 3). After the completion of five years of tamoxifen, women from this group were then invited to be rerandomized to either continue indefinitely ($n = 173$) or to stop therapy ($n = 169$). Like NSABP B14, both premenopausal and postmenopausal women with node-negative disease were included in the study, but unlike the NSABP trial, postmenopausal women with node-positive disease were enrolled as well. Of particular importance is that ER status was *not* required for enrollment.

At a median of 6.2 years following rerandomization (11.2 years vs. 5 years of tamoxifen), the results show no statistical difference in overall survival between the two groups. Since the trial is of very limited size, it clearly will not be able demonstrate that continuation of tamoxifen beyond five years is beneficial. The NCI clinical alert states that 'the data do suggest that, if there is a disease-free survival or overall survival benefit to be derived (with greater

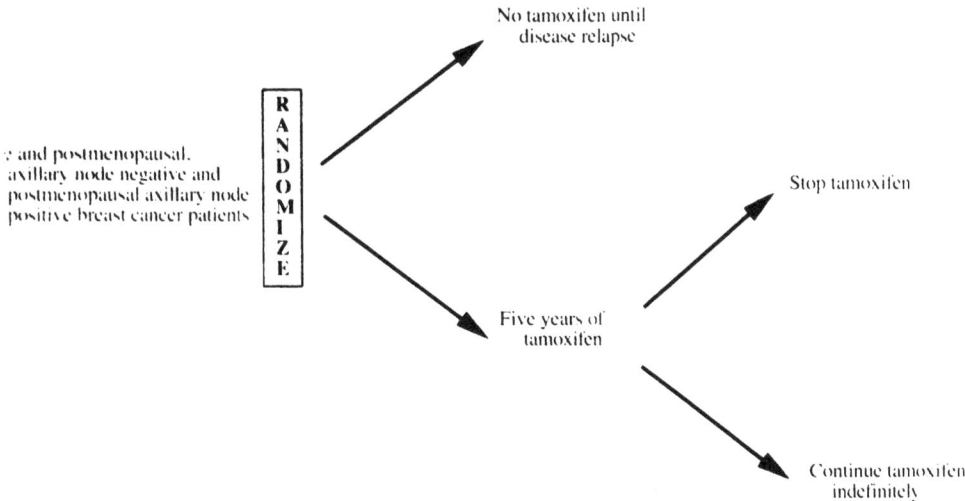

Figure 3. Study protocol of the Scottish Tamoxifen Trial.

than five years of tamoxifen) it would likely be small.' This conclusion appears reasonable, but small differences could prove to be important to breast cancer patients. It is clear that small benefits with tamoxifen therapy multiplied by the almost 100,000 women per year who develop breast cancer and receive tamoxifen can make a profound impact on lives saved. A 1% difference in survival would result in 1000 lives extended each year.

As with the NSABP trial, there are no data available about differences between the two trial groups with respect to tumor size and menopausal status. This trial, also, contains two additional confounding variables in that the ER status of all the women in the trial is not known and there is inclusion of node-positive postmenopausal women in the study. Clearly, meaningful conclusions from this study cannot be obtained without a closer investigation into the impact these variables have on the two study groups. For example, if it was discovered that the patients who received tamoxifen for more than five years were originally ER negative, then this finding would erode the significance of the study. Obviously, tamoxifen would not be expected to benefit these women in the long term.

Finally, there is one benefit of tamoxifen therapy that has been noted as a direct result of the Scottish Tamoxifen Trial. In 1991, in a retrospective review, McDonald and Stewart [25] noted that 10 of 200 women in the tamoxifen-treated arm had died of myocardial infarction, while 25 of 251 had died of the same disease in the control group. An update of their patient data in 1995 showed that women in the tamoxifen-treated arm of the study had 14 myocardial infarctions per 1000 years of risk compared to 23 myocardial infarctions per 1000 years of risk for the control group [26]. Others have also found that longer durations of tamoxifen have a greater benefit upon cardiovascular disease. Rutqvist et al. [27], upon analysis of the Stockholm randomized trial, found that hospital admissions for cardiac disease were statistically lower for women taking five years of tamoxifen as opposed to women on only two years of therapy.

The benefit towards cardiovascular risk obtained from tamoxifen use appears to be associated with a lowering of total cholesterol by 13% and low-density lipoprotein by 19% [1]. This finding clearly can account for the benefit, since it has been recognized that a 1% drop in serum cholesterol can lead to a 2% drop in coronary heart disease [28]. Another possible mechanism for the cardioprotective effects of tamoxifen lies in the finding that tamoxifen-treated patients have a statistically significant reduction in serum lipoprotein(a) levels. Indeed, several epidemiologic and clinical studies have shown that increased lipoprotein(a) levels are an independent risk factor for coronary heart disease [29–31]. Although the exact mechanism remains unclear, what is clear is that tamoxifen users maintain the cardioprotective effects of tamoxifen, a benefit that would be reduced when their tamoxifen use is terminated. The implication is that certain patients, in this instance postmenopausal women with risk factors for coronary heart disease, may have survival benefits from longer than five years of tamoxifen therapy.

Table 1. Trials of five years of tamoxifen therapy versus longer

Trial	Year started	Entry criteria	Background therapy	Design (years)	Size
NSABP B14	1981	N−, ER−	None	5 vs. 10	1166
Scottish Trial	1978	Pre N−, Post any N	None	5 vs. life	342
ECOG 4181	1982	Post N+	CMFP	5 vs. life	87+
ECOG 5181	1982	Pre N+	CMFP	5 vs. life	100+

Abbreviations: N, axillary node; ER, estrogen receptor; Pre, premenopausal; Post, postmenopausal; CMFP, cyclophosphamide, methotrexate, flurouracil, prednisone.

6. Eastern Cooperative Oncology Group trials

The idea that long-term tamoxifen use as an adjuvant therapy may benefit patients has been known to the clinical community for nearly 20 years. Regrettably, few studies have evaluated long-term adjuvant tamoxifen in node-positive breast cancer patients. The Eastern Cooperative Oncology Group (ECOG) trials 4181 and 5181 both compare five years of tamoxifen therapy versus indefinite therapy in node-positive breast cancer patients [32,33]. ECOG trial 4181 made this comparison in postmenopausal node-positive patients, while ECOG trial 5181 used the same treatment strategy with tamoxifen for premenopausal node-positive patients.

Table 1 lists the current trials comparing five years of tamoxifen with longer therapy. The ECOG trials currently have fewer patients (approximately 200 patients) than either the NSABP B14 (1166 patients) or the Scottish trial (342 patients). Though no definitive results of the ECOG trials have been published, it is clear that the limited power of the studies will not allow a statistically significant finding. Clearly, large randomized trials of long-term tamoxifen therapy that analyze the treatment groups with respect to tumor size, menopausal status, ER status, and nodal status are needed.

7. ATLAS trial and ATTOM trial

Despite the recommendation of the National Cancer Institute, trials designed to determine the efficacy of more than five years of tamoxifen are currently under way in the United Kingdom. In the Adjuvant Tamoxifen — Longer Against Shorter (ATLAS) trial, women who have been on tamoxifen for at least two years and who, in conjunction with their physician, are unsure of whether to continue are randomized either to stop tamoxifen or to continue for an additional five years. Most importantly, some patients are projected to be enrolled into a group using tamoxifen for more than 10 years (figure 4).

The trial, which is centered in Oxford, is randomizing 20,000 breast cancer

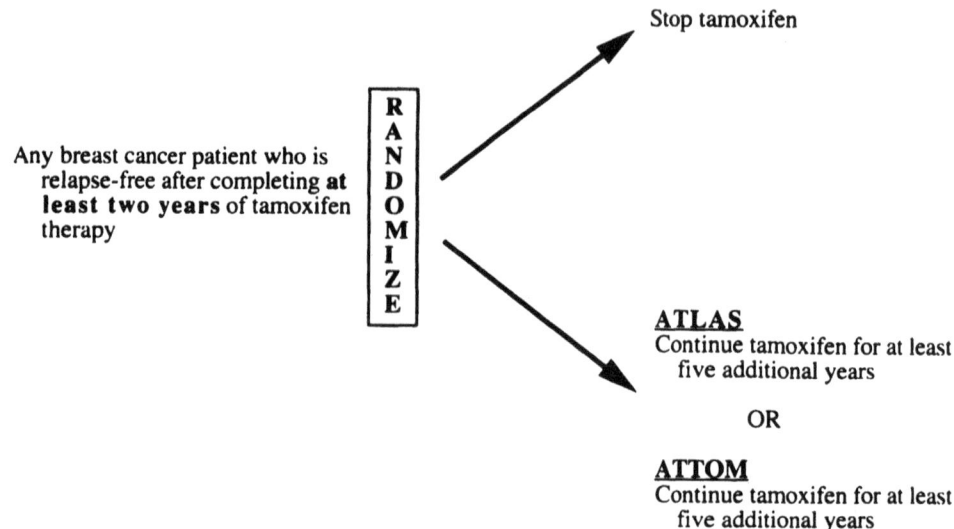

Figure 4. Study protocol of the Adjuvant Tamoxifen — Longer against Shorter(ATLAS) trial and the Adjuvant Tamoxifen — Treatment Offer More? (ATTOM) trial.

patients. Interestingly, the researchers cite this number as being crucial to their study in that they will need this enrollment of patients in order to have a 95% chance of detecting a 2%–3% difference in survival at $2p < 0.05$ and an 85% chance of doing so at $2p < 0.01$. By comparison, the NSABP B14 trial had about one twentieth the projected enrollment of the United Kingdom study. It is clear that only through trials like ATLAS can any true assessments about the proper duration of tamoxifen therapy be made.

Additionally, the Adjuvant Tamoxifen — Treatment Offer More? (ATTOM) trial, is currently under way in England. The trial, centered in Birmingham, is designed such that breast cancer patients with any node status and any ER status who have been on tamoxifen therapy for at least two years are randomized either to stop tamoxifen or to continue for at least another five years (figure 4). The trial estimates that in order to detect a 2% difference in absolute survival, 20,000 patients will need to be randomized to have an 80% chance of detecting the difference. The ATLAS and ATTOM trials will each provide a huge database to answer the question about the appropriate duration of tamoxifen therapy.

8. Conclusion

Twenty years ago, clinical trials were only considering one-year treatment regimens with tamoxifen. The cooperation between the laboratory and the clinic has established the principle through clinical trials that longer therapy is better. Despite this important advance, that has resulted in the increased survival of tens of thousands of women with breast cancer, there are no definitive data to aid the physician on a case-by-case basis. There is no answer to the central question: How long is long enough? The National Cancer Institute's clinical alert has focused current concerns on the duration of tamoxifen therapy. Many clinicians may be reassured by the NCI's recommendation that node-negative, ER-positive women may not benefit from more than five years of adjuvant tamoxifen. However, there are serious concerns about the appropriateness of applying these preliminary findings to all women with breast cancer. Very large patient numbers are vital to make such statements to the clinical community because the history of clinical trials in the last decade demonstrates that individual results can be flawed or misleading. A major analysis of differences in menopausal status or tumor size would be helpful in a large patient population to identify subgroups of patients who might receive benefit from longer than five years of therapy. Receptor status of the primary tumor is vital to consider, and the additional risk factors for coronary heart disease must not be ignored. Until a valid analysis and database exist, an individualized approach to the duration of tamoxifen use for patients should be employed [1].

Ongoing are trials trying to determine whether more than five years of tamoxifen therapy is better than five years or less. Despite the clinical alert released by the NCI with respect to the NSABP B14 trial, the ongoing ATLAS and ATTOM clinical trials demonstrate that many in the clinical community still regard the length of tamoxifen therapy in different categories and stages of breast cancer as an open question.

Acknowledgments

We are grateful to the Lynn Sage Breast Cancer Foundation for their generous support.

Note added in proof: Recent publications of ECOG clinical trials data demonstrate that in their small study ER positive patients benefit from more than five years of tamoxifen [34].

References

1. Bilimoria MM, Assikis VJ, Jordan VC. 1996. Should adjuvant tamoxifen therapy be stopped at 5 years? Cancer J Sci Am 2:140–150.
2. Ludwig Breast Cancer Study Group. 1984. Randomized trial of chemoendocrine therapy, endocrine therapy, and mastectomy alone in postmenopausal patients with operable breast cancer and axillary node metastasis. Lancet 1:1256–1260.
3. Ribeiro G, Swindell R. 1985. The Christie Hospital tamoxifen (Nolvadex) adjuvant trial for operable breast carcinoma — 7 year results. Eur J Cancer Clin Oncol 21:897–900.
4. Rose C, Thorpe SM, Andersen KW, et al. 1985. Beneficial effects of adjuvant tamoxifen therapy in primary breast cancer patients with high oestrogen levels. Lancet 1:16–19.

5. Hubay CA, Gordon NH, Crowe JP, et al. 1984. Antiestrogen-cytotoxic chemotherapy and bacillus Calmatte–Guerin vaccination in Stage II breast cancer: seventy-two month followup. Surgery 96:61–72.
6. Jordan VC, Allen KE. 1980. Evaluation of the antitumor activity of the nonsteroidal antioestrogen monohydroxytamoxifen in the DMBA-induced rat mammary carcinoma model. Eur J Cancer 16:239–251.
7. Jordan VC. 1978. Use of DMBA induced rat mammary carcinoma system for the evaluation of tamoxifen as a potential adjuvant therapy. Rev Endocr Rel Cancer (Oct) 49–55.
8. Jordan VC, Dix CJ, Allen KE. 1979. The effectiveness of long-term tamoxifen treatment in a laboratory model for adjuvant hormone therapy of breast cancer. In Salmon SE, Jones SE, eds. Adjuvant Therapy of Cancer II. New York: Grune & Stratton, pp. 19–26.
9. Jordan VC, Naylor KE, Dix CJ, Prestwich G. 1980. Antioestrogen action in experimental breast cancer. In Endocrine Treatment of Breast Cancer. Recent Results Cancer Res 71:30–44.
10. Nolvadex Adjuvant Trial Organization. 1985. Controlled trial of tamoxifen as a single agent in the management of early breast cancer. Lancet 1:836–839.
11. Cancer Research Campaign, Adjuvant Breast Trial Working Party. 1988. Cyclophosphamide and tamoxifen as adjuvant therapies in the management of breast cancer. Br J Cancer 57:604–607.
12. Breast Cancer Trials Committee, Scottish Cancer Trials. 1987. Adjuvant tamoxifen in the management of operable breast cancer: The Scottish Trial. Lancet 2:171–175.
13. Fisher B, Costantino J, Redmond C, et al. 1989. A randomized clinical trial evaluating tamoxifen in the treatment of patients with node-negative breast cancer who have estrogen-receptor positive tumors. N Engl J Med 320:479–484.
14. Early Breast Cancer Trialists' Collaborative Group. 1992. Systemic treatment of early breast cancer by hormonal, cytotoxic, or immune therapy. Lancet 339:1–15, 71–85.
15. Gottardis MM, Robinson SP, Jordan VC. 1988. Estradiol-stimulated growth of MCF-7 tumors implanted in athymic mice: a model to study the tumoristatic action of tamoxifen. J Steroid Biochem 20:311–314.
16. Jordan VC. 1983. Laboratory studies to develop general principles for the adjuvant treatment of breast cancer with antiestrogens: problems and potential for future clinical applications. Breast Cancer Res Treat 3:S73–S86.
17. Gottardis MM, Jordan VC. 1988. Development of tamoxifen stimulated growth of MCF-7 tumors in athymic mice after long-term antiestrogen administration. Cancer Res 48;5183–5187.
18. Gottardis MM, Wagner RJ, Borden EC, Jordan VC. 1989. Differential ability of antiestrogens to stimulate breast cancer cell (MCF-7) growth in vivo and in vitro. Cancer Res 49:4765–4769.
19. Wakeling AE, Dukes M, Bowler J. 1991. A potent specific pure antiestrogen with clinical potential. Cancer Res 15:3867–3873.
20. Howell A, DeFriend D, Robertson J, Blamey R, Walton P. 1995. Response to a specific antiestrogen (ICI182,780) in tamoxifen-resistant breast cancer. Lancet 345:29–30.
21. Wolf DM, Jordan VC. 1993. A laboratory model to explain the survival advantages observed in patients taking adjuvant tamoxifen therapy. Recent Res Cancer Res 53:533–535.
22. Aubele M, Auer G, Voss A, et al. 1995. Different risk groups in node-negative breast cancer: prognostic value of cytophotometrically assessed DNA, morphometry and texture. Int J Cancer 63:7–12.
23. Assikis VJ, Jordan VC. 1995. Gynecological effects of tamoxifen and the association with endometrial carcinoma. Int J Gynecol Obstet 49:241–257.
24. Rutqvist LE, Johansson H, Signomklao T, et al. 1995. Adjuvant tamoxifen therapy for early stage breast cancer and second primary malignancies. J Natl Cancer Inst 87:645–651.
25. McDonald CC, Stewart HJ. 1991. Fatal myocardial infarctions in the Scottish adjuvant tamoxifen trial. Br Med J 303:435–437.
26. McDonald CC, Alexander FE, Whyte BW, et al. 1995. Cardiac and vascular morbidity in

women receiving adjuvant tamoxifen for breast cancer in a randomised trial. Br Med J 311:977–980.
27. Rutqvist LE, Mattsson A. 1993. Cardiac and thromboembolic morbidity among postmenopausal women with early stage breast cancer in a randomized trial of adjuvant tamoxifen. J Natl Cancer Inst 85:1398–1406.
28. Castelli WP. 1988. Cholesterol and lipids in the risk of coronary artery disease — the Farmingham Heart Study. Can J Cardiol 4:5A–10A.
29. Loscalzo J. 1990. Lipoprotein(a): a unique risk factor for atherothrombotic disease. Arteriosclerosis 10:672–679.
30. Utermann G. 1990. Lipoprotein(a): a genetic risk factor for premature coronary heart disease. Curr Opin Lipidol 1:404–410.
31. Sandholzer C, Saha N, Kark JD, et al. 1992. Apo(a) isoforms predict risk for coronary heart disease. A study in six populations. Arterioscler Thromb 12:1214–1226.
32. Tormey DC, Gray R, Abeloff MD, et al. 1992. Adjuvant therapy with a doxorubicin regimen and long-term tamoxifen in premenopausal breast cancer patients: an Eastern Cooperative Oncology Group trial. J Clin Oncol 10:1848–1856.
33. Falkson HC, Gray R, Wolberg WH, et al. 1990. Adjuvant trial of 12 cycles of CMFPT followed by observation or continuous tamoxifen versus four cycles of CMFPT in postmenopausal women with breastcancer: an Eastern Cooperative Oncology Group phase III study. J Clin Oncol 8:599–607.
34. Tormey DC, Gray R, Falkson HC. 1996. Postchomotherapy adjuvant tamoxifen therapy beyond five years in patients with lymph node positive breast cancer. J. Natl. Cancer Inst. 88:1828–1833.

11. Tamoxifen and the endometrium

Richard R. Barakat

1. Introduction

Tamoxifen, a nonsteroidal antiestrogen, was first approved by the Food and Drug Administration in 1978 for the treatment of patients with breast cancer. Large clinical trials involving over 75,000 patients have demonstrated an improved recurrence-free and overall survival benefit in both premenopausal and postmenopausal women. Long-term adjuvant tamoxifen is the endocrine treatment of choice for selected patients with breast cancer, and there are currently large-scale trials to evaluate its role as a chemopreventative agent in healthy women at risk for breast cancer. Consequently, a large number of women, including healthy young patients with no history of cancer, will be subjected to the long-term effects of tamoxifen. One of the most significant complications of long-term tamoxifen use is the possible development of endometrial cancer. The purpose of this chapter is to review the current literature regarding tamoxifen use in breast cancer patients and associated benign and malignant uterine neoplasia. In addition, the role of screening for endometrial cancer in tamoxifen-treated breast cancer patients is explored.

2. Laboratory data

Tamoxifen is believed to exert its main effect by blocking the binding of estrogen to the estrogen receptor. While acting primarily as an antiestrogen, tamoxifen may also exhibit some mild estrogenic effects. Although there is no evidence that tamoxifen induces endometrial cancer in laboratory animals, several preclinical studies have indicated that tamoxifen may indeed exert an estrogenic effect on the endometrium. Satyaswaroop et al. [1] transplanted both estrogen receptor-positive and estrogen receptor-negative human endometrial cancer cell lines into nude mice and evaluated the effect of both tamoxifen and 17-β-estradiol on tumor growth. Although the estrogen receptor-negative tumor grew rapidly, there was no difference in the rate of tumor growth between tamoxifen or estrogen-treated animals compared with controls. In contrast, the rate of growth of the estrogen receptor-positive cell

Kenneth A. Foon and Hyman B. Muss (eds), BIOLOGICAL AND HORMONAL THERAPIES OF CANCER. Copyright © 1998. Kluwer Academic Publishers, Boston. All rights reserved.

line was significantly accelerated in the tamoxifen-treated animals compared to controls, although to a lesser degree than was seen with estrogen treatment. In addition, tamoxifen increased the levels of functional progesterone receptors, lending further evidence to the estrogenic potential of tamoxifen. Gottardis et al. [2] demonstrated in athymic mice the contrasting actions of tamoxifen on the growth of estrogen receptor-positive breast and endometrial cancer cell lines. While stimulating the growth of the endometrial tumor, tamoxifen had no effect on the breast tumor growth and had an antagonistic action on the estradiol-stimulated growth of breast tumors.

The etiology of tamoxifen-associated endometrial stimulation has not been established. There are, however, some metabolites of tamoxifen that may act primarily as estrogen agonists and some investigators favor this mechanism as a possible hypothesis for the development of endometrial neoplasia. Metabolite E is formed by the removal of the aminoethane side chain from tamoxifen. This compound is a weak estrogen agonist that binds the estrogen receptor with low affinity [3]. The presence of a hydroxyl group in this compound destabilizes the ethylene bond, allowing isomerization of the compound to its E isomer, a potent estrogen agonist. The clinical significance of metabolite E is controversial, and its role in endometrial neoplasia remains to be determined.

The mechanisms of tamoxifen-associated endometrial carcinogenesis remain undetermined. Chemical substances may exert their carcinogenic effect through a direct genotoxic mechanism. Conventional methods such as the Ames assay and the human lymphocyte chromosome test used to screen chemicals for potential carcinogenicity have proved negative for tamoxifen [4]. Tamoxifen has been shown to cause DNA adduct formation in rodent liver [5,6], but in vivo DNA adduct formation in tamoxifen-treated women does not appear to differ from that in untreated patients [7]. Recently, Pongracz et al. [8] demonstrated that metabolite E of tamoxifen, which is found in the plasma of tamoxifen-treated patients, can be microsomally activated to form DNA adducts. Carmichael et al. [9] examined in vitro and in vivo the potential of tamoxifen to induce genotoxic damage (DNA adducts) in the human endometrium. No evidence for any DNA adducts induced by tamoxifen was found.

3. Clinical studies

Tamoxifen has been demonstrated clinically to have estrogenic effects on the female genital tract. Boccardo et al. [10] noted the estrogen-like effect of tamoxifen on the vaginal epithelium by means of exfoliative vaginal cytology using the karyopyknotic index (KPI), which is the relation of mature superficial cells to intermediate cells. Postmenopausal estrogen replacement therapy generally induces increased cellular maturity and, consequently, increases the KPI. Following tamoxifen treatment of at least eight weeks, these researchers noted a significantly higher KPI than for untreated patients, suggesting an estrogenic effect of tamoxifen on the vaginal epithelium.

4. Endometrial polyps and hyperplasia

Several recent reports have implicated tamoxifen treatment in the development of endometrial polyps and hyperplasia (table 1). Lahti et al. [11] performed transvaginal sonography, hysteroscopy, and endometrial curettage on 103 postmenopausal breast cancer patients, 51 of whom had received tamoxifen at 20–40 mg/day for a median of 30 months and 52 of whom had not received any hormonal treatment. The patients were matched with respect to age, parity, time since menopause, body mass index, and concomitant medical conditions. Compared with control subjects, the tamoxifen-treated patients were found to have a significantly thicker mean endometrial width (10.4 mm vs. 4.2 mm) and a larger uterine volume as determined by transvaginal sonography. However, they also had a higher incidence of uterine fibroids.

A significantly higher percentage of endometrial polyps was found in the tamoxifen-treated group compared with controls (36% vs. 10%). Of the 43 patients in the tamoxifen-treated group who were found to have an endometrial thickness of 5 mm or more, 17 (39.5%) were found to have endometrial polyps; however, 22 (51.2%) had no abnormal pathologic findings. Two patients in the tamoxifen group were found to have endometrial hyperplasia, and one patient had endometrial cancer at the time of curettage. Two patients in the control group were also found to have endometrial cancer. All significant endometrial pathology was found in asymptomatic patients with an endometrial width greater than 5 mm on transvaginal sonography. If transvaginal sonography were used as a screening method for endometrial cancer, with the abnormal cutoff limit being set at 5 mm, approximately 50% of patients would undergo endometrial sampling unnecessarily.

Since endometrial polyps often contain hyperplastic endometrial glands,

Table 1. Studies reporting on tamoxifen-associated endometrial pathology

Author [ref]	No. of patients	Daily dose	Duration	Polyps	Hyperplasia	Carcinoma
Neven [13]	16	20 mg	Mean 21 mos	4 (25%)	0 (0%)	1 (6%)
Lahti [11]	51	20–40 mg	Median 30 mos	17 (33%)	2 (4%)	1 (2%)
Cohen [14]	93	20–30 mg	Mean 22 mos	5 (5.4%)	2 (2%)	3 (3%)
Gal [15]	49	20 mg	>12 mos	Unknown	10 (20%)	0 (0%)
Gibson [16]	75	20 mg	Mean 26 mos	10 (13%)	1 (1%)	6 (8%)
Kedar [17]	61	20 mg	Median 22 mos	5 (8%)	10 (16%)	0 (0%)
Total	345			36 (12%)[a]	25 (7.2%)	11 (3%)

[a] Does not include [18].

their etiology is thought to be the presence of endogenous or exogenous estrogenic activity. The authors therefore concluded that long-term tamoxifen use is associated with estrogenic side effects manifested by an increased occurrence of polyps. This study failed to demonstrate any increase in precancerous or cancerous endometrial lesions associated with tamoxifen treatment.

Other authors have also reported a higher incidence of endometrial polyps and hyperplasia in tamoxifen-treated breast cancer patients. Corley et al. [12] reported on four tamoxifen-treated patients who developed unusual endometrial polyps characterized by cystically dilated glands and stromal decidualization. These findings were not confirmed in the 17 cases of endometrial polyps reported by Lahti et al. [11]. Neven et al. [13] reported that 7 of 16 patients who had an atrophic endometrial biopsy prior to the initiation of tamoxifen therapy developed proliferative endometrium on subsequent hysteroscopic biopsy 6–36 months later, while four developed endometrial polyps and one developed adenocarcinoma. Cohen et al. [14] noted that 35.5% of 93 tamoxifen-treated patients had positive histological findings compared to 20.0% of 20 patients not receiving tamoxifen. Gal et al. [15] reported an 18% incidence of endometrial hyperplasia on random endometrial biopsies obtained from 38 breast cancer patients who had received tamoxifen at a dose of 20 mg/day for at least 12 months. Thirty-two patients (46%) who were initially eligible for study could not participate, since endometrial samples could not be obtained due to atrophic changes. In the second phase of the study, the authors performed endometrial biopsies prospectively on 11 patients at 4–6-month intervals. Three of these patients (28%) developed endometrial hyperplasia following 6, 10, and 12 months of tamoxifen use, respectively, while 40% of the patients initially eligible for study could not participate secondary to inability to undergo an endometrial biopsy.

The 20% overall incidence of endometrial hyperplasia reported by Gal et al. [15] was higher than the 4% incidence of endometrial hyperplasia noted by Lahti et al. [9] in 51 tamoxifen-treated breast cancer patients. Gibson et al. [16] reported the results of a retrospective review of endometrial pathology found at dilatation and curettage (D&C) performed in 240 breast cancer patients. Seventy-five (31%) of these patients had received tamoxifen for a mean duration of 27 months as therapy for their breast cancer. Patients in this study were stratified as symptomatic (abnormal bleeding) or asymptomatic (curettage performed as part of another procedure or dur to the presence of a thickened endometrial stripe on ultrasound examination). Among tamoxifen users who were symptomatic at the time of D&C, the incidence of endometrial polyps was 15%, hyperplasia 2%, and adenocarcinoma 11%, compared to an incidence of 13%, 4%, and 11%, respectively, for nonusers. Among asymptomatic patients receiving tamoxifen, the incidence of polyps, hyperplasia, and adenocarcinoma was 9%, 0%, and 0%, while nonusers had an incidence of 5%, 4%, and 0%, respectively. All the cases of endometrial carcinoma in this study were associated with abnormal vaginal bleeding. The 11% incidence of endometrial carcinoma in this study was comparable to what has been reported for all patients presenting with postmenopausal bleeding in the general population [18].

The dose of tamoxifen used by the patients in this study was 20 mg/day. The mean duration of tamoxifen use in those patients found to have adenocarcinoma was 44 months, compared to 18 months in those patients with polyps and 19 months in the patient with hyperplasia. This difference was not statistically significant, possibly due to small numbers. The authors concluded that short-term tamoxifen use at the 20 mg/day dose level was not associated with a higher incidence of abnormal pathology as detected at the time of D&C in breast cancer patients. Overall, it appears that tamoxifen may cause increased endometrial proliferation in 30% to 40% of patients and results in a threefold increase in endometrial polyps.

5. Endometrial carcinoma

Following the initial report by Killackey et al. [19] of endometrial cancer occurring in three breast cancer patients receiving antiestrogens, approximately 250 additional tamoxifen-associated uterine cancers have been reported [20]. The anecdotal nature of many of these small series, while suggesting an association between tamoxifen treatment for breast cancer and the subsequent development of endometrial cancer, fail to provide conclusive evidence for its occurrence. Perhaps the strongest data initially implicating tamoxifen use and the subsequent development of endometrial cancer were published in 1989 by Fornander et al. [21]. The authors reviewed the frequency of new primary cancers as recorded in the Swedish Cancer Registry for a group of 1846 postmenopausal women with early breast cancer who were included in a randomized trial of adjuvant tamoxifen. They noted a 6.4-fold increase in the relative risk of endometrial cancer in 931 tamoxifen-treated patients, compared to 915 patients in the control group. The dose of tamoxifen in this study was 40 mg/day, and the greatest cumulative risk of developing endometrial cancer was after five years of tamoxifen use.

Fisher et al. [22] recently published the most compelling data to date regarding the association between tamoxifen use and the development of endometrial cancer when they reported the findings of the National Surgical Adjuvant Breast and Bowel Project (NSABP) B14 trial. Data regarding the rates of endometrial and other cancers were analyzed on 2843 patients with node-negative, estrogen receptor-positive, invasive breast cancer randomly assigned to placebo or tamoxifen (20 mg/day) and on 1220 tamoxifen-treated patients registered in NSABP B14 subsequent to randomization. Two of the 1424 patients assigned to receive placebo developed endometrial cancer; however, both had subsequently received tamoxifen for treatment of breast cancer recurrence. Fifteen patients randomized to tamoxifen treatment developed endometrial cancer. One of these patients never actually accepted tamoxifen therapy. Eight additional cases of uterine cancer occurred in the 1220 tamoxifen-treated patients. Seventy-six percent of the endometrial cancers occurred in women age 60 or older. The mean duration of tamoxifen therapy was 35 months, with 36% of the endometrial cancers developing within two yeas of therapy and six occurring less than nine months after treatment was initiated, suggesting that some of the cancers may have been present prior to starting tamoxifen therapy.

The average annual hazard rate for endometrial cancer in the placebo group was 0.2/1000 and 1.6/1000 for the randomized tamoxifen-treated group. The relative risk of an endometrial cancer occurring in the randomized, tamoxifen-treated group was 7.5. Similar results were seen in the 1220 registered patients who received tamoxifen. The authors point out, however, that while the findings indicate that the average annual and cumulative hazard rates of occurrence of endometrial cancer are greater in tamoxifen-treated patients than in those receiving placebo, several caveats need to be mentioned. First, there may have been a bias in detection, since tamoxifen-treated patients are more often symptomatic and more likely therefore to seek gynecologic consultation. Secondly, the rate of endometrial cancer in the placebo-treated group appeared to be unusually low. Results from SEER data [23] would predict that 6.9 cancers would occur in the placebo group. This outcome would result in a relative risk of endometrial cancer of 2.2 in the randomized tamoxifen-treated group. In addition, findings from the NSABP B06 trial noted seven endometrial cancers occurring in 1159 breast cancer patients with negative lymph nodes who did not receive systemic therapy. This outcome yielded an average annual hazard rate for endometrial cancer of 0.7/1000. Comparing this with the rate of 1.7/1000 for endometrial cancer in the randomized tamoxifen-treated group from the B14 trial, the relative risk for endometrial cancer is 2.3, similar to that obtained using SEER data.

Any conclusions regarding the risks of tamoxifen treatment inducing endometrial cancer must weigh the benefits of tamoxifen in reducing breast cancer recurrence and new contralateral breast cancers. In the B14 trial, the cumulative rate per 1000 cases of breast cancer relapse was reduced from 227.8 in the placebo group to 123.5 in the randomized tamoxifen-treated group. In addition, the cumulative rate of contralateral breast cancer was reduced from 40.5 to 23.5, respectively, in the two groups. Taking into account the increased cumulative rate of endometrial cancer, there was a 38% reduction in the five-year cumulative hazard rate in the tamoxifen-treated group. These results led the authors to conclude that the benefit of tamoxifen therapy for breast cancer outweighs the potential increase in endometrial cancer being reported. Recent results from three large Scandinavian breast cancer trials have further confirmed the relationship between tamoxifen use and the development of endometrial cancer [24]. These studies, which included a total of 4914 patients with a median follow-up of 8–9 years, were analyzed for the occurrence of second primary cancers. There were statistically significant increases in endometrial cancers among the tamoxifen-treated patients [RR = 4.1].

6. Histology of tamoxifen-associated uterine cancer

It is well established that unopposed estrogen administration is associated with an increased risk of developing endometrial carcinomas. These tend to be predominantly early-stage, low-grade, minimally invasive lesions that have a favorable prognosis [25]. If the effect of tamoxifen on the endometrium is that of a weak estrogen agonist, one could expect associated endometrial cancers to have clinical characteristics comparable to those associated with unopposed estrogen. A recent report from the Yale Tumor Registry by Magriples et al. [26] suggested that uterine cancers occurring in breast cancer patients on tamoxifen may behave more aggressively and carry a worse prognosis. The authors identified 53 patients with invasive or in situ breast cancer who subsequently developed uterine cancer. Fifteen of the patients had received adjuvant tamoxifen at a dose of 40 mg/day for a mean of 4.2 years, while 38 had not received tamoxifen. The mean patient age was 72.3 years for tamoxifen users, which was not statistically different from those not receiving tamoxifen (68.5 years). The interval between the diagnosis of breast and endometrial cancer was significantly lower in the tamoxifen-treated group compared to those not receiving tasmoxifen (5.3 vs. 12.3 years). Sixty-seven percent of the uterine cancers occurring in the tamoxifen-treated patients had high-grade lesions (grade 3 adenocarcinoma) or high-risk histologies (papillary serous, clear cell, mixed mesodermal tumor), compared to 28% of those developing in the 38 breast cancer patients who had not received tamoxifen. In addition, patients in the tamoxifen-treated group were statistically more likely to die of endometrial cancer (33.3% vs. 2.6%).

These findings led the authors to conclude that 'women receiving tamoxifen as treatment for breast cancer are at risk for high-grade endometrial cancers that have a poor prognosis.' In addition, the presence of a high percentage of poor-prognosis histologies, including poorly differentiated adenocarcinoma, papillary serous cancers, and clear-cell cancers, along with mixed mesodermal tumors in the tamoxifen-treated group, led the authors to speculate that the mechanism of tamoxifen-induced endometrial neoplasia may be different than that of exogenous estrogen, which is associated with more favorable histologies. Silva et al. [27] reviewed the data from M.D. Anderson Cancer Center of 72 breast cancer patients who subsequently developed malignant uterine neoplasms. Fifth-seven patients had not received tamoxifen as part of their treatment, while 15 patients had. Among tamoxifen-treated patients, 33% of the tumors had papillary serous histology, which was significantly higher than the 7% incidence occurring in patients who had not received tamoxifen. No mention is made by the authors, however, as to the type or duration of chemotherapy given to either group of patients for treatment of their breast cancer.

Table 2. Clinicopathologic data from recent series reporting on tamoxifen-associated uterine cancer

	Author [ref]						
Data	Magriples [26]	Barakat [28]	Silva [27]	Fisher [22]	Fornander [29]	van Leeuwen [30]	Total (%)
No. pts.	15	23	15	25	17	23	118
FIGO stage							
I	7	15	10	21	14	17	84 (71.2%)
II	0	2	1	1	2	3	9 (7.6%)
III	2	5	2	1	0	0	10 (8.5%)
IV	0	1	1	1	1	0	4 (3.4%)
Unstaged	6	0	1	1	0	3	11 (9.3%)
Histology							
Endometrioid	9	17	3	18	16	17	80 (67%)
High-risk[a]	6	6	12	7	1	6	38 (32%)
Grade (adenocarcinoma)							
Low (grade 1–2)	5	13	3	18	15	Not given	54 (74.0%)
High (grade 3)	10	4	0	5	0	Not given	19 (26.0%)
Deaths from uterine cancer	5 (33%)	5 (22%)	1 (7%)	4 (16%)	3 (18%)	0 (0%)	18 (15.3%)

[a] Includes papillary serous, clear cell, and sarcoma.

A high incidence of leiomyosarcomas was noted in both tamoxifen-treated and untreated patients — 14% vs. 17%, much higher than the 1% to 2% incidence of sarcomas that one would expect to find. Other reports of uterine sarcomas occurring in tamoxifen-treated breast cancer patients have been published, but these essentially consist of anecdotal case reports.

Several recent studies, however, have not been able to confirm that tamoxifen use is associated with the development of high-risk endometrial cancers (table 2). Barakat et al. [28] reported the Memorial Sloan-Kettering Cancer Center experience in 73 patients with a history of breast cancer who subsequently developed uterine cancer. Twenty-three (32%) had received tamoxifen for at least one year, with a median duration of use of 4.5 years, while 50 (68%) did not receive tamoxifen. There was no significant difference in age, mean weight, or median survival following hysterectomy between the two groups of patients. The median interval between diagnosis of breast and uterine cancer was less in those receiving tamoxifen (4.6 vs. 6.7 years), but this finding was not statistically significant. There was no significant difference in the FIGO stage of the uterine cancers occurring in those patients who had received tamoxifen compared with nonusers. Seventy-four percent of the corpus cancers occurring in the tamoxifen-treated group were endometrial adenocarcinomas, while 26% consisted of high-risk histologic subtypes, including papillary serous and clear-cell carcinomas, as well as uterine sarcomas. This distribution was identical to that seen in the group not receiving tamoxifen. Five women (22%) from the tamoxifen group died of uterine cancer, as did 13 (26%) of those who did not receive tamoxifen. The authors concluded that there was no difference in the stage, grade, or histologic subtype of corpus cancers that develop in breast cancer patients based on tamoxifen use.

Other authors have reported similar results. Fornander et al. [29] recently reported the clinicopathologic findings of endometrial cancers occurring as second primaries in 931 tamoxifen-treated patients with early breast cancer from the Stockholm Adjuvant Tamoxifen Trial. The median duration of tamoxifen use was 24 months, given at a dose of 40 mg/day. On histologic review of these cancers, 82% were FIGO stage I, and all were histologic grade 1 or 2. Three deaths (18%) were attributable to endometrial cancer. Van Leeuwen et al. [30] recently reported the results of a case–control study from the Netherlands Cancer Registry. There was no difference in the FIGO stage or histologic distribution of endometrial cancers that occurred in 23 breast cancer patients who received tamoxifen compared to 75 who did not. None of the tamoxifen-treated patients died of endometrial cancer, whereas four of those who did not receive tamoxifen died. Finally, the results of the NSABP B14 trial [22] also confirmed that uterine cancers occurring in tamoxifen-treated breast cancer patients are not associated with a higher incidence of adverse histologic features. Eighty-eight percent of the tamoxifen-associated endometrial cancers were FIGO stage I. In addition, 71% were endometrioid adenocarcinomas and 78% were low-grade lesions. Four deaths (16.7%) were attributed to endometrial cancer.

7. Screening for endometrial cancer

7.1. Endometrial sampling

To date, there is no proven method of screening for endometrial cancer in breast cancer patients on tamoxifen. The expected annual risk of endometrial cancer in these patients is approximately 2 out of 1000, as defined by the B14 trial [22]. A screening program may detect premalignant endometrial precursors, such as atypical hyperplasia, or benign endometrial conditions including polyps, the incidence of which will be higher than 2 in 1000. The best method for screening, however, remains to be determined. Some authors have proposed annual endometrial sampling, although this is not without its difficulties. Gal et al. [15] were unable to perform office endometrial biopsies with a Novak curette in 44% of 89 postmenopausal patients due to atrophic changes. Should asymptomatic patients who cannot undergo an office endometrial biopsy be subjected to the inherent morbidity of a fractional D&C under general anesthesia? Certainly all patients with abnormal bleeding should seek immediate gynecologic evaluation. As reported by Gibson et al. [16], all cases of endometrial carcinoma detected by D&C in tamoxifen-treated breast cancer patients presented with abnormal bleeding.

Barakat et al. [31] presented the preliminary results of a prospective endometrial screening study in tamoxifen-treated breast cancer patients at the 1995 Annual Meeting of the American Society of Clinical Oncology. One hundred twenty-six patients with a mean age of 51 years were entered in the study; six (4.8%) could not undergo the biopsy procedure due to a stenotic cervix. Of the remaining 120 patients, seven (5.8%) were noncompliant, four were removed from the study due to progression of breast cancer, four discontinued use of tamoxifen, and four were considered protocol violations. The remaining 101 evaluable patients underwent a total of 296 biopsies (mean 3) that utilized a Pipelle endometrial biopsy device (Unimar; Wilmington, Connecticut), with a median surveillance time of 16.2 months. Four (4%) biopsies were abnormal, including two complex hyperplasias, one atypical hyperplasia, and one with an abnormal amount of histiocytes. All abnormal biopsies were confirmed by fractional D&C. Six (6%) additional patients required D&C for persistent bleeding despite benign biopsies. The findings at D&C included polyps (three), normal (two), and pseudodecidualization (one). Three patients underwent hysterectomy. The first developed complex atypical hyperplasia following 12 months of tamoxifen. The second underwent a hysterectomy for a pelvic mass following 15 months of tamoxifen that on final pathology revealed a high-grade leiomyosarcoma. A third patient underwent hysterectomy for complex hyperplasia with extensive mucinous change after 13 months of tamoxifen. The authors concluded that office endometrial biopsies can be used to monitor the endometrium in the majority (95%) of breast cancer patients on tamoxifen. Six percent of patients may require a D&C for persistent bleeding. Significant pathology was detected by endometrial biopsy in two (2%) patients and by close surveillance in a third. However, longer follow-up will be required to determine the value of routine endometrial biopsies in tamoxifen-treated breast cancer patients.

7.2. Transvaginal sonography

Transvaginal sonography may provide a noninvasive means of screening for endometrial pathology in tamoxifen-treated breast cancer patients. The definition of an abnormal endometrial stripe in tamoxifen-treated breast cancer patients remains undefined. Lahti et al. [11] reported that if a cutoff of 5 mm or more was used to define an abnormal endometrial echo, 22 (51.2%) patients had no abnormal endometrial pathology. Similar findings were reported by Cohen et al. [32], who prospectively performed endometrial biopsies following vaginal sonography in 72 tamoxifen-treated breast cancer patients. Among the patients with an endometrial stripe greater than 5 mm, approximately 70% had no endometrial tissue identifiable, and only one patient was found to have endometrial cancer. Kedar et al. [17] reported a predictive value of 100% (16 of 16) for atypical hyperplasia or polyps with an endometrial stripe of 8 mm or more. These findings suggest that premalignant changes can be detected with transvaginal sonography, and the use of ultrasound and/or endometrial sampling to screen for endometrial neoplasia needs to be evaluated in large prospective trials before recommendations for screening can be made.

There is, however, a risk in overinterpreting the ultrasonographic findings of the endometrium in tamoxifen-treated patients. Goldstein [33] recently reported five postmenopausal tamoxifen-treated patients who on routine surveillance with vaginal probe ultrasonography were described as having heterogeneous, bizarre-appearing endometria with multiple sonolucent areas suggestive of a polyp. Because of concerns regarding tamoxifen use and endometrial neoplasia, the first patient was referred for a curettage and hysteroscopy. Minimal tissue was obtained, and hysteroscopic evaluation revealed a smooth atrophic endometrium. When the abnormal sonographic appearance persisted, the patient underwent a sonohysterogram, which involves the instillation of 3–10 mL of saline at the time of sonography. The fluid enhancement revealed that the changes originally interpreted as endometrial were actually subendometrial in origin. Four additional patients with similar abnormal sonographic findings were actually found to have subendometrial abnormalities on sonohysterogram. It is unclear what these abnormal areas represent, since none of the patients have undergone hysterectomy, although it was speculated that they may represent adenomyomatous-like changes. Further studies regarding the sonographic appearance of the endometrium in tamoxifen-treated patients are warranted.

The ultimate goal of any cancer screening program is to detect disease at an earlier stage, when it is more curable. Since tamoxifen-associated endometrial cancers appear to have a stage, grade, and histology similar to endometrial cancers occurring in the general population, their prognosis is generally good, and early detection will probably not improve outcome significantly. A very small number of tamoxifen-treated breast cancer patients could be expected to benefit from screening for endometrial cancer. Since the annual risk of endometrial cancer is 2 in 1000 in this population, and since approximately 15% of these cancers will result in the patient's death, annual screening could potentially decrease mortality in only $0.002 \times 0.15 = 0.0003$, or 0.03%, of all tamoxifen-treated patients. Since approximately 80,000 women begin tamoxifen treatment annually, the cost to undertake screening for endometrial cancer in this population may be prohibitively high. For now, all women with breast cancer, whether or not they are receiving tamoxifen, should be encouraged to undergo an annual gynecologic evaluation. Endometrial sampling should be reserved for patients with any sign of abnormal vaginal bleeding, including spotting or brownish vaginal discharge.

8. Future directions

Barakat et al. [34] evaluated the status of c-Ki-*ras* mutations in endometrial cancers occurring in breast cancers patients. Using DNA-SSCP screening, they noted a higher incidence of mobility shifts consistent with mutation in 14 tamoxifen-associated cancers compared with the 13 cancers that occurred in patients not receiving tamoxifen. Direct sequencing, however, revealed that there were six Ki-*ras* mutations in each group. The mean interval between the diagnosis of breast and endometrial cancer was not significantly shorter in the tamoxifen-treated group compared to the group not receiving tamoxifen (4.9 vs. 6.8 years). However, among patients whose endometrial cancers contained Ki-*ras* mutations, the mean interval between the diagnosis of breast and endometrial cancer was 2.4 times shorter in the tamoxifen-treated group compared with the group that had not received tamoxifen (4.9 vs. 11.7 years). These preliminary results need to be confirmed in a larger number of cases. In addition, it may be valuable to evaluate the status of other proto-oncogenes and tumor-suppressor genes in tamoxifen-associated endometrial cancers, as well as endometrial cancers occurring in breast cancer patients who have not received tamoxifen. Studies such as these may ultimately increase our understanding of the mechanisms involved in tamoxifen-induced endometrial carcinogenesis. For now, all women with breast cancer, whether or not they are receiving tamoxifen, should be encouraged to undergo annual gynecologic evaluation, which should include endometrial sampling in the presence of abnormal vaginal bleeding.

References

1. Satyaswaroop PG, Zaino RJ, Mortel R. 1984. Estrogen-like effects of tamoxifen on human endometrial carcinoma transplanted into nude mice. Cancer Res 44:4006–4010.
2. Gottardis MM, Robinson SP, Satyaswaroop PG, et al. 1988. Contrasting actions of tamoxifen on endometrial and breast tumor growth in the athymic mouse. Cancer Res 48:812–815.
3. Wolf DM, Jordan VC. 1992. Gynecologic complications associated with long-term adjuvant tamoxifen therapy for breast cancer. Gynecol Oncol 45:118–128.
4. Tucker MJ, Adams HK, Patterson JS. 1984. In Laurence DR, Mclean AEM, Weatherall M, eds. *Safety Testing of New Drugs*. New York: Academic Press, pp. 125–161.
5. Han XL, Liehr JG. 1992. Induction of covalent DNA adducts in rodents by tamoxifen. Cancer Res 52:1360–1363.
6. White IN, De Matteis F, Davies A, et al. 1992. Genotoxic potential of tamoxifen and analogues in female Fischer F344/n rats, DBA/2 and C57BL/6 mice and in human MCL-5 cells. Carcinogenesis 13:2197–2203.
7. Martin EA, Rich KJ, White INH, et al. 1995. ^{32}P-Postlabeled DNA adducts in liver obtained from women treated with tamoxifen. Carcinogenesis 16:1651–1654.
8. Pongracz K, Pathak DN, Nakamura T, et al. 1995. Activation of the tamoxifen derivative metabolite E to form DNA adducts: comparison with the adducts formed by microsomal activation of tamoxifen. Cancer Res 55:3012–3015.
9. Carmichael PL, Ugwumanda AHN, Neven P, et al. 1996. Lack of genotoxicity of tamoxifen in the human endometrium. Cancer Res 56:1475–1479.
10. Boccardo F, Bruzzi P, Rubagotti A, et al. 1981. Estrogen-like action of tamoxifen on vaginal epithelium in breast cancer patients. Oncology 38:281–285.
11. Lahti E, Blanco G, Kauppila A, et al. 1993. Endometrial changes in postmenopausal breast cancer patients receiving tamoxifen. Obstet Gynecol 81:660–664.
12. Corley D, Rowe J, Curtis MT, et al. 1992. Postmenopausal bleeding from unusual endometrial polyps in women on chronic tamoxifen therapy. Obstet Gynecol 79:111–116.

13. Neven P, De Muylder X, Van Belle Y, Vanderick G, De Muylder Y. 1990. Hysteroscopic follow up during tamoxifen treatment. Eur J Obstet Gynecol Reprod Biol 35:235–238.
14. Cohen I, Rosen DJD, Shapira J, et al. 1994. Endometrial changes with tamoxifen: comparison between tamoxifen-treated and non-treated asymptomatic, postmenopausal breast cancer patients. Gynecol Oncol 52:185–190.
15. Gal D, Kopel S, Bashevkin M, et al. 1991. Oncologic potential of tamoxifen on endometria of postmenopausal women with breast cancer: preliminary report. Gynecol Oncol 42:120–123.
16. Gibson LE, Barakat RR, Venkatraman ES, et al. 1995. Endometrial pathology at dilatation and curettage in breast cancer patients: comparison of tamoxifen users and nonusers. Cancer J Sci Am 2:35–38.
17. Kedar RP, Bourne TH, Powles TJ, et al. 1994. Effects of tamoxifen on uterus and ovaries of postmenopausal women in a randomised breast cancer prevention trial. Lancet 343:1318–1321.
18. Hacker NF, Moore JG, eds. 1992. Essentials of Obstetrics and Gynecology, 2nd ed. Philadelphia: WB Saunders, p. 577.
19. Killackey MA, Hakes TB, Pierce VK. 1985. Endometrial adenocarcinoma in breast cancer patients receiving antiestrogens. Cancer Treat Rep 69:237–238.
20. Assikis VJ, Jordan VC. 1995. Gynecologic effects of tamoxifen and the association with endometrial carcinoma. Int J Gynecol Obstet 49:241–257.
21. Fornander T, Cedermark B, Mattsson A, et al. 1989. Adjuvant tamoxifen in early breast cancer: occurrence of new primary cancers. Lancet 1:117–120.
22. Fisher B, Costantino JP, Redmond CK, et al. 1994. Endometrial cancer in tamoxifen-treated breast cancer patients: findings from the National Surgical Adjuvant Breast and Bowel Project (NSABP) B-14. J Natl Cancer Inst 86:527–537.
23. National Cancer Institute. 1993. SEER Cancer Statistics Review 1973–1990. Document #93–2789. Bethesda, MD: NCI.
24. Rutqvist LE, Johansson H, Signomklao T, et al. 1995. Adjuvant tamoxifen therapy for early stage breast cancer and second primary malignancies. J Natl Cancer Inst 87:645–651.
25. Elwood JM, Boyes DA. 1980. Clinical and pathological features and survival of endometrial cancer patients in relation to prior use of estrogens. Gynecol Oncol 10:173–187.
26. Magriples U, Naftolin F, Schwartz PE, et al. 1993. High-grade endometrial carcinoma in tamoxifen-treated breast cancer patients. J Clin Oncol 11:485–490.
27. Silva EG, Tornos CS, Follen-Mitchell M. 1994. Malignant neoplasms of the uterine corpus in patients treated for breast carcinoma: the effects of tamoxifen. Int J Gynecol Pathol 13:248–258.
28. Barakat RR, Wong G, Curtin JP, et al. 1994. Tamoxifen use in breast cancer patients who subsequently develop corpus cancer is not associated with a higher incidence of adverse histologic features. Gynecol Oncol 55:164–168.
29. Fornander T, Hellstrom A-C, Moberger B. 1993. Descriptive clinicopathologic study of 17 patients with endometrial cancer during or after adjuvant tamoxifen in early breast cancer. J Natl Cancer Inst 85:1850–1855.
30. Van Leeuwen FE, Benraadt J, Coebergh JWW, et al. 1994. Risk of endometrial cancer after tamoxifen treatment of breast cancer. Lancet 343:448–452.
31. Barakat RR, Gilewski TA, Saigo PE, et al. 1995. The effect of adjuvant tamoxifen on the endometrium in women with breast cancer: an interim analysis of a prospective study (abstract). Proc ASCO 779.
32. Cohen I, Rosen D, Tepper R, et al. 1993. Ultrasonographic evaluation of the endometrium and correlation with endometrial sampling in postmenopausal patients treated with tamoxifen. J Ultrasound Med 5:275–280.
33. Goldstein SR. 1994. Unusual ultrasonographic appearance of the uterus in patients receiving tamoxifen. Am J Obstet Gynecol 170:447–451.
34. Barakat RR, Adhikari D, Saigo PE, O'Connor B, Banerjee D, Bertino JR. In press. Mutation of c-Ki-*ras* in tamoxifen-associated endometrial carcinoma. Accepted for presentation, Society of Gynecologic Oncologists' Annual Meeting, 1996.

12. Hormone replacement therapy and nonhormonal control of menopausal symptoms in breast cancer survivors

Melody A. Cobleigh

1. Introduction

Postmenopausal women often experience annoying and sometimes debilitating menopausal symptoms, and breast cancer survivors are no exception. Hot flashes, dyspareunia, atrophic vaginitis with attendant urinary tract symptoms, sleep disturbance, and mood change are among these symptoms. Estrogen replacement therapy (ERT) has been shown to ameliorate these problems [1,2], and as informed consumers, breast cancer survivors are increasingly inquiring about and/or requesting ERT.

Tamoxifen can precipitate or worsen vasomotor and vaginal symptoms. Some women discontinue tamoxifen adjuvant therapy because they find these symptoms intolerable. Some women request estrogen to alleviate their symptoms, and some physicians prescribe it. There has never been a prospective, randomized trial of hormone replacement therapy (HRT) in breast cancer survivors.

Coronary artery disease is a more insidious but potentially fatal consequence of menopausal estrogen decline. The magnitude of the reduction of coronary heart disease reported in ERT users who undergo natural menopause is large and in general ranges between 30% and 70% [3–5].

Osteoporosis is another potential cause of morbidity and mortality among postmenopausal women. A reduction in the rate of subsequent fracture in ERT users has been reported to range between 30% and 60% [3,6].

There are more breast cancer survivors alive now than ever before, so their nononcologic health problems are a growing concern. A dramatic rise in the incidence rates of breast cancer occurred in the United States between 1982 and 1987, presumably because of increased screening [7]. The incidence of both noninvasive and small, invasive, axillary node-negative breast cancers rose concurrently [8]. Five-year survival rates for breast cancer patients also have been rising since 1979 [8].

Prohibition of HRT may diminish quality of life in breast cancer survivors. Furthermore, it is possible that the prohibition of HRT could reduce overall survival in such women by leaving them at increased risk of coronary heart disease, stroke, and osteoporotic fracture.

Kenneth A. Foon and Hyman B. Muss (eds), BIOLOGICAL AND HORMONAL THERAPIES OF CANCER.
Copyright © 1998. Kluwer Academic Publishers, Boston. All rights reserved.

Of greater concern is the precipitation of premature menopause in women treated for breast cancer. Adjuvant chemotherapy is prescribed more often now, based on favorable outcomes for women with small invasive but node-negative disease. Along with the rising incidence of small, prognostically favorable cancers, the indications for adjuvant therapy have expanded. In 1989, the results of Four major, prospective, randomized clinical trials were published. These studies compared treatment with no treatment and documented the benefit of adjuvant therapy in women with node-negative, invasive breast cancers larger than 1 cm [8–11]. Chemotherapy was the intervention used in three of the studies [9–11]. Since then, chemotherapy has increasingly been prescribed for this favorable subset of breast cancer patients.

Adjuvant chemotherapy causes premature ovarian failure [12]. The incidence of amenorrhea is both age and drug dependent. For CMF, the most commonly prescribed regimen, amenorrhea occurs in 53% of women under age 35, 84% age 35–44, and 94% over age 45 [13]. Of those with ovarian failure, it is permanent in 86% of women under age 40 and in 96% over age 40 [14].

This outcome is of concern, since most studies that have examined the role of premature menopause on coronary heart disease have found an increased risk in women with early menopause (reviewed in [4]). Evidence that ERT can reduce this effect of early menopause comes from the Harvard Nurses' Health Study, where nurses who underwent surgical menopause and received ERT had a significantly lower risk of cardiovascular disease compared with those with surgical menopause who did not receive ERT. The age-adjusted relative risk of major coronary disease for ERT users was 0.40 (95% confidence intervals 0.22–0.73) [15].

Death from nonneoplastic conditions is common among node-negative breast cancer survivors, and cardiovascular disease is the most common cause [16]. These data are derived from patients who did not receive chemotherapy and thus did not undergo premature menopause. As more node-negative women receive adjuvant chemotherapy, the possibility exists that early chemotherapy-mediated gains in survival from breast cancer may be overshadowed by higher mortality from cardiovascular and osteoporotic events later on. That is, women may survive their breast cancers only to succumb to these other more common but delayable afflictions. Concern for quality of life as well as longevity in our patients justifies a trial of HRT in breast cancer survivors.

The Eastern Cooperative Oncology Group (ECOG) plans a double-blind, placebo-controlled phase III trial of HRT for breast cancer survivors on tamoxifen, who have menopausal symptoms for which they seek medical intervention. This chapter describes the standard of care for prescribing HRT. It focuses on the effects of combining HRT and tamoxifen on menopausal symptoms and end organs. Nonestrogenic methods of controlling menopausal symptoms are examined. Finally, theoretical detrimental effects of HRT on breast cancer survivors are analyzed.

2. The standard of care

The standard of care in the United States is to discourage prescription of HRT in breast cancer survivors. Although there are theoretical justifications for this position, the limited number of studies offer little support for such concern (vide infra). This lack of study is not because of indifference [17–27]; physicians are increasingly calling for clinical trials, and some have published guidelines for administration of ERT to breast cancer survivors [27]. Further, we know of many clinicians who will treat breast cancer survivors with HRT in the absence of evidence showing a harmful effect. A distinguished investigator has stated '... it is no longer justifiable to deprive those women who have received treatment for breast cancer of hormonal treatment which can relieve symptoms which are making their lives intolerable' [28]. Nonetheless, the practicing physician who follows breast cancer survivors currently has no official justification to offer HRT to his/her patients, since the opinions of many professional societies are either ambiguous or opposed to such treatment.

The American College of Physicians has recently published guidelines for counseling postmenopausal women about preventive hormone therapy [29]. The authors support HRT in women with or at increased risk for coronary heart disease. They speculate that the risks of HRT in women who are at increased risk for breast cancer *might* outweigh the benefits of HRT. For other women, the best course of action is unclear, but they suggest describing the probable risks and benefits of HRT.

The American College of Obstetrics and Gynecology supports the use of HRT in postmenopausal women but considers breast cancer a contraindication [1]. The Science Advisory Committee of the American Heart Association recommends ERT for women who have a high risk of cardiovascular disease because of adverse lipid profiles or preexisting cardiovascular disease [30].

3. The role of tamoxifen in breast cancer treatment and its potential hazards and benefits as they relate to the potential hazards and benefits of HRT

A discussion of HRT in breast cancer survivors must consider the increasing prescription of tamoxifen. The window of opportunity to study the impact of HRT on the natural history of breast cancer, independent of tamoxifen, has closed.

Tamoxifen is recommended adjuvant therapy for an increasing number of women with breast cancer. A recent world overview suggested that all women with invasive tumors might benefit from tamoxifen and that longer durations of treatment may be superior to shorter durations [31]. Currently, adjuvant tamoxifen is prescribed for five years in node-negative women. The optimal duration of therapy in node-positive patients is not known but is at least five years.

A clinical trial to evaluate the efficacy of tamoxifen in ductal carcinoma in situ (DCIS), NSABP B24, completed accrual rapidly. If results are favorable, tamoxifen will become standard therapy for the large numbers of women diagnosed with DCIS each year on the basis of screening mammography.

In the future, tamoxifen may also be widely used not only in breast cancer survivors but also in women who are considered at risk of breast cancer. Three breast cancer prevention trials evaluating tamoxifen prophylaxis in healthy women at high risk for breast cancer are currently under way; one in the U.S./Canada, one in Italy, and one in the U.K./Australia. If the results of these trials are positive, tamoxifen may be recommended as a chemopreventive agent for large numbers of premenopausal and postmenopausal women.

ERT and tamoxifen have been administered simultaneously to postmenopausal patients, apparently without ill effect [32]. In the British Breast Cancer Prevention Trial, which uses tamoxifen as the preventive agent, postmenopausal women who experience hot flashes are given ERT for relief. However, carefully controlled studies of combined ERT or HRT and tamoxifen have not been performed.

A logical concern over the administration of ERT/HRT and tamoxifen together is that estrogen might antagonize the effect of tamoxifen on breast cells or on tumor cells. However, premenopausal women have high levels of estradiol circulating on sex-hormone-binding globulin; yet they respond to tamoxifen, and therefore postmenopausal women on ERT should also.

Postmenopausal women receiving ERT have serum concentrations of estradiol that are not significantly different from estradiol levels in premenopausal women during the follicular phase of the menstrual cycle. Premenopausal patients have much higher levels through the rest of their cycle (table 1; [33–35]).

Tamoxifen stimulates estrogen secretion in premenopausal women [34–36].

Table 1. Estradiol levels in premenopausal and postmenopausal women, in postmenopausal women taking ERT, and in premenopausal women taking tamoxifen

Clinical state [ref]	pg/mL	pM/L
Postmenopausal [33]	15	51.4
Postmenopausal on Premarin®, 0.625 mg/day	80–100	294–367
Premenopausal, follicular phase [34]	199	731
Premenopausal, follicular phase after two months of tamoxifen [34]	506	1860
Premenopausal, luteal phase [34]	197	725
Premenopausal, taking tamoxifen [35]	190 **over baseline**	700 **over baseline**
Premenopausal, luteal phase after two months of tamoxifen [34]	586	2154

The rise in sex-hormone-binding globulin observed in these women, a normal hepatic response to hyper-estrogenemia, suggests that premenopausal women experience a physiologically hyper-estrogenemic state corresponding to their high estrogen levels [36]. Mean estradiol levels in tamoxifen-treated premenopausal patients are 2 to 3 times those seen throughout a normal menstrual cycle [35]. Despite such high levels of estradiol, these premenopausal women experience tumor regression when tamoxifen is administered.

Tamoxifen's mechanism of action was initially thought to be mediated solely through the estrogen receptor. If this were true, high levels of endogenous estrogen should competitively inhibit binding of tamoxifen to the estrogen receptor, thereby diminishing or eliminating the drug's effectiveness in premenopausal women.

More recent research has shown that tamoxifen influences other physiologic processes. For example, tamoxifen decreases secretion of stimulatory growth factors such as *tumor* growth factor-alpha (TGF-α), insulin-like growth factors I and II (IGF-I and IGF-II), and PDGF and increases secretion of inhibitory growth factors such as TGF-beta [37,38]. It inhibits the mitogenic effect of growth factors on breast cancer cells in the total absence of estrogens [39]. Tamoxifen can block protein kinase C and calmodulin activation, alter cell membrane permeability, and modulate immunoregulatory function [40–43]. It is reasonable to presume that these effects would be independent of serum estrogen levels.

Observations suggesting that ERT will not reduce tamoxifen's therapeutic effect include its efficacy in premenopausal women with metastatic and operable breast cancer. Premenopausal women with metastatic breast cancer experience remission when treated with tamoxifen [44–53]. For most physicians, tamoxifen has replaced oophorectomy as the initial treatment of choice for premenopausal women with metastatic breast cancer in whom a hormone manipulation is indicated. The FDA has approved the use of tamoxifen in premenopausal women.

Adjuvant therapy trials comparing tamoxifen alone with placebo also show that tamoxifen benefits both premenopausal and postmenopausal women. In the largest trial with that design, NSABP B14, node-negative, estrogen receptor-positive breast cancer patients were randomly assigned to five years of tamoxifen or placebo. In that trial, premenopausal women derived a greater benefit from tamoxifen than postmenopausal women [8], suggesting that the combination of (endogenous) estrogen and tamoxifen is not antithetical and may be beneficial. Yet when these same premenopausal women undergo menopause, they will be denied HRT.

In order to elucidate a potential negative interaction between HRT and tamoxifen, the Eastern Cooperative Oncology Group (ECOG) trial of HRT in breast cancer survivors will monitor serum IGF-I levels in women who take tamoxifen and HRT. Breast cancer cells are mitogenically responsive to IGFs [54]. Receptors for IGF-I are present in breast cancer biopsy specimens and in breast cancer cell lines [55,56]. The mitogenic effects of IGFs on ER-positive breast cancer cells are enhanced by estrogens [57]. Antiestrogens attenuate the actions of IGF-I on breast cancer cells in the absence of estrogen [58]. Tamoxifen lowers serum IGF-I levels [59]. A rise in IGF-I levels after beginning HRT in patients receiving tamoxifen would be of concern.

As the twenty-first century approaches, an era in which tamoxifen may be prescribed for nearly all breast cancer survivors and for women at high risk (all women?), it is reasonable to ask whether tamoxifen and HRT can be administered safely together. Furthermore, it is reasonable to study the combined impact of HRT and tamoxifen on menopausal symptoms, breast cancer outcome, and medical problems that accelerate after menopause.

4. The role of nonestrogenic medications in alleviating vasomotor and vaginal symptoms

4.1. Vasomotor symptoms

Clonidine decreases the frequency and severity of hot flashes in women receiving tamoxifen. Although statistically significant, the clinical benefit is modest and is achieved at the expense of significant increases in constipation, dry mouth, and drowsiness [60].

Another alpha$_2$-adrenoceptor agonist, methyldopa, reduces the frequency of hot flashes significantly but is also associated with unpleasant side effects (tiredness and dry mouth) [61]. Neither of these compounds affects vaginal symptoms.

Megestrol acetate (MA) ameliorates hot flashes. In an unblinded study, it reduced vasomotor symptoms by 80%, 89%, and 98% in daily doses of 20, 40, and 80 mg, respectively [62]. A prospective, randomized, double-blind, placbo-controlled trial confirmed these results [63]. Importantly, most of the women were taking tamoxifen.

Medroxyprogesterone acetate (MPA) has also been shown to lessen hot flashes [64–68]. However, MPA is not expected to alleviate vaginal symptoms [64–68]. Women who received a single 50 mg does of I.M. depo-MPA experienced significant relief of vasomotor symptoms for eight weeks [66].

The placebo effect observed in these trials was substantial (table 2). Another important lesson learned from one trial was that early improvements in quality of life are not necessarily maintained and that trials evaluating efficacy of compounds against vasomotor symptoms should be conducted for at least 12 weeks [69].

Some investigators have suggested that progestogens should be used to relieve vasomotor symptoms in breast cancer survivors [63]. However, the effect of low-dose MA or of MPA on normal and malignant breast cells is unknown.

In striking contrast to the endometrium, where progesterone is associated

Table 2. Reduction in frequency of hot flashes according to intervention in placebo-controlled, double-blind, randomized trials

Author [ref]	Number	Medication	Placebo
Nesheim [61]	40	Methyldopa 65% (45–75)	38% (0–59)
Goldberg [60]	110	Clonidine patch 44%	27%
Loprinzi [63]	80	MA 73%	26%
Morrison [65]	34	MPA 68%	20%
Bergmans [69]	38	Bellergal 85%[a]	85%
Albrecht [66]	6	MPA 87%	25%
Schiff [68]	32	MPA 74%	26%
Bullock [64]	57 MPA 12 placebo	MPA 90%[b]	25%[a]

[a] Reported either elimination or a significant decrease of their hot flashes.
[b] After eight weeks of treatment.

with reduced proliferation, mitotic activity in breast epithelium peaks during days 23–25 of the menstrual cycle. This is shortly after the progesterone and second estradiol peak and suggests that progesterone or possibly combined estrogen and progesterone are responsible [70–72]. Progestins have been implicated in the development of breast cancer in humans [73] and in the growth of breast cancer, both in experimental animals [74–77] and in vitro [77–79]. MPA reduces the proliferative effect of estrogen on the endometrium, and it is expected to protect the endometrium from the stimulatory effects of tamoxifen as well [80].

Likewise, interactions between progestational agents and tamoxifen have not been studied in breast cancer survivors. Clinically, the combination of progestins and tamoxifen is less effective than tamoxifen alone in metastatic breast cancer [81]. That progesterone, given for only one week per month, has been shown to reverse the protective effect of tamoxifen in a rat mammary carcinoma model is of concern [82].

4.2. Vaginal symptoms

Some postmenopausal women who take tamoxifen experience atrophic changes in the vulva, vagina, urethra, and bladder. These changes can result in recurring infections, shortening and narrowing of the vagina, dyspareunia, pevic relaxation, urinary frequency, and incontinence. Estrogen relieves these symptoms and has been approved by the FDA for treatment of atrophic vaginitis, but not for women with a history of breast cancer.

Oncologists may be more willing to prescribe vaginal estrogen-containing creams than oral estrogens for symptomatic patients, not realizing that vaginal administration raises serum estrogen levels 16–20-fold compared with oral administration of the same dose [83–85].

5. The role of nonhormonal medications in alleviating vaginal symptoms

A prospective, randomized, open-label trial compared a nonhormonal local bioadhesive vaginal moisturizer (Replens®) with vaginal extrogen cream (Premarin®) [86]. Replens® improved vaginal health, though to a lesser extent than did Premarin® cream.

Replens® improved vaginal moisture, fluid volume, elasticity, and pH, despite a lack of cornification. No quality-of-life instruments were employed, so it is not known how these changes in the vagina correlated with symptom relief.

5.1. Measurement of vaginal effect

The maturation value (MV) gives different weights to parabasal, intermediate, and superficial cells. The percent of superficial cells is multiplied by 1, intermediate cells by 0.5, and parabasal cells by zero. The MV is the sum of these values. The higher the MV, the greater the cornification. Vaginal smears are performed by drawing a wooden spatula down the upper half of both lateral vaginal walls. The smears are fixed in 95% alcohol and the slides stained by the Papanicolaou method.

MVs increased from a median value of 52 (0–95) to 58 (25–88) after one year of ERT [87,88]. What is clear from these studies, and has been reported previously, is that indices in exfoliative cytology are meaningful only when they relate to a previous index on the same patient.

We are unaware of MVs among women taking tamoxifen, or among women who take tamoxifen and ERT/HRT. We believe that the maturation value is the most objective measure of vaginal health, since the cell types used in the evaluation are well established in the cytology literature. Another tool is the vaginal health index [87] (table 3).

Table 3. Vaginal health index

	1	2	3	4	5
Vaginal moisture (coating)	None, surface inflamed	None surface not inflamed	Minimal	Moderate	Normal
Vaginal fluid volume (pooling of secretions)	None	Scant amount, vault partially covered	Superficial amount, vault fully covered	Moderate amount	Normal amount
Elasticity	None	Poor	Fair	Good	Excellent
Epithelial integrity (mucosa)	Petichiae noted before contact	Bleeds with light contact	Bleeds with scraping	Nonfriable, thin	Normal
Vaginal pH[a]	≥6.1	5.6–6	5.1–5.5	4.7–5	≤4.6

[a] Vaginal fluid pH is measured with pH indicator strips (colorpHast; EM Science, Gibbstown, NJ).

6. End organ effects

6.1. The skeletal system

Tamoxifen protects spinal bone to a lesser extent than estrogen, but it does not appear to preserve bone mineral density at the radius [89]. The risk of fracture has not been assessed among tamoxifen users, and tamoxifen has not been approved by the FDA for this indication. The Breast Cancer Prevention Trial (BCPT) in the U.S./Canada will record bone fracture in all participants and will assess bone mineral density in a smaller cohort.

ERT/HRT preserves bone at the spine, hip, and distal radius [90]. The FDA has approved ERT for the prevention of osteoporosis. It is possible that the protective effects of tamoxifen and HRT may be accentuated by combined treatment.

6.2. The cardiovascular system

Conjugated equine estrogen has been shown to improve blood lipid profiles significantly [83]. In particular, it causes a meaningful rise in HDL-C, the best predictor of cardiovascular health among women [80]. While tamoxifen has been shown to lower LDL cholesterol, it does not increase HDL-C, and this finding is of concern [91,92]. It is possible that the HRT and tamoxifen will show important increases in HDL-C and reductions in LDL-C, amplifying the protective effect of each medication on cardiovascular health.

6.3. The coagulation system

Tamoxifen increases the risk of vascular thrombosis slightly [8]; however, there is no clear epidemiologic evidence of estrogen-mediated hypercoagulability among HRT users [93]. Thus, combining HRT and tamoxifen is not expected to worsen this toxicity.

Importantly, the safety of combined tamoxifen and (endogenous) estrogen has been demonstrated in clinical trials. Premenopausal women who take tamoxifen have a lower risk of thromboembolism compared with postmenopausal women on tamoxifen [8]. This finding is true despite that fact that premenopausal women on tamoxifen experience hyperestrogenemia.

6.4. The endometrium

Unopposed estrogen causes atypical or adenomatous endometrial hyperplasia in one third of women [80]. Both tamoxifen and unopposed estrogen cause a small but significant increase in endometrial cancer [94–96].

Progestogens protect the uterus from the proliferative effect of estrogen [80]. Therefore, the standard approach to HRT in women is to use estrogen and progesterone in women who have a uterus and estrogen alone in those who have undergone hysterectomy.

6.5. The breast

6.5.1. ERT/HRT and mammographic detection of breast cancer.
HRT might increase breast density and thus potentially delay diagnosis of breast cancer. The literature on the subject is limited. Most studies were retrospective [97–99]. The duration and type of HRT varied. Baseline studies were often unavailable. Radiologists were not blinded as to the HRT status of the patient. Technique varied; some women underwent film screen, others xeromammography.

HRT probably causes increased parenchymal density in a minority of women [97,98,100]. Parenchymal density was increased in 17% of 30 women in one study [97] and in 24% of 50 in another [100]. Increased parenchymal density has not been uniformly observed. A matched-cohort study of 405 women who underwent screening xeromammography demonstrated no increase in breast density among HRT users [99].

There is conflicting information on duration of HRT and parenchymal patterns. Significant differences in the proportion of high- and low-risk parenchymal patterns were not observed as the duration of HRT increased in one study [98]. However, duration of HRT did matter in another [99]. High-risk patterns were observed significantly more often among 194 women who had taken HRT for more than five years compared with 216 nonusers.

Mammography before and after treatment, evaluated by an observer blinded to the assigned treatment (placebo vs. ERT vs. HRT), would provide valuable prospective information. The study of mammographic parenchymal changes should be included in any clinical trial of HRT in breast cancer survivors.

6.5.2. ERT/HRT and second breast cancers.
Concern over ERT/HRT-induced new breast cancers must be addressed in any trial of replacement therapy for breast cancer survivors. A personal history of breast cancer is a strong risk factor for subsequent development of primary breast cancers [101]. The annual incidence of new primary breast cancers among breast cancer survivors is 14 per 1000, compared to an incidence of 2 per 1000 in the general population [102]. The association between ERT/HRT and risk of breast cancer remains controversial, although 25 studies and six meta-analyses have been published since 1980 [103–132] (table 4).

Collectively, the studies do not consistently demonstrate an increased risk of breast cancer among women who have ever used ERT/HRT [133]. Studies that controlled for screening showed no difference in relative risk between cases and controls [133]. This finding suggests that there may be a detection bias operating in some studies that have reported an increased risk of breast

Table 4. Meta-analyses of breast cancer incidence among HRT users vs. nonusers

Author [ref]	RR any use (95% CI)	Longer vs. shorter RR (95% CI)
Dupont [127]	1.07 (1.0–1.15)	Can't conclude
Steinberg [128]	1.0	1.3 (1.2–1.6 after 15 yrs)
Armstrong [129]	1.01 (0.95–1.08)	No effect
Grady & Ernster [130]	No increase	1.25
Sillero-Arenas [131]	1.06 (1.0–1.12)	
Colditz [132]	1.02 (0.93–1.12)	

cancer among ERT/HRT users. Importantly, low-dose (0.625 mg daily) conjugated ERT for several years did not appreciably increase the risk of breast cancer [127].

Although having ever used ERT/HRT does not appear to substantially increase the risk of breast cancer, there remains a concern that selected subgroups of the population will be adversely affected. For example, some studies have suggested that long-term estrogen use (10–15 years or more) does increase the risk of breast cancer in women using replacement doses [129]. Although these results are based on small numbers of cases (since relatively few women have used HRT for 15 or more years), these findings are of concern.

Raising serum levels of estradiol slightly in breast cancer survivors who receive HRT may be not be detrimental, however, since the postmenopausal breast has the capacity to concentrate (or manufacture) estrogen. Estradiol levels in ductal fluid that bathes the breast epithelium are 50-fold higher than serum levels. Breast fluid estradiol levels are comparable in premenopausal and postmenopausal women.

Postmenopausal women who are using HRT do not have significantly higher breast fluid estradiol levels than nonusers [33]. Studies of breast tissue confirm these results. Despite considerable differences in plasma estradiol levels between premenopausal and postmenopausal women, it is striking that tissue levels are very similar, regardless of age, in normal breast tissue. Breast cancers from postmenopausal women have even higher estradiol levels, and these levels do not correlate with estrogen receptor levels [134].

Despite the preponderance of evidence that short-term use (less than 10 years) of ERT/HRT does not appear to cause breast cancer in healthy women, it is possible that women with a personal history of breast cancer may be more susceptible to the tumor-promoting effects of estrogen. Tamoxifen reduces the risk of contralateral breast cancers in women with a history of breast cancer (reviewed in [135]). Among eight prospective, randomized trials of tamoxifen vs. no therapy, the relative risk reduction was 35% for women receiving tamoxifen. Thus, it is possible that tamoxifen, if administered with ERT or HRT, may attenuate any potential cancer-promoting effect of estrogen on breast cells.

6.5.3. HRT and breast cancer relapse/survival. A major concern over prescribing HRT for women with a history of breast cancer is that dormant tumor cells might be activated. There is surprisingly little clinical information to substantiate such concern. If endogenous estrogen stimulated breast cancer growth, women diagnosed with breast cancer after menopause should have a better prognosis than women diagnosed premenopausally. This outcome does not occur. Instead, there is rapid prognostic deterioration in breast cancers diagnosed after menopause [136]. Such deterioration could be explained by an interaction between endogenous hormones and the metastatic process [137]. Counterintuitive though it may seem, endogenous hormones might somehow inhibit microscopic tumor deposits.

If HRT were injurious for patients with breast cancer, one would expect that women who developed breast cancer while taking estrogen would have a worse prognosis. In fact, the prognosis of women with breast cancer who took HRT before diagnosis is better than that of women with no recorded exposure [73,103,138–141], and women who were diagnosed within a year of taking HRT enjoy a longer relative survival than women with no recorded exposure or those whose exposure has been more than a year from diagnosis [73] (table 5).

Bergkvist et al. studied survival among women with breast cancer in a cohort exposed to ERT before diagnosis. These women were then compared with women of the background population diagnosed with breast cancer during the same time [73]. Women with a history of ERT exposure had significantly better observed and relative survival rates compared with those who had no recorded history of ERT use.

Gambrell conducted a prospective study of postmenopausal breast cancer patients and evaluated the impact of hormone use on breast cancer survival [140]. At the time of he analysis, 102 of 256 women had died. The mortality rate was 22% among those diagnosed with breast cancer while using hormones

Table 5. Relative risk of mortality from breast cancer among HRT users compared with never users in cohort studies

Author [ref]	Breast cancers[a]	Relative risk	p-value
Bergkvist [73]	261	0.68 (0.52–.087)	<0.01
Gambrell [140]	50	0.53	<0.007
Hunt [103]	50	0.55 (0.28–0.96)	<0.05
Henderson [138]	ns	0.81	>0.05
Criqui [139]	42	0.73 (0.44–1.22)[b]	>0.05
Colditz [141]	359	0.8 (0.6–1.07)[c]	>0.05
Colditz [139]	359	1.14 (0.85–1.51)[d]	>0.05

[a] In estrogen users.
[b] All cancer mortality.
[c] Prior users.
ns: not stated.

and 46% among those not using hormones ($p < 0.002$). Fifty-seven percent of the hormone users had negative nodes; 42% of the nonusers were node negative. Within this node-negative group, the mortality rate was 8% for hormone users and 25% for nonusers ($p < 0.05$).

Hunt et al. reported on mortality from breast cancer among 4544 ERT users [103]. Their cohort experienced a relative risk of 0.55 compared with national rates. Screening mammography was rarely if ever used to diagnose breast cancer.

Another study confirms the above reports. Henderson et al. observed a 19% reduction in the mortality from breast cancer among 4988 ERT users vs. 3865 nonusers who subsequently developed breast cancer [138].

The recently published trial by Colditz et al. is the only one to report (in subset analysis) that *current* consumers of more than five years of ERT/HRT have a significantly increased risk of death from breast cancer. The relative risk was 1.45 (C.I. 1.01–2.09). The number of women who fell into this category was not stated but must have been small.

There are potential confounding variables that might explain these protective findings, including the supposition that ERT might promote development of estrogen-dependent breast cancers that wither upon estrogen withdrawal. Nevertheless, the data are coherent in that they suggest that ERT may have a beneficial impact on survival of women with breast cancer.

7. Reactivation of dormant tumor cells

Dao et al. found a significant increase in tritiated thymidine incorporation in skin metastasis among women treated with 'physiological doses' of intramuscular estradiol and progrogesterone for three days [142]. The labeling index (LI) increased in 7 of 10 tumors, and receptor status did not correlate with changes in LI. The menopausal status of the patients was not reported, nor were changes in serum levels of estrogen and progesterone. It is not possible to know whether the effect observed was due to the addition of estrogen or progesterone or the combination. Concurrent use of tamoxifen could protect dormant tumor cells from stimulation by exogenous hormones.

Dhodapkar et al. recently reported that ERT withdrawal resulted in regression of metastatic breast cancer, suggesting that ERT was capable of stimulating metastatic breast cancer deposits [143]. Three women with a history of stage I breast cancer relapsed while receiving ERT. All were reported to have experienced 'regression' of metastatic disease upon withdrawal of ERT.

The interval between starting ERT and presentation with metastatic breast cancer was 5, 7, and 17 years for the women with stage I disease. This long interval between prescription of ERT and diagnosis of metastatic disease suggests that these relapses were unrelated to ERT. The hormone might just as likely have kept their disease under control for a period of time.

The first patient relapsed with a pleural effusion and 'diffuse osteoblastic metastases involving the entire skeleton.' Her *response* was 'substantial resolution of her pleural effusion (after thoracentesis) and improvement in her bone survey.' Patients with pleural effusions and purely osteoblastic bone disease are ineligible for clinical trials that evaluate new agents because they are considered to have neither measurable nor evaluable disease.

The second patient relapsed with 'an asymptomatic lung nodule near the right hilum' and had 'an excellent response with near resolution of the nodule' after ERT withdrawal. The term *response* was not defined. Radiographs were not presented.

The third patient relapsed with bone-only disease. Her response consised of 'significant improvement in bone pain.' Symptom relief does not fulfill the classic definition of response.

The final patient presented de novo with metastatic disease to bone, including at least one lytic lesion. Her response consisted of 'significant clinical improvement with resolution of bone pain and improvement in her bone survey showing evidence of healing.' Response was not defined, and radiographs were not presented.

Counterbalancing these few reports is a larger body of evidence suggesting that ERT/HRT will not harm, and might actually benefit, breast cancer survivors.

8. Clinical trials of HRT in breast cancer survivors

Proponents of ERT in breast cancer survivors bolster their argument by stating that estrogen has been and is used as a treatment for breast cancer [24]. It must be remembered, however, that the doses of estrogen used for treatment of breast cancer are pharmacologic, not physiologic, and in vitro studies show that low-dose estrogen stimulates and high-dose estrogen inhibits breast cancer cell growth [144]. However, contradictory human evidence exists.

Stoll treated postmenopausal breast cancer patients with Lyndiol®, an oral contraceptive pill containing estrogen (17-alpha-ethynyl-estradiol, 0.15 mg) and a progestin (17-alpha-ethynyl-estrenol, 5 mg) [145]. Patients had measurable soft tissue metastases. Nearly complete resolution of disease was observed in a significant proportion of patients. A dose response was not observed. One tablet daily (the normal oral contraceptive dose) was as effective as 3 or 6 tablets per day. Menopausal symptoms were relieved [25].

Clinical series of HRT use in breast cancer survivors have been published. Neither demonstrated a striking adverse outcome. However, these reports were essentially anecdotal and not formal clinical trials with clearly defined objectives, eligibility criteria, and endpoints.

Stoll gave conjugated equine estrogens, 0.625 mg and norgestrel 0.15 mg daily. The women were suffering severe sweats or hot flashes, unrelieved by clonidine [28]. Patients were followed for two years; no relapses occurred.

Wile et al. conducted a case–control study of 25 breast cancer survivors who received HRT [146]. The average duration between diagnosis and beginning HRT was two years. Each patient was matched with two non-HRT users for stage, age, and duration of observation. The average duration of observation of patients receiving HRT was two years. There was one cancer-related death in the treated group, and there were two in the control group. A subsequent report by these authors revealed that the type of HRT varied [147]. At the time of the second report, patients had been observed for a mean of 35 months; three women who received HRT had relapsed.

A case–controlled study of 901 breast cancer survivors, 90 of whom took HRT after their diagnosis of breast cancer for relief of menopausal symptoms, demonstrated significantly fewer tumor recurrences in the HRT group using combined continuous estrogen–moderate-dose progestogen, compared with the non-HRT matched controls [148]. Matching criteria included age at diagnosis, number of involved nodes, size of primary tumor, and disease-free interval prior to starting HRT.

Sellin et al. are conducting a prospective clinical trial of ERT in breast cancer survivors. Eligibility criteria for the trial include a disease-free interval of two years for women with estrogen receptor-negative and 10 years for those with estrogen receptor-unknown tumors [149].

This trial is an important step in the study of ERT in breast cancer survivors. However, it cannot detect less than a 10% increase in relapse rate that could be caused by ERT. In a disease as common as breast cancer, even a small difference in effect can affect many lives. Additionally, the women in the trial are not receiving tamoxifen. Whether the results can be generalized to a population of women taking tamoxifen is not known.

9. Conclusions

Ultimately, the question of impact of HRT on all-cause mortality among breast cancer survivors can only be answered by a prospective, randomized trial requiring thousands of women. Many questions regarding such a trial exist, and it is premature to mount such a trial without pilot data.

For example, it will be important to know if breast cancer survivors will participate in trials of HRT. Likewise, whether oncologists will accept such trials is not known. What are the baseline quality-of-life measurements in these women, and how are they changed by ERT/HRT among tamoxifen-users? What is the proper dose of ERT/HRT in tamoxifen users? These questions should be answered before larger trials are planned.

The benefits of HRT on quality of life for women are indisputable. The effect on overall health appears to be favorable as well and is the subject of The Womens' Health Initiative. Theoretical concern over reactivating dormant tumor cells is not supported by existing clinical evidence. The National Cancer Institute approved concepts on HRT trials in breast cancer survivors that were submitted by cooperative groups in 1995. Clinical protocols are under review and, hopefully, will begin in 1997.

References

1. American College of Obstetricians and Gynecologists. 1992. Hormone Replacement Therapy. Washington, DC: ACOG Technical Bulletin, April, no.166.
2. Wiklund I, Holst J, Karlberg J, et al. 1992. A new methodological approach to the evaluation of quality of life in postmenopausal women. Maturitas 14:211–224.
3. Grady D, Rubin SM, Petitti DB, et al. 1992. Hormone therapy to prevent disease and prolong life in postmenopausal women. Ann Intern Med 15:1016–1037.
4. Barrett-Connor E, Bush TL. 1991. Estrogen and coronary heart disease in women. Clin Cardiol 265:1861–1867.
5. Editorial. 1990. Cardiovascular implications of estrogen replacement therapy. Obstet Gynecol 75 (Suppl 4):18S–25S.
6. Kiel DP, Felson DT, Anderson JJ, et al. 1987. Hip fracture and the use of estrogens in postmenopausal women. N Engl J Med 317:1169–1174.
7. Miller BA, Feuer EJ, Hankey BF, et al. 1993. Recent incidence trends for breast cancer in women and the relevance of early detection: an update. Cancer 43:27–41.
8. Fisher B, Costantino J, Redmond C, et al. 1989. A randomized clinical trial evaluating tamoxifen in the treatment of patients with node-negative breast cancer who have estrogen-receptor-positive tumors. N Engl J Med 320:479–484.
9. Mansour EG, Gray R, Shatila AH, et al. 1989. Efficacy of adjuvant chemotherapy in high-risk node-negative breast cancer. N Engl J Med 320:485–490.
10. The Ludwig Breast Cancer Study Group. 1989. Prolonged disease-free survival after one course of perioperative adjuvant chemotherapy for node-negative breast cancer. N Engl J Med 320:491–496.
11. Fisher B, Redmond C, Dimitrov NV, et al. 1989. A randomized trial evaluating sequential methotrexate and fluorouracil in the treatment of patients with node-negative breast cancer who have estrogen-receptor-negative tumors. N Engl J Med 320:474–478.
12. Bines J, Oleske DM, Cobleigh MA. 1996. Ovarian function in premenopausal women treated with adjuvant chemotherapy for breast cancer. J Clin Oncol 14:1718–1729.
13. Mehta RR, Beattie CW, Das Gupta. 1991. Endocrine profile in breast cancer patients receiving chemotherapy. Breast Cancer Res Treat 20:125–132.
14. Bonadonna G, Valagussa P, Rossi A, et al. 1979. CMF adjuvant chemotherapy in operable breast cancer. In Jones SE, Salmon SS, eds. Adjuvant Therapy of Cancer II. New York: Grune and Stratton, pp. 227–235.
15. Stampfer MJ, Colditz GA, Willett WC, et al. 1991. Postmenopausal estrogen therapy and cardiovascular disease. Ten-year follow-up from the Nurses' Health Study. N Engl J Med 325:756–762.
16. Rosen PP, Groshen S, Kinne DW, et al. 1993. Factors influencing prognosis in node-negative breast carcinoma: analysis of 767 T1N0M0/T2N0M0 patients with long-term follow-up. J Clin Oncol 11:2090–2100.
17. Merill JM. 1992. Questions and answers. Estrogen replacement therapy after breast cancer. JAMA 267:568.
18. Creasman WT. 1991. Estrogen replacement therapy: is previously treated cancer a contraindication? Obstet Gynecol 77:308–311.
19. Hutchinson-Williams KA, et al. 1991. Yale J Biol Med 64:607–626.
20. Theriault RL, Sellin RV. 1991. A clinical dilemma: estrogen replacement therapy in postmenopausal women with a background of primary breast cancer. Ann Oncol 2:709–717.
21. Davidson JA. 1991. The need for a randomized trial of hormone replacement therapy in women with breast cancer. Med J Aust 157:429.

22. DiSaia PJ. 1984. Invited discussion. Am J Obstet Gynecol 150:129.
23. Henderson IC. 1993. Risk factors for development of breast cancer. Cancer (Suppl) 71:2127–2140.
24. Eden JA. 1992. General practice, common problems: oestrogen and the breast. 1. Myths about oestrogen and breast cancer. Med J Aust 157:175–176.
25. Stoll BA, Parbhoo S. 1988. Treatment of menopausal symptoms in breast cancer patients. Lancet 1(8597):1278–1279.
26. Marchant DJ. 1993. Estrogen-replacement therapy after breast cancer. Cancer 71:2169–2176.
27. Eden J. 1992. General practice, common problems: oestrogen and the breast. 2. The management of the menopausal woman with breast cancer. Med J Aust 157:247–250.
28. Stoll A. 1989. Hormone replacement therapy in women treated for breast cancer. Eur J Cancer Clin Oncol 25:1909.
29. American College of Physicians. 1992. Guidelines for counseling postmenopausal women about preventive hormone therapy. Ann Intern Med 117:1038–1041.
30. Eaker ED, Chesebro JH, Sacks FM, Wenger NK, Whisnant JP, Winston M. 1993. Cardiovascular disease in women. Circulation 88:1900–2009.
31. Early Breast Cancer Trialists' Collaborative Group. 1992. Systemic treatment of early breast cancer by hormonal, cytotoxic, or immune therapy. 133 randomized trials involving 31,000 recurrences and 24,000 deaths among 75,000 women. Lancet 339:1–15.
32. Powles TJ. 1990. Tamoxifen and oestrogen replacement. Lancet 336(8706):48.
33. Ernster VL, Wrensch MR, Petrakis NL, King EB, Miike R, Mural J, Goodson WH III, Siiteri PK. 1987. Benign and malignant breast disease: initial study results of serum and breast fluid analyses of endogenous estrogens. J Natl Cancer Inst 79:949–960.
34. Jordan VC, Fritz NF, Tormey DC. 1987. Endocrine effects of adjuvant chemotherapy and long-term tamoxifen administration on node-positive patients with breast cancer. Cancer Res 47:624–630.
35. Powles TJ, Hardy JR, Ashley SE, et al. 1989. Chemo-prevention of breast cancer. Breast Cancer Res Treat 14:23–31.
36. Sherman BM, Chapler FK, Crickard K, et al. 1979. Endocrine consequences of continuous antiestrogen therapy with tamoxifen in premenopausal women. J Clin Invest 64:398–404.
37. Sunderland MC, Osborne CK. 1991. Tamoxifen in premenopausal patients with metastatic breast cancer: a review. J Clin Oncol 9:1283–1297.
38. Pollack M, Polychronakos C, Blauer S, et al. 1990. Effect of tamoxifen on serum insulin-like growth factor I (IGF-I) levels of stae I breast cancer patients. Proc Annu Meet Am Soc Clin Oncol 9:A70.
39. Vignon F, Bouton M-M, Rochefort H. 1987. Antiestrogens inhibit the mitogenic effect of growth factors on breast cancer cells in the total absence of estrogens. Biochem Biophys Res Commun 146:1502–1508.
40. O'Brien CA, Liskamp RM, Solomon DH, et al. 1985. Inhibition of protein kinase C by tamoxifen. Cancer Res 45:2462–2465.
41. Lam H-YP. 1984. Tamoxifen is a calmodulin antagonist in the activation of cAMP phosphodiesterase. Biochem Biophys Res Commun 118:27–32.
42. Hug V, Hortobagyi GN, Drewinka B, et al. 1985. Tamoxifen-citrate counteracts the antitumor effects of cytotoxic drugs in vitro. J Clin Oncol 3:1672–1677.
43. Mandeville R, Ghali SS, Chausseau J-P. 1984. In vitro stimulation of human NK activity by an estrogen antagonist (tamoxifen). Eur J Cancer Clin Oncol 20:983–985.
44. Heuson JC. 1976. Current overview of EORTC clinical trials with tamoxifen. Cancer Treat Rep 60:1463–1466.
45. Manni A, Pearson OH. 1980. Antiestrogen-induced remissions in premenopausal women with stage IV breast cancer: effects on ovarian function. Cancer Treat Rep 64:779–785.
46. Sawka CA, Pritchard KI, Paterson AHG, et al. 1986. Role and mechanism of action of tamoxifen in premenopausal women with metastatic breast carcinoma. Cancer Res 46:3152–3156.

47. Pritchard KI, Thomson DB, Myers RE, et al. 1980. Tamoxifen therapy in premenopausal patients with metastatic breast cancer. Cancer Treat Rep 64:787–796.
48. Wada T, Koyama H, Terasawa T. 1981. Effect of tamoxifen in premenopausal Japanese women with advanced breast cancer. Cancer Treat Rep 65:728–729.
49. Yoshida M, Murai H, Miura S. 1982. Tamoxifen therapy for premenopausal and postmenopausal Japanese females with advanced breast cancer. Jpn J Clin Oncol 12:57–64.
50. Hoogstraten B, Fletcher WS, Grad-el-Mawia N, et al. 1982. Tamoxifen and oophorectomy in the treatment of recurrent breast cancer. A Southwest Oncology Group study. Cancer Res 42:4788–4791.
51. Hoogstraten B, Gad-el-Mawla N, Maloney TR, et al. 1984. Combined modality therapy for first recurrence of breast cancer. A Southwest Oncology Group study. Cancer 54:2248–2256.
52. Margrieter R, Wiegele J. 1984. Tamoxifen for premenopausal patients with advanced breast cancer. Cancer Res Treat 4:45–49.
53. Planting AST, Alexieva-Figusch J, Blonk-v.d. Wijst J, et al. 1985. Tamoxifen therapy in premenopausal women with metastatic breast cancer. Cancer Treat Rep 69:363–368.
54. Krywicki RF, Yee D. 1992. The insulin-like growth family family of ligands, receptors and binding proteins. Breast Cancer Res Treat 22:7–19.
55. Peyrat JP, Bonneterre J. 1992. Type I IGF receptor in human breast diseases. Breast Cancer Res Treat 22:59–67.
56. Pollak MN, Polychronakos C, Yousefi S, et al. 1988. Characterization of insulin-like growth factor (IGF-1) receptors of human breast cancer cells. Biochem Biophys Res Commun 154:326–331.
57. Thorsen T, Lahooti H, Rasmussen M, et al. 1992. Oestradiol treatment increases the sensitivity of MCF-7 cells for the growth stimulatory effect of IGF-I. J Steroid Biochem Mol Biol 41:537–540.
58. Vignon F, Bouton MM, Rochefort H. 1987. Antiestrogens inhibit the mitogenic effect of growth factors on breast cancer cells in the total absence of estrogens. Biochem Biophys Res Commun 146:1502–1508.
59. Friedl A, Jordan VC, Pollak M. 1993. Suppression of serum insulin-like growth factor-1 levels in breast cancer patients during adjuvant tamoxifen therapy. Eur J Cancer 29A(10):1368–1372.
60. Goldberg RM, Loprinzi CL, O'Fallon JR, Veeder MH, Miser AW, Mailliard JA, Michalak JC, Dose A, Rowland KM, Burnham NL. 1994. Transdermal clonidine for ameliorating tamoxifen-induced hot flashes. J Clin Oncol 12:155–158.
61. Nesheim BI, Saetre T. 1981. Reduction of menopausal hot flushes by methyldopa. Eur J Clin Pharmacol 20:413–416.
62. Erik Y, Meldrum DR, Lagasse LD, Judd HL. 1981. Effect of megestrol acetate on flushing and bone metabolism in postmenopausal women. Maturitas 3:167–172.
63. Loprinzi CL, Michalak JC, Quella SK, et al. 1994. Megestrol acetate for the prevention of hot flashes. N Engl J Med 331:347–352.
64. Bullock JL, Massey FM, Cambrell RD Jr. 1975. Use of medroxyprogesterone acetate to prevent menopausal symptoms. Obstet Gynecol 46:165–168.
65. Morrison JC, Martin DC, Blair RA, et al. 1980. The use of medroxyprogesterone acetate for relief of climacteric symptoms. Am J Obstet Gynecol 138:99–104.
66. Albrecht BG, Schiff I, Tulchinsky D, Ryan KJ. 1981. Objective evidence that placebo and oral medroxyprogesterone acetate therapy diminish menopausal valomotor flushes. Am J Obstet Gynecol 139:631–635.
67. Young RL, Kumar NS, Goldzieher JW. 1990. Management of menopause when estrogen cannot be used. Drugs 40:220–230.
68. Schiff I, Tuschinsky D, Cramer D. 1980. Oral medroxyprogesterone acetate in the treatment of postmenopausal symtoms. JAMA 244:1443–1445.
69. Bergmans MGM, Merkus JMWM, Corbey RS, Schellekens LA, Ubach JM. 1987. Effect of bellergal Retard on climacteric complaints: a double-blind, placebo-controlled study. Maturitas 9:227–234.

70. Longacre TA, Bartow SA. 1986. A correlative morphologic study of human breast and endometrium in the menstrual cycle. Am J Surg Pathol 10:382–393.
71. Potten CS, Watson RJ, Williams GT, Tickle S, Roberts SA, Harris M, Howell A. 1988. The effect of age and menstrual cycle upon proliferative activity of the normal human breast. Br J Cancer 58:163–170.
72. Anderson TJ, Battersby S, King RJB, McPherson K, Going JJ. 1989. Oral contraceptive use influences resting breast proliferation. Hum Pathol 20:1139–1144.
73. Bergkvist L, Adami Ho, Person I, et al. 1992. Prognosis after breast cancer diagnosis in women exposed to estrogen and estrogen-progestogen replacement therapy. Am J Epidemiol 130:221–228.
74. Huggins C, Yang NC. 1962. Induction and extinction of mammary cancer. Science 137:257–262.
75. Diamond JE, Hollander VP. 1979. Progesterone and breast cancer. Mt Sinai J Med 46:225–235.
76. Jordan VC, MK, Langan-Fahey S. 1991. Suppression of mouse mammary tumorigenesis by long term tamoxifen therapy. J Natl Cancer Inst 83:492–496.
77. Kordon E, Lanari C, Meiss R, Elizalde P, Charreau E, Pasqualini CD. 1990. Hormone dependence of a mouse mammary tumor line induced in vivo by medroxyprogesterone acetate. Breast Cancer Res Treat 33–43.
78. Hissom JR, Moore MR. 1987. Progestin effects on growth in the human breast cancer cell line T47D. Possible therapeutic implications. Biochem Biophys Res Commun 45:706–711.
79. Braunsberg H, Coldham NG, Wong W. 1986. Hormonal therapies for breast cancer: can progestogens stimulate growth? Cancer Let 30:213–218.
80. The Writing Group for the PEPI trial. 1995. Effects of estrogen or estrogen/progestin regimens on heart disease risk factors in postmenopausal women. JAMA 273:199–208.
81. Mouridsen HT, Elleman K, Mattsson W. 1979. Therapeuic effect of tamoxifen vs tamoxifen combined with medroxyprogesterone acetate in advanced breast cancer in postmenopausal women. Cancer Treat Rep 63:171–175.
82. Gibson DFC, Johnson DA, Langan-Fahey SM, Lababidi MK, Wolberg WH, Jordan VC. 1993. The effects of intermittent progesterone upon tamoxifen inhibition of tumor growth in the 7,12-dimethylbenzanthracene rat mammary tumor model. Breast Cancer Res and Treat 27:283–287.
83. Schiff I, Wentworth B, Koos B, Tulchinsky D, Ryan KJ. 1978. Effect of estriol administration on the hypogonadal woman. Fertil Steril 30:278–282.
84. Mattsson LA, Cullberg G. 1983. Vaginal absorption of two estriol preparations. Asta Obstet Gynecol Scand 62:393–396.
85. Heimer GM. 1987. Estriol in the menopause. Acta Obstet Gynecol Scand Suppl 139:23P.
86. Nachtigall LE. 1994. Comparative study: Replens versus local estrogen in menopausal women. Fertil Steril 61:178–180.
87. Mattsson LA, Cullberg G, Eriksson O, Knutsson F. 1989. Vaginal administration of low-dose estradiol — effects on the endometrium and vaginal cytology. Maturitas 11:217–222.
88. Rymer J, Chapman MG, Fogelman I, Wilson POG. 1994. A study of the effect of tibolone on the vagina in postmenopausal women. Maturitas 18:127–133.
89. Love RR, Mazess RB, Barden HS, et al. 1992. Effects of tamoxifen on bone mineral density in postmenopausal women with breast cancer. N Engl J Med 326:852–856.
90. Aloia JF, Vaswani A, Yeh JK, et al. 1994. Calcium supplementation with and without hormone replacement therapy to prevent postmenopausal bone loss. Ann Intern Med 120:97–103.
91. Love RR, Newcomb PA, Wiebe DA, Surawicz TS, Jorhan VC, Carbone PP, DeMets DL. 1990. Effects of tamoxifen therapy on lipid and lipoprotein levels in postmenopausal patients with node-negative breast cancer. J Natl Cancer Inst 82:1327–1332.
92. Love RR, Wiebe DA, Newcomb PA, Cameron L, Leventhal H, Jorhan VC, Feyzi J, DeMets. 1991. Effects of tamoxifen on cardiovascular risk factors in postmenopausal women. Ann Intern Med 115:860–864.

93. Devor M, Barrett-Connor E, Ranvall M, et al. 1992. Estrogen replacement therapy and the risk of venous thrombosis. Am J Med 92:275–282.
94. Smith DC, Prentice R, Donovan JT, et al. 1975. Association of exogenous estrogen and endometrial carcinoma. N Engl J Med 293:1164–1167.
95. Henderson BE, Casagrande JT, Pike MC, et al. 1983. The epidemiology of endometrial cancer in young women. Br J Cancer 47:749–756.
96. Fornander T, Rutqvist LE, Cedermark B, et al. 1989. Adjuvant tamoxifen in early breast cancer: occurrence of new primary cancers. Lancet 1:117–120.
97. Berkowitz JE, Gatewood OM, Goldblum LE, et al. 1990. Hormonal replacement therapy: mammographic manifestations. Radiology 174:199–201.
98. Kaufman Z, Garstin WI, Hayes R, et al. 1991. The mammographic parenchymal patterns of women on hormonal replacement therapy. Clin Radiol 43:389–392.
99. Bland KI, Buchanan JB, Weisberg BF, et al. 1980. The effects of exogenous estrogen replacement therapy of the breast: breast cancer risk and mammographic parenchymal patterns. Cancer 45:3027–3033.
100. Stomper PC, Van Voorhis BJ, Ravnikar VA, et al. 1990. Mammographic changes associated with postmenopausal hormone replacement therapy: a longitudinal study. Radiology 174:487–490.
101. Kelsey JL, Berkowitz GS. 1988. Breast cancer epidemiology. Cancer Res 48:5615–5623.
102. Harvey EB, Brinton LA. 1985. Second cancer following cancer of the breast in Connecticut, 1935–1982. In Boice JD Jr, Storm HH, Curtis RE, eds. Multiple primary cancers in Connecticut and Denmark. National Cancer Institute Monograph 68. Washington, DC: Government Printing Office, pp. 99–112 (NIH publication no. 85-2714).
103. Hunt K, Vessey M, McPherson K, Coleman M. 1987. Long-term surveillance of mortality and cancer incidence in women receiving hormone replacement therapy. Br J Obstet Gynecol 94:620–635.
104. Palmer JR, Rosenbert L, Clarkey EA, et al. 1991. Breast cancer risk after estrogen replacement therapy: results from the Toronto Breast Cancer Society. Am J Epidemiol 134:1386–1395.
105. DuPont WD, Page DL, Roges LW, et al. 1989. Influence of exogenous estrogens, proliferative breast disease and other variables on breast cancer risk. Cancer 643:948–957.
106. Brownson RC, Blackwell CW, Pearson DK, et al. 1988. Risk of breast cancer relation to cigarette smoking. Arch Intern Med 148:140–144.
107. Rohan TE, McMichael AJ. 1988. Non-contraceptive exogenous oestrogen therapy and breast cancer. Med J Aust 148:217–221.
108. Wingo PQ, Layde PM, Lee NC, et al. 1987. The risk of breast cancer in postmenopausal women who have used estrogen replacement therapy. JAMA 257:209–215.
109. Buring JE, Hennekens CH, Lipnick RJ. 1987. A prospective cohort study of postmenopausal hormone use and risk of breast cancer in US women. Am J Epidemiol 125:939–947.
110. Brinton LA, Hoover R, Fraumeni JF Jr. 1986. Menopausal oestrogens and breast cancer risk: an expanded case–control study. Br J Cancer 54:825–832.
111. Nomura AM, Kolonel LN, Hirohata T, et al. 1986. The association of replacement estrogens with breast cancer. Int J Cancer 37:49–53.
112. Horwitz RI, Stewart KR. 1984. Effect of clinical features on the association of estrogens and breast cancer. Am J Med 76:192–198.
113. Kaufman DW, Miller DR, Rosenberg L, et al. 1984. Noncontraceptive estrogen use and the risk of breast cancer. JAMA 252:63–67.
114. Hiatt RA, Bawol R, Friedman GD, et al. 1984. Exogenous estrogen and breast cancer after bilateral oophorectomy. Cancer 54:139–144.
115. Sherman B, Wallace R, Bean J. 1983. Estrogen use and breast cancer: interaction with body mass. Cancer 51:1527–1531.
116. Gambrell RD, Maier RC, Sanders BI. 1983. Decreased incidence of breast cancer in postmenopausal estrogen–progestogen users. Obstet Gynecol 62:435–443.

117. Kelsey JL, Fischer DB, Holford TR, et al. 1981. Exogenous estrogens and other factors in the epidemiology of breast cancer. J Natl Cancer Inst 67:327–333.
118. Kaufman DW, Palmer JR, deMouzon J, et al. 1991. Estrogen replacement therapy and the risk of breast cancer: results from the case–control surveillance study. Am J Epidemiol 134:1375–1385.
119. Colditz GA, Stampfer MJ, Willett WC, et al. 1990. Prospective study of estrogen replacement therapy and risk of breast cancer in pmp women. JAMA 264:2648–2653.
120. Bergkvist L, Adami HO, Person I, et al. 1989. The risk of breast cancer after estrogen and estrogen–progestin replacement. N Engl J Med 321:293–297.
121. Mills PK, Beeson WL, Phillips RL, et al. 1989. Prospective study of exogenous hormone use and breast cancer in Seventh-Day Adventists. Cancer 64:591–597.
122. Ewertz M. 1988. Influence of non-contraceptive exogenous and endogenous sex hormones on breast cancer risk in Denmark. Int J Cancer 42:832–838.
123. Hulka BS, Chambless LE, Deubner DC, et al. 1982. Breast cancer and estrogen replacement therapy. Am J Obstet Gynecol 143:638–644.
124. Thomas DB, Persing JP, Hutchinson WB. 1982. Exogenous estrogens and other risk factors for breast cancer in women with benign breast diseases. J Natl Cancer Inst 69:1017–1025.
125. Hoover R, Glass A, Finkle WD, et al. 1981. Conjugated estrogens and breast cancer risk in women. J Natl Cancer Inst 67:815–820.
126. Ross RK, Paganini-Hill, Gerkins VR, et al. 1980. A case–control study of menopausal estrogen therapy and breast cancer. JAMA 243:1635–1639.
127. DuPont WD, Page DL. 1991. Menopausal estrogen replacement therapy and breast cancer. Arch Intern Med 151:67–72.
128. Steinberg KK, Thacker SB, Smith SJ, et al. 1991. A meta-analysis of the effect of estrogen replacement therapy on the risk of breast cancer. JAMA 265:1985–1990.
129. Armstrong BK. 1988. Oestrogen therapy after the menopause -- boon or bane? Med J Aust 148:213–214.
130. Grady D, Ernster V. 1991. Invited commentary: does postmenopausal hormone therapy cause breast cancer? Am J Epidemiol 134:1396–1400.
131. Sillero-Arenas M, Delgado-Rodriguez M, Rodrigues-Canteras R, et al. 1992. Menopausal hormone replacement therapy and breast cancer; a meta-analysis. Obstet Gynecol 79:286–294.
132. Colditz GA, Egan KM, Stampfer MJ. 1993. Hormone replacement therapy and risk of breast cancer; results from epidemilogic studies. Am J Obstet Gynecol 168:1473–1480.
133. Henrich JB. 1992. The postmenopausal estrogen/breast cancer controversy. JAMA 268:1900-1902.
134. Thijssen JHH, Van Landeghem AAJ, Poortman J. 1986. Uptake and concentration of steroid hormones in mammary tissues. Ann N Y Acad Sci 464:106–116.
135. Nayfield SG, Karp JE, Ford LG, et al. 1991. Potential role of tamoxifen in prevention of breast cancer. J Natl Cancer Inst 83:1450–1458.
136. Adami HO, Malker B, Holmberg L, et al. 1986. The relation between survival and age at diagnosis in breast cancer. N Engl J Med 315:559–563.
137. Adami HO, Holmberg L, Malker B, et al. 1987. Letter. N Engl J Med 316:752.
138. Henderson BE, Paganini-Hill A, Ross RK. 1991. Decreased mortality in users of estrogen replacement therapy. Arch Intern Med 151:75–78.
139. Criqui MH, Suarez L, Barrett-Connor E, et al. 1988. Postmenopausal estrogen use and mortality. Am J Epidemiol 128:606–614.
140. Gambrell DR. 1984. Proposal to decrease the risk and improve the prognosis in breast cancer. Am J Obstet Gynecol 150:119–128.
141. Colditz GA, Hankinson SE, Hunter DJ, Willett WC, Manson JE, Stampfer MJ, Hennekens C, Rosner B, Speizer FE. 1995. The use of estrogens and progestins and the risk of breast cancer in postmenopausal women. N Engl J Med 332:1589–1593.
142. Dao TL, Sinha DI, Nemoto T, Patel J. 1982. Effect of estrogen and progesterone on cellular replication of human breast tumors. Cancer Res 42:359–362.

143. Dhodapkar MV, Ingle JN, Ahmann DL. 1995. Estrogen replacement therapy withdrawal and regression of metastatic breast cancer. Cancer 75:43–46.
144. Lippman M, Bolan G, Huff K. 1976. The effects of estrogens and antiestrogens on hormone responsive human breast cancer in long-term tissue culture. Cancer Res 36:4595–4601.
145. Stoll BA. 1967. Effect of Lyndiol, an oral contraceptive, on breast cancer. Br Med J 1:150–153.
146. Wile AG, Opfell DA, Hoda AC. 1991. Hormone replacement therapy does not affect breast cancer outcome. Proc Am Soc Clin Oncol 10:58.
147. Wile AG, Opfell RW, Margileth DA. 1993. Hormone replacement therapy in previously treated breast cancer patients. Am J Surg 165:372–375.
148. Eden JA, Bush T, Nand S, Wren BG. 1995. The Royal Hospital for Women Breast Cancer Study — a case-controlled study of combined continuous hormone replacement therapy amongst women with a personal history of breast cancer. Menopause 2:67–72.
149. Theriault RV, Sellin RV. 1994. Estrogen-replacement therapy in younger women with breast cancer. Monogr Natl Cancer Inst (16):149–152.

13. Endocrine therapy in metastatic breast cancer

Gretchen G. Kimmick and Hyman B. Muss

1. Introduction

Breast cancer is the most common cancer diagnosis and the second leading cancer-related cause of death in American women. In 1996, it is estimated that there will be 185,700 new diagnoses of and 44,560 deaths due to breast cancer [1]. At diagnosis, approximately 5% of women have metastatic disease. Unfortunately, treatment of advanced disease is currently only palliative.

Endocrine therapy generally is well tolerated and because of the favorable therapeutic index, it is the treatment of choice for women with advanced breast cancer. In fact, randomized trials show no adverse effect on survival for patients initially treated with endocrine therapy rather than chemotherapy, although initial rates of response to chemotherapy tend to be somewhat higher [2–4].

Hormonal manipulation is a very effective treatment for metastatic breast cancer. Responses are seen in approximately one third of unselected patients and in at least 50% of patients with estrogen receptor- (ER-) positive tumors [5]. Well-defined factors associated with greater likelihood of response to endocrine therapy include 1) ER and progesterone receptor (PR) positivity, 2) late premenopausal or postmenopausal status, 3) older age, 4) a long interval from diagnosis to first recurrence (disease-free interval), 5) disease limited to sites outside viscera, such as bone and soft tissue, and 6) previous response to endocrine therapy [4].

The standard, first-line endocrine agent is tamoxifen. Second-line therapy includes progestins and aromatase inhibitors that have similar response rates but more side effects than tamoxifen.

2. The biologic basis of endocrine therapy

In 1896, Beatson first described a patient in whom oophorectomy caused regression of skin metastases [6]. This was the first hormonal-change manipulation noted to affect breast cancer progression. Indeed, ovarian ablation results in an overall response rate of about 35% in premenopausal women with metastatic breast cancer [7]. Various treatments have since been developed to suppress gonadal and/or peripheral estrogen production or to antagonize the stimulative effects of estrogens on breast cancer cells [8,9].

In the 1940s and 1950s, other ablative therapies, including bilateral surgical adrenalectomy and hypophysectomy, were developed. These treatments, although effective, had significant morbidity and occasional mortality. Moreover, 'medical' forms of endocrine ablation were found that were as effective as surgical ablation [10,11]. Randomized trials have confirmed similar response rates for adrenalectomy and tamoxifen and aromatase inhibitors [12,13]. Small randomized trials have been done comparing hypophysectomy with tamoxifen and with aminoglutethimide (AG) [14,15]. All yielded similar results. Less radical procedures to achieve hypophysectomy, such as the transsphenoid approach or radioactive implants, carry less morbidity and mortality but are still fraught with more complications than medical hormonal manipulation.

Breast cancer cells have steroid receptors for estrogens, progestins, glucocorticoids, and androgens. Treatment of breast cancer in premenopausal women traditionally has involved removal of the ovaries, the source of estrogen, and, in postmenopausal patients, administration of pharmacological doses of estrogen. (In postmenopausal women, large doses of estrogen can cause tumor regression.) The exact mechanism of these treatment modalities and the effects of estrogens and antiestrogens on the breast cancer cell are not fully defined. Our current understanding is that estrogen downregulates ERs, decreasing the hormone's effects [16].

Breast cancer cells also secrete other growth factors that are autostimulatory (autocrine) and/or are stimulated by substances secreted by surrounding cells (paracrine) (figure 1). Receptors for epidermal growth factor (EGFR) and c-*erb*B2 (Her-2/*neu*) are found on breast cancer cells. EGF and transforming growth factor alpha (TGF-alpha) interact with the EGFR and activate tyrosine kinase, a signal transduction pathway shown to induce proliferation of breast cancer cell lines in nude mice [17].

TGF-alpha can act as an autocrine or paracrine growth factor, and some breast cancer cells produce TGF-alpha in response to estrogens. Receptors for TGF-beta also are present on breast cancer cells (primarily those that are ER negative). Using antibodies against TGF-alpha or EGFR to block TGF-alpha's effects can inhibit the growth of some breast cancer cells. Insulin-like growth factor (IGF) also is produced by breast cancer cells in vitro and may result in both autocrine and paracrine mitogenic effects [18]. Factors that increase IGF production include estrogen, TGF-alpha, EGF, and insulin. Antiestrogens, TGF-beta, and glucocorticoids inhibit its secretion [17].

Currently available additive therapies include androgens, progestins, gonadotropin-releasing hormone (GnRH) agonists, corticosteriods, and estrogens. Androgens, which were discovered to be effective in the 1940s, cause tumors to regress in approximately 20% of patients but are poorly tolerated because of virilization and other major toxicities. Physiologic doses of estrogen (hormone replacement therapy) are generally avoided in women with breast can-

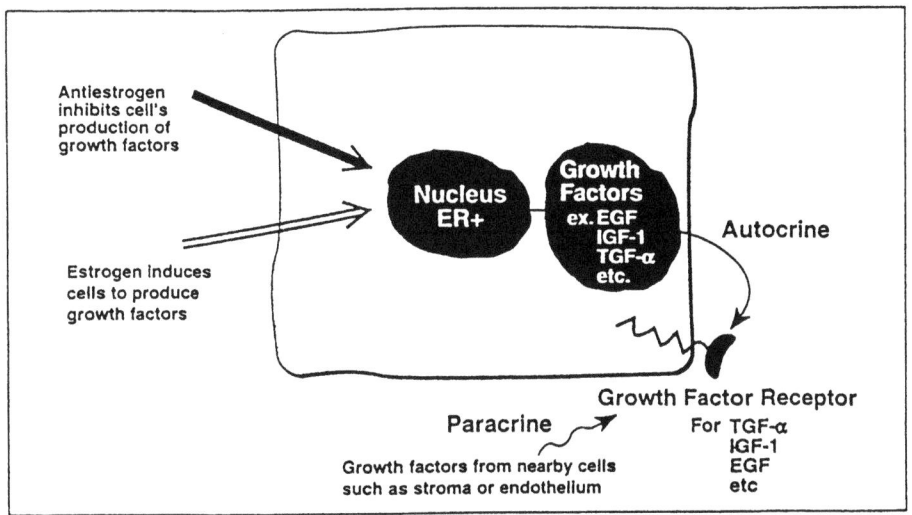

Figure 1. Autocrine and paracrine effects of growth factors on breast cancer cells.

cer because of theoretical concerns that estrogens might stimulate breast cancer cell growth. Higher doses yield response rates in postmenopausal women similar to those produced by other available agents, but estrogen therapy is frequently associated with nausea, vomiting, and other side effects [19,20]. Response rates of 20% to 25% also were reported for corticosteroid therapy alone [21]. For example, in elderly patients in whom endocrine therapy has failed, 15 mg prednisolone administered daily caused tumor regression in 14% and tumor stabilization lasting six months or longer in 21% [22]. Corticosteroids also can improve sense of well-being, appetite, and functional status in seriously ill cancer patients [23]. However, because of their long-term undesirable toxicities, corticosteroids typically are reserved for reducing inflammation and swelling associated with intracranial metastases and superior vena cava syndrome.

Tamoxifen is the prototypic hormonal agent used in breast cancer. It is one of several antiestrogens now available and falls into the broad category of *hormone antagonists or ablative therapies*. Other groups of hormone antagonists only recently introduced into the armamentarium of breast cancer therapy include antiandrogens, antiprogestins, and aromatase inhibitors.

3. Hormone antagonists

3.1. Antiestrogens

Antiestrogens inhibit the growth of hormone-responsive human breast cancer cells in vitro, an effect modulated through the estrogen receptor (ER) (figure

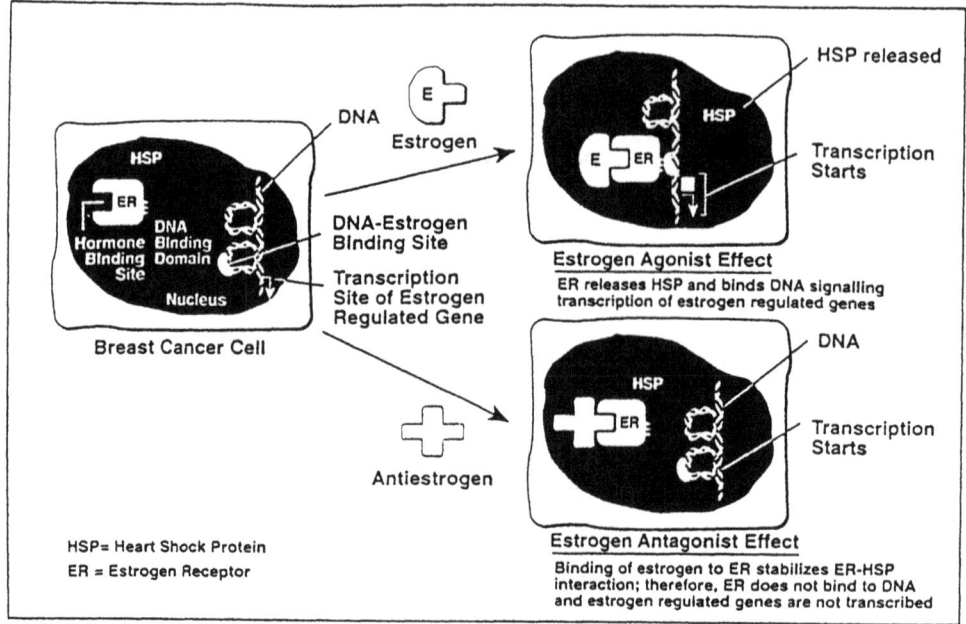

Figure 2. Estrogen/antiestrogen effects on breast cancer cells.

Table 1. Estrogen antagonists

Tamoxifen	Gold Standard
Trioxifene mesylate	Similar in efficacy to but more toxic than tamoxifen
Toremifene	Similar toxicities to tamoxifen but may be more efficacious
Droloxifene (4-OH tamoxifen)	Less estrogenic and more antiestrogenic than tamoxifen
Idoxifene (pyrrolidine-4-iodotamoxifen)	Under clinical investigation
Zindoxifene	Marginal therapeutic activity
'Pure antiestrogens' ICI 164,384 ICI 182,780	Currently being developed, may be more efficacious and less toxic than tamoxifen

2) [24]. Antiestrogens that are currently available or under investigation are listed in table 1.

Most antiestrogens have both estrogen agonist and estrogen antagonist effects. Some newer antiestrogens with fewer agonist properties than tamoxifen, and therefore proportionally greater antiestrogenic activity, theoretically should be more effective in ablating the mitogenic action of estrogens on breast tumor growth. Pure antiestrogens might also work faster and for longer periods of time than antiestrogens with partial agonist action and should be less detrimental to other tissues such as the uterus and liver. Moreover, concentrations of pure antiestrogen needed to block the ER in breast cancer cells might not affect the central nervous system's ERs, leading to fewer vasomotor symptoms. The increase in follicle stimulating hormone (FSH), luteinizing hormone (LH), and circulating estrogen frequently noted in premenopausal patients using tamoxifen might be avoided [25].

The most popular endocrine treatment for advanced breast cancer, tamoxifen (Nolvadex, ICI 46,474), is appropriate initial endocrine treatment in both premenopausal and postmenopausal patients [26]. In randomized trials, it is as effective as other available endocrine therapies [21,27,28]. As initial therapy, tamoxifen elicits complete and partial responses in 30%–40% of unselected patients, with response durations averaging about one year. Half of those with ER+ breast tumors respond [28]. The withdrawal of therapy also yields responses in as many as 20% of patients whose tumors initially regressed and then later progressed on tamoxifen [29].

Due to isomerization and metabolism, tamoxifen exists in both *trans* and *cis* configurations in vitro [30]. *Trans*-4-hydroxytamoxifen, although a minor metabolite, has a higher affinity for the ER and is a more potent antiestrogen than the parent compound, but can isomerize to *cis*-4-hydroxytamoxifen, which is a less potent antiestrogen with weak estrogenic properties [31]. The *trans* isomer is available commercially as tamoxifen citrate.

Tamoxifen competitively binds to the ER, blocking estrogen binding and inhibiting estrogen-dependent cell growth [30]. Eventually, however, cells develop resistance, for which several mechanisms have been postulated: 1) alterations in tumor and cellular heterogeneity, such as loss of the ER; 2) alteration in ER structure and function, which is rare and unlikely to be a major factor in tamixifen resistance [32]; 3) changes in paracrine interactions; 4) pharmacologic alteration in cellular uptake, retention, and/or metabolism; and 5) reflex increases in extraovarian estrogen production [33,34] (figure 3). Isomerization of tamoxifen may also occur in vivo [35,36]. Osborne and colleagues showed that tamoxifen-resistant human breast cancer cells had lower tamoxifen concentrations and contained higher levels of the less antiestrogenic *cis*-isomer of 4-hydroxytamoxifen [37]. This finding suggests that tumor resistance may be partly related to the decreased cellular tamoxifen's uptake or tamoxifen's conversion to a less antiestrogenic metabolite. (Recent research confirmed that breast cancer cells can metabolize tamoxifen to the more estrogenic compounds [38]). Other investigators, however, have not been able to confirm this hypothesis in vitro [39].

In approximately 5% of patients with skin or bone metastases, tamoxifen causes a tumor 'flare' manifested by an increase in size, number, and discomfort of skin lesions and by increasing bone pain and/or hypercalcemia. Such reactions generally occur within days or weeks of treatment initiation [40,41]. Flare reactions may occur in association with other hormonal therapies such as estrogens, androgens, progestins, and ablative therapies [40].

Other antiestrogens with less estrogenic activity than tamoxifen have been evaluated. Clinical studies show that trioxifene mesylate, a potent antiestrogen with low intrinsic estrogenic activity and higher affinity for the ER than

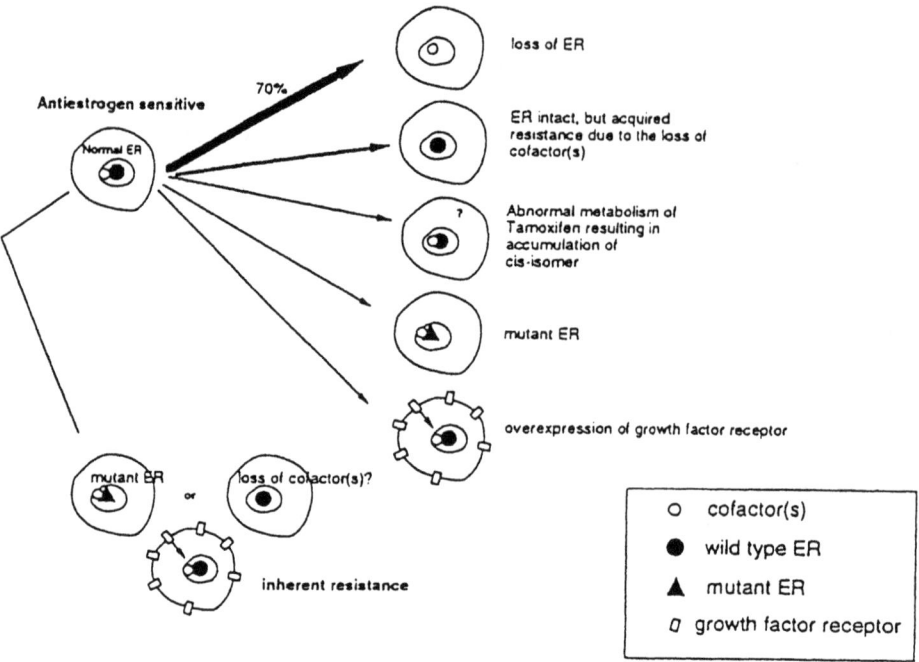

Figure 3. Postulated mechanisms of antiestrogen resistance.

tamoxifen, has antitumor effects comparable to tamoxifen's. However, further study of this agent has been abandoned because of unacceptable toxicity [42–44].

A triphenylethylene antiestrogen, toremifene, has an antiestrogenic/estrogenic ratio five times greater than tamoxifen's. It is well absorbed after oral dosing and the elimination half-life is about 5–6 days [45,46]. Phase I clinical trials in healthy postmenopausal women showed antiestrogenic activity at daily doses of 20, 40, and 60 mg but not 10 mg. Side effects occurred with the same frequency as with tamoxifen. Rarely, dizziness, tremor, hypercalcemia, and allergic reactions were encountered [46]. Phase II trials showed toremifene to be effective and safe for treating postmenopausal women with advanced ER+ breast cancer [47]. In more recent trials, however, toremifene and tamoxifen have been found similar in efficacy and, in fact, exhibit cross-resistance [48,49].

Several other antiestrogens have undergone limited clinical testing, including droloxifene (4-hydroxytamoxifen), idoxifene (pyrrolidine-4-iodotamoxifen), and zindoxifene. Of these, droloxifene has the most promise. Droloxifene is less estrogenic and more antiestrogenic than tamoxifen and has been shown to inhibit breast cancer cell growth in vitro and in vivo [50]. Phase I and II studies of droloxifene in ER+, postmenopausal patients with metastatic breast cancer have demonstrated overall response rates of 30%–40% with minimal toxicity [51–54]. In patients who have previously been treated with tamoxifen, the response rate is 15% [55]. Larger clinical trials are under way. Zindoxifene, an indole derivative of tamoxifen, has shown only marginal therapeutic activity [56]. Idoxifene, when compared to tamoxifen, was found to have a greater affinity for the ER, less estrogenic effect, and greater activity in vitro [57]. Idoxifene is currently under clinical investigation.

Two 'pure antiestrogens' have recently been introduced, and comparison of their clinical activity to that of tamoxifen is of interest. ICI 164,384 [N-*n*-butyl-N-Methyl-11-(3,17-*beta*-dihydroxyestra-1,3,5(10)-triene-7-*alpha*-yl)undecanamide] is a novel 7-alpha-analogue of 17-beta-estradiol that produces complete blockade of endogenous and exogenous estrogens and produces castration-like effects on adult rats without affecting the hypothalamic–pituitary–ovarian axis [58]. When studied in human breast cancer cell lines in vitro, ICI 164,384 was 100 times more potent than tamoxifen without the growth stimulatory effect [59–61]. In addition, it appears to be associated with less resistance, suggesting that it may be more effective than tamoxifen in breast cancer [62]. In fact, ICI 164,384 inhibits tamoxifen-stimulated breast tumor growth [63].

ICI 182,780 [7-alpha-(9-(4,4,5,5,5-pentafluoro-pentyl-sulfinyl)nonyl)estra-1,3,5(10)-triene-3,17-beta-diol], another new pure antiestrogen, is substantially more potent than ICI 164,384 [64]. Oral bioavailability, however, is low, and depot formulations are being tested. One study of ICI 182,780 found that tumor growth ceased for at least one month after a single injection [65]. In a trial of postmenopausal women with primary breast cancer, short-term administration of ICI 182,780 was well tolerated and produced demonstrable antiestrogenic effects in breast tumors in vivo without demonstrating estrogen agonist activity [66]. A small trial assessed the use of ICI 182,780 in patients with tamoxifen-resistant disease [67]. Nineteen patients were treated with intramuscular ICI 182,780. Sixty-nine percent responded (seven partial and six stable disease) with a minimum 18 months of response before progression.

3.2. Antiprogestins

Mifepristone (RU486), the only antiprogestin currently in clinical trials, also has antiglucocorticoid activity that can result in adrenal insufficiency. A study in 11 postmenopausal women with metastatic breast cancer showed an objective response in one, stable tumors in six, and progressive disease in four [68]. Because treatment resulted in increased plasma estradiol levels, mifepristone combined with an antiestrogen or GnRH agonist may be more successful. Major side effects of mifepristone are related to its antiglucocorticoid properties.

Other progesterone antagonists are under investigation in mammary tumor models. Onaprostone (ZK 98,299) and ZK112993, for example, have less antiglucocorticoid activity than mifepristone [68,69]. In hormone-dependent rat mammary tumors, these antiprogestins have shown some promise. Gestrinone, another antiprogestin, had previously been tested and was found to have no antitumor activity in endocrine-sensitive breast cancer [70].

3.3. Antiandrogens

Antiandrogens such as flutamide and cyproterone acetate in breast cancer have undergone only limited investigation in breast cancer. In one study by Perrault and colleagues, 750 mg of flutamide daily produced noted only one response in 29 women with advanced breast cancer [71]. Most patients had ER negative tumors and/or received prior hormonal therapy, however, lowering their likelihood for response.

3.4. Aromatase inhibitors

Extraovarian conversion of adrenal androstenedione to estrone is the primary source of estrogen production in postmenopausal women. Aromatase, concentrated mainly in the adipose tissue, muscle, and liver, is the major enzyme responsible for this conversion [72–75] (figure 4). Inhibitors of aromatase decrease breast cancer cell growth by decreasing the peripheral concentration of estradiol. In addition, about two thirds of breast tumors show aromatase activity, which appears to provide a local source of estrogens [76]; theoretically, aromatase inhibitors block estrogen synthesis within breast tumors, too. Table 2 lists aromatase inhibitors currently in clinical trials.

By blocking cholesterol side chain cleavage, 11-beta-hydroxylase, and aromatase, aminoglutethimide (AG) causes medical adrenalectomy and effectively eliminates estrogen production in postmenopausal women [77]. Many studies have confirmed its effectiveness in metastatic breast cancer in this population [21,72–74]. Randomized trials have confirmed that response rates to aminoglutethimide are similar to tamoxifen [28,72]. (Few responses have been observed in premenopausal women, and aromatase inhibitors may cause a reflex increase in gonadotropin levels in premenopausal women, potentially causing ovarian hyperstimulation [75,78]) AG may even yield a higher response rate than tamoxifen when used as first-line therapy in metastatic breast cancer. In a study of 216 postmenopausal patients, the overall response rates were 27% and 45% to tamoxifen and AG, respectively [34]. After disease progression, patients were crossed over to the other agent, and response rates were still better for AG (19% versus 36%). Overall survival between the two groups, however, was identical, and toxicity was greater with AG.

As second-line therapy after failure of tamoxifen, AG had an overall response rate of 34% in one study of 120 patients, with a median response duration of 9.5 months [79]. Twenty-five percent of patients whose tumors failed to respond to tamoxifen responded to AG.

Side effects of AG are considerable; they occur in about 35% of patients and require discontinuation of drug in 5% [75]. The major toxicities are

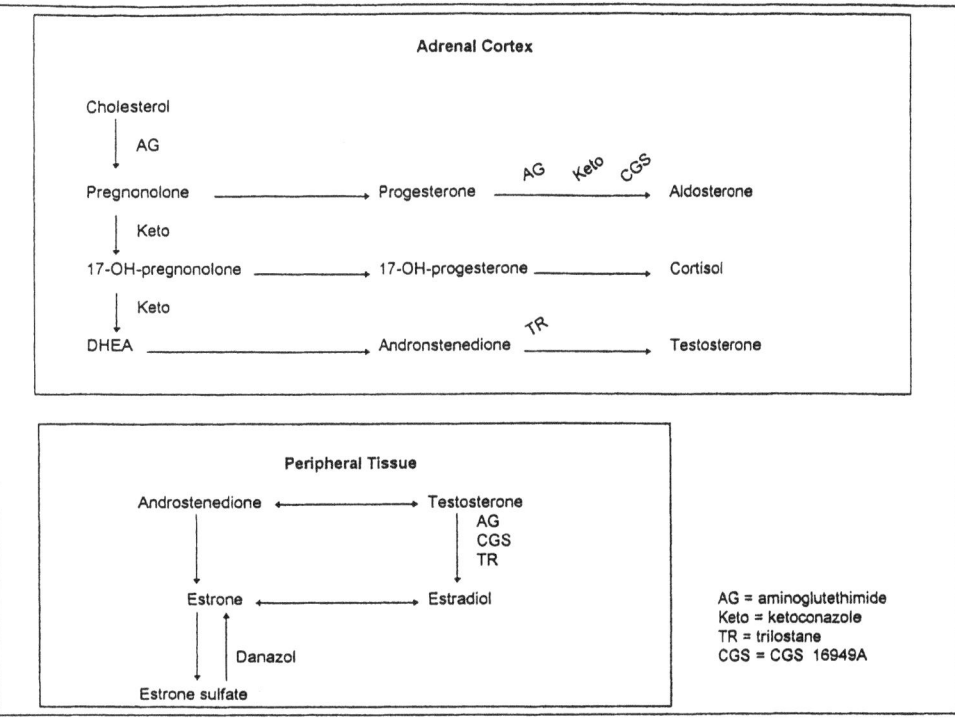

Figure 4. Sites of inhibition of steroidogenic enzyme inhibitors for metastatic breast cancer.

Table 2. Aromatase inhibitors

Glutethimide derivatives
Aminoglutethimide (Cytadren)
Pyridoglutethimide (rogletimide)
Anastrozole (Armidex, ICI-D1033)

Steroids
Trilostane
4-hydroxyandrostenedione (Lentaron, Formestane)
Exemestane (FCE24304)
Testololactone
Atamestane
1-methyl-1,4-androstadiene-3,7-dione (MAD)

Imidazoles
Ketoconazole
Fadrazole (CGS 16,949A)
Letrozole (CGS 20,267)
Vorozole (R 83,842)

lethargy (36%), a transient maculopapular rash (25%), dizziness (15%), and nausea and vomiting (10%), with severe myelosuppression reported in less than 1% of patients [80]. Severity and frequency of these side effects have made aminoglutethimide less desirable than tamoxifen or progestins for palliation [74]. Steroid supplementation with hydrocortisone generally is used to prevent hypoadrenalism that can arise with standard AG dosage of 250 mg four times daily. Randomized trials have shown that lower doses — 250 mg twice daily — are as effective as higher doses and can be given without steroid supplementation [28].

Formed by AG modification, pyridoglutethimide [pyridylglutarimide-3-ethyl-3-(4-pyridyl)piperidine-2,6-dione] displays similar capacity for inhibiting aromatase but, unlike AG, it does not inhibit cholesterol side-chain cleavage [81]. Pyridoglutethimide was shown to suppress plasma estradiol concentrations in postmenopausal women with breast cancer [82]. Early clinical studies have shown few responses with significant toxicity unrelated to dose [75].

Anastrozole (Armidex, ICI-D1033) is an orally active, potent, and selective benzyltriazole derivative in preclinical and clinical trials [83]. It suppresses estradiol production without affecting cortisol or aldosterone secretion. Two doses of anastrozole (1 mg and 10 mg orally once daily) were compared with megestrol acetate (40 mg orally four times daily) in a recent randomized trial of 378 postmenopausal women who had progressed after prior tamoxifen therapy [84]. After a median follow-up of 192 days, response rates and time to progression were similar in all treatment groups. Anastrozole was well tolerated at both dose levels and caused fewer side effects than megestrol acetate. This effective and minimally toxic aromatase inhibitor may be a logical second-line choice in women with metastatic breast cancer.

Several other steroidal aromatase inhibitors are being studied. Trilostane, an inhibitor of 3-beta-hydroxysteroid-dehydrogenase-isomerase, also inhibits aromatase with low potency [85]. Trilostane has been compared to AG in a multicenter crossover study of 72 postmenopausal patients with metastatic breast cancer [86]. Both drugs were similar in efficacy and did not demonstrate cross-resistance. Because of its inherent suppression of cortisol synthesis, trilostane must be administered with a glucocorticoid, and its use has been supplanted by other drugs.

4-hydroxyandrostenedione, the first androstenedione derivative to be used in clinical practice, binds irreversibly to and inhibits aromatase in vivo and is more potent than aminoglutethimide in vitro [87]. It must be given in parenteral form because it is not well absorbed orally and is rapidly and extensively cleared by the liver. Phase II trials have shown objective response rates ranging from 23% to 39% and stabilization of disease in 14% to 29% of women [88–90]. At doses of 500 mg given intramuscularly every two weeks, responses are seen in approximately one quarter of patients when used as second-line hormonal therapy [91]. As first-line endocrine therapy in postmenopausal women, response rates are similar to those seen with tamoxifen

[92,93]. In one trial of women who had received previous adjuvant therapy (42% had received adjuvant hormonal therapy), 4-hydroxyandrostenedione was extremely well tolerated and yielded long-lasting complete responses (median 14 months) [92]. Generally, 4-hydroxyandrostenedione has been better tolerated than aminoglutethimide [75]. Side effects include pain at the injection site, hot flashes, lethargy, rash, transient leukopenia, facial swelling, and, rarely, anaphylaxis [94]. Intramuscular depot forms are being tested in phase III trials; oral preparations, however, are still in the early stages of development.

Exemestane (FCE 24304), an orally active, irreversible aromatase inhibitor, is also a derivative of androstenedione. It has been studied in postmenopausal patients with metastatic breast cancer whose tumor had progressed on tamoxifen and was shown to reduce estrogen levels and elicit an objective response rate of 18% [95]. The drug was well tolerated, causing nausea and dyspepsia in only 16% of patients. Phase II trials are under way.

Other steroidal aromatase inhibitors worthy of clinical investigation include atamestane, 1-methyl-1,4-androstadiene-3,7-dione (MAD), and testololactone. Testololactone yields tumor regression without significant masculinizing or feminizing side effects, but response rates are inferior to those achieved with AG [75].

Another class of aromatase inhibitors, imidazoles, also decrease estrogen synthesis. This class includes ketoconazole, fadrozole (CGS 16949A), letrozole (CGS 20,267), vorozole. Fadrazole (CGS 16949A), a tetrahydroimidazopyridine, is a nonsteroidal competitive inhibitor of aromatase that prevents conversion of testosterone to estradiol and androstenedione to estrone. In one phase I trial, fadrozole was 500 times more potent than aminoglutethimide and had minimal toxicity [96]. It is readily absorbed after oral dosing and effectively maintains estradiol suppression when given twice daily [97]. In clinical studies, fadrozole achieved response rates of approximately 20% in postmenopausal patients with advanced breast cancer [75,98,99]. Toxicity included hot flashes, nausea and vomiting, fatigue, and loss of appetite. Fadrozole is now being tested in phase III clinical trials in postmenopausal patients with metastatic breast cancer.

Letrozole (CGS 20,267) is a nonsteroidal aromatase inhibitor that has the advantage of inhibiting estrogen synthesis but not adrenal steroidogenesis when used at low doses [100,101]. It is more potent than fadrozole in vitro and has undergone phase I and II testing, showing responses in about one third of patients with minimal toxicity [75,102]. The main side effects are headache and gastrointestinal (nausea, vomiting, constipation, and heartburn) [103]. Letrozole is also undergoing phase III testing.

Vorozole (R 83842) is a powerful nonsteroidal competitive stereospecific inhibitor of the cytochrome P450-dependent aromatase enzyme. Phase II trials recently reported response rates of 25%–35% as second-line therapy after tamoxifen failure [104–106].

In summary, AG and anastrozole are the aromatase inhibitors that are currently available for clinical use. Pyridoglutethimide more specifically inhibits estradiol production compared to AG but has significant toxicity. Formestane's toxicity profile is good, but it must be administered parenterally. Fadrozole is a very potent inhibitor of aromatase but is not specific and may also cause postural hypotension. Oral aromatase inhibitors with more specificity include letrozole, exemestane, and vorozole. All show promise and are undergoing clinical testing.

3.5. Androgens

Use of androgenic agents such as testosterone, fluoxymestrone, testololactone, and calusterone in metastatic breast cancer is associated with response rates in the range of 20% [28]. However, unacceptable side effects occur in many patients; 60%–70% of patients note masculinization with deepening of the voice and hirsutism, and 20%–40% have hair loss, acne, and increased libido [21]. Tumor flare and hypercalcemia are also encountered more frequently than with any other hormonal agents [40].

An effective androgen that has no masculinizing effects has not been found [107,108]. Danazol, a weak androgen with no primary estrogenic or progestational action, also inhibits pituitary gonadotropin secretion and has weak antiprogestogenic activity [109]. Its use as second-line hormonal therapy in advanced breast cancer is associated with response rates of approximately 25% [110–113]. Coombes and colleagues noted responses in 17% of 41 postmenopausal women with advanced breast cancer treated with the drug [110]. No responses were seen in premenopausal patients. Toxicities, which occurred in 22%, included lethargy, peripheral edema, and hot flashes. Generally mild, these side effects decreased when the dose was lowered; no patient discontinued therapy due to toxicity. Response to danazol in other studies has not been as promising. Pronzato and colleagues claimed response in only 3 of 21 patients, and Brodovsky and coworkers reported only 2 partial responses in 35 postmenopausal women [112,113]. A later study by Coombes and colleagues found responses in only 10 of 69 patients (14.9%) with advanced breast cancer [111]. This favorable therapeutic profile may make danazol a viable salvage agent.

3.6. Progestins

Progestational agents have been shown to abrogate the trophic effects of estrogen [17]. During the 1950s, progestins were found to yield response rates of 30% in unselected patients with breast cancer [114]. Randomized trials have shown that progestins are equal in efficacy to tamoxifen and other endocrine agents [115–119]. Toxicity is minimal in standard doses, and weight gain is the only significant consideration with long-term use. Progestational agents currently available include medroxyprogesterone acetate (MPA) and megestrol acetate (MA). Phase II trials showed high doses to be superior to lower doses of MPA, but randomized trials have been inconclusive, and it is unclear whether there is a dose–response effect for progestins [120–125]. An overview analysis of randomized clinical trials of progestins versus tamoxifen suggested that MPA may be more efficacious than tamoxifen in postmenopausal women [119].

MA, an oral progestin, is the progestin most often used in treatment of metastatic breast cancer in the United States [126]. Because of its low toxicity, it is often used as second-line hormonal treatment for metastatic breast cancer, although response rates may be poor. One study of MA (160 mg/day) given after tamoxifen or AG failure found no complete responses and only 4% partial responses, with a median of nine months [127]. Forty-eight percent of patients had stable disease of a median of eight months. In addition, responses were only seen in bone and pleural sites of metastatic disease. MA, therefore, is a reasonable second-line treatment for asymptomatic patients with bone or pleural metastases.

The dose of MA has also been of some debate. Serum levels achieved with oral doses of 160 mg daily are similar to those at MPA doses of 1000 mg daily. In one randomized trial, 160 mg of MA produced a higher response rate than 800 mg but no convincing improvement in survival [128]. Preliminary results from a similar Cancer and Leukemia Group B trial have not confirmed these observations. High-dose progestins may be more effective than lower doses or tamoxifen in causing regression of bone metastases [128,129].

3.7. Gonadotropin releasing factors (LHRH agonists)

Gonadotropin analogues cause pituitary-gonadal axis suppression similar to surgical or radiotherapeutic castration, but without serious side effects. In 1976, DeSombre and colleagues demonstrated that rat mammary tumors could be reduced by a luteinizing hormone releasing hormone (LHRH) analogue [130]. Since then, a series of experimental studies in rodents has defined the effects of chronic LHRH agonist treatment at pharmacologic doses: 1) decreased gonadotropin and prolactin secretion; 2) a striking fall in plasma sex steroids preceding a reduction in weight of accessory sex organs; 3) inhibition of enzymes involved in steroidogenesis; and 4) direct effects on extrapituitary tissues such as breast tumor cells [131].

Pituitary gonadotropin secretion is dependent on the intermittent, pulsating GnRH secretion from the hypothalamic neurons [132]. Continuous stimulation of the pituitary by GnRH or the long-acting GnRH agonists results in desensitization of gonadotropin secretion and subsequent gonadal suppression [133]. The clinical utility of the GnRH analogues in premenopausal women rests in the continuous stimulation of these agents. GnRH analogues bind to the GnRH receptors in the pituitary with an affinity 10 times that of natural GnRH and block the effects of normal hypothalamic GnRH. This process results in long-term inhibition of FSH and LH secretion and estrogen

Table 3. Gonadotropin releasing hormone analogues

Goserelin (Zolodex)
Leuprolide (Leupron)
  Buserelin
  Nafarelin
  Deslorelin
  Histrelin

suppression in premenopausal women [131]. In postmenopausal women, LH and FSH levels are suppressed, but estrogen levels remain relatively unchanged, accounting for the limited clinical effect of GnRH analogues in postmenopausal patients [134]. GnRH analogues may also have a direct antitumor effect. Low-affinity binding sites for GnRH have been demonstrated on human breast cancer cells; in vitro, growth of these cells in the presence of GnRH agonists is inhibited [135,136].

Because LHRH analogues are small peptides susceptible to digestion in the gastrointestinal tract, they are unsuitable for oral use and must be administered via nasal spray or subcutaneous or intramuscular injections. Newly available depot forms offer greater efficacy and administrative ease. GnRH analogues cause hypogonadism, and their side effects include hot flashes (usually transient), decreased libido, and depression. Interestingly, tumor flare has not yet been described with these agents [8].

Results of phase II studies with GnRH analogues in premenopausal women with metastatic breast cancer have been encouraging. Response rates have approximated 40%, with little variation among different agents [131,137]. Patients with receptor-positive tumors had an objective response rate of 50%, whereas those with receptor-negative tumors responded less frequently (7%–33%) [138]. Response duration has been approximately one year. Table 3 lists GnRH analogues currently in clinical trial.

4. Combination endocrine therapy

Investigational approaches include combinations of hormonal agents, hormonal agents and biologics, and hormonal and antiproliferative agents (for example, fenretinide). Theoretically, hormonal agent combinations may further reduce estrogen levels and/or decrease estrogen's effect on breast cancer cells. To date, however, no hormonal agent combination has been shown to be convincingly superior to single-agent therapy. Some trials have shown higher response rates, but longer survival or response duration generally has not been seen [28,139]. In other trials, the combinations' toxicity was prohibitive [140–142].

Interferon-alpha increases ER expression and potentiates tamoxifen inhibition of breast cancer cell growth in vitro [143]. In vivo, studies of the combination have shown complex effects, and clinical trials have been inconclusive [144].

Fenretinide, a vitamin A analogue, displays chemopreventive properties against carcinogen-induced mammary cancer in rodents. Combined with tamoxifen, it recently was tested in women with metastatic breast cancer [145]. In 12 of 15 patients, disease improved or stabilized and side effects were minimal; phase III trials are in development.

Studies of vitamin D analogues combined with tamoxifen are ongoing. Vitamin D has an antiproliferative effect on breast cancer cells in vivo, but its in vitro use is haltered by its calcemic side effects. Vitamin D analogues have been developed that do not cause hypercalcemia but still inhibit breast cancer cell growth. It is thought that these compounds will be useful in tamoxifen-resistant breast cancer [146].

Somatostatin has also been used with tamoxifen. There is evidence that this combination leads to decreased levels of IGF1 and/or leads to apoptosis [147]. Clinical trials are under way.

Recent studies have found that the pineal hormone melatonin may modulate estrogen receptor expression and inhibit breast cancer cell growth. In fact, melatonin combined with tamoxifen in patients with metastatic breast cancer that progressed on or was resistant to tamoxifen alone produced partial response in 28.5% of patients [148].

5. Summary

Endocrine therapy represents a mainstay of effective, minimally toxic, palliative treatment for metastatic breast cancer. Research focusing on the mechanism of action of endocrine agents will provide new insights leading to new hormonal approaches in breast cancer treatment. Development of new agents, especially the 'pure' antiestrogens, is of great interest. Combining endocrine therapy with biologic agents, especially antiproliferative compounds, may lead to more effective treatment in the adjuvant as well as the advanced setting.

Tables 4 and 5 summarize response rates to the different groups of endocrine agents used in metastatic breast cancer and doses of commonly used agents, respectively. At present, tamoxifen is the drug of choice as first-line endocrine therapy for metastatic breast cancer with no or minimal symptoms in premenopausal or postmenopausal women. Second-line therapy usually consists of megace. Aromatase inhibitors may be used as second- or third-line therapy in postmenopausal women. In premenopausal women, LHRH analogues are a reasonable choice. The other hormonal agents may be beneficial as salvage therapy. More effective endocrine approaches are under development.

Table 4. Metastatic breast cancer standard hormonal treatment modalities

	Response rates [ref]	Major Toxicity
Premenopausal		
Oophorectomy	30% [149]	Hot flashes, amenorrhea, osteoporosis
LHRH Agonists	35–40% [28]	Hot flashes, amenorrhea, nausea, vomiting
Postmenopausal		
Estrogens	20–40%	Nausea, vomiting, sodium retention, uterine bleeding, breast tenderness and engorgement, nipple pigmentation
Androgens	5–20% [28]	Masculinization, nausea, vomiting, cholestatic jaundice, fluid retention
Aromatase inhibitors	30–40% [8]	Nausea, vomiting, skin rash, lethargy
Corticosteroids	20–25% [21]	Mood disturbance, proximal muscular weakness, osteoporosis, bone loss, Cushingoid appearance, immunosuppression
Pre- or postmenopausal		
Antiestrogens	30–40% [29]	Hot flashes, menstrual irregularities, vaginal discharge, uterine cancer
Progestins	20–40% [115]	Weight gain, withdrawal bleeding, fluid retention

Table 5. Dose schedules of commonly used hormonal agents

Agent	Dose	Schedule
Estrogens		
Stilbestrol (DES)	5 mg po	tid
Ethinyl estradiol	0.5–1.0 mg po	tid
Premarin™	0.625 mg po	qd
Antiestrogens		
Tamoxifen	20 mg po	qd
Progestins		
Medroxyprogesterone	400 mg po	qd
Megestrol	40 mg po	qid
Aromatase inhibitors		
Aminoglutethimide	250 mg po	bid–qid
Anastrozole	1 mg po	qd
Androgens		
Fluoxymesterone	10 mg po	bid–tid
LHRH agonists		
Leuprolide	Depot 7.5 mg IM	q month
Goserelin	Depot 3.6 mg IM	q month
Corticosteroids		
Prednisone	15–40 mg po	qd

References

1. Parker SL, Tong T, Bolden S, Wingo PA. 1996. Cancer Statistics, 1996. CA 65:5–27.
2. Taylor SG, Gelman RS, Falkson G, Cummings FJ. 1986. Combination chemotherapy compared to tamoxifen as initial therapy for stage IV breast cancer in elderly women. Ann Intern Med 104:455–461.
3. Anonymous. 1986. A randomized trial in postmenopausal patients with advanced breast cancer comparing endocrine and cytotoxic therapy given sequentially or in combination. The Australian and New Zealand Breast Cancer Trials Group, Clinical Oncological Society of Australia. J Clin Oncol 4:186–193.
4. Muss HB. 1992. Endocrine therapy for advanced breast cancer: a review. Breast Cancer Res Treat 21:15–26.
5. Kimmick G, Muss HB, 1995. Current status of endocrine therapy for metastatic breast cancer. Contemp Oncol 9:877–890.
6. Beatson GT. 1896. On the treatment of inoperable cases of carcinoma of the mamma: suggestions for a new method of treatment, with illustrative cases. Lancet 2:104–107.
7. Davidson NE. 1994. Ovarian ablation as treatment for young women with breast cancer (review). Monogr Nat cancer Inst ••:95–99.
8. Santen RJ, Manni A, Harvey H, Redmond C. 1990. Endocrine treatment of breast cancer in women (review). Endocrine Rev 11:221–265.
9. Dowsett M. 1990. Novel approaches to the endocrine therapy of breast cancer (review). Eur J Cancer 26:989–992.
10. Cash R, Brough AJ, Cohen MN, Satoh PS. 1967. Aminoglutethimide (Elipten-Ciba) as an inhibitor of adrenal steroidogenesis: mechanism of action and therapeutic trial. J Clin Endocrinol Metab 27:1239–1248.
11. Griffiths CT, Hall TC, Saba Z, Barlow JJ, Nevinny HB. 1973. Preliminary trial of aminoglutethimide in breast cancer. Cancer 32:31–37.
12. Nemoto T, Patel J, Rosner D, Dao TL. 1984. Tamoxifen (Nolvadex) versus adrenalectomy in metastatic breast cancer. Cancer 53:1333–1335.
13. Santen RJ, Worgul TJ, Samojlik E, Interrante A, Boucher AE, Lipton A, Harvey HA, White DS, Smart E, Cox C, Wells SA. 1981. A randomized trial comparing surgical adrenalectomy with aminoglutethimide plus hydrocortisone in women with advanced breast cancer. N Engl J Med 305:545–551.
14. Kiang DT, Frenning DH, Vosika GJ, Kennedy BJ. 1980. Comparison of tamoxifen and hypophysectomy in breast cancer treatment. Cancer 45:1322–1325.
15. Harvey HA, Santen RJ, Osterman J, Samojlik E, White DS, Lipton A. 1979. A comparative trial of transsphenoidal hypophysectomy and estrogen suppression with aminoglutethimide in advanced breast cancer. Cancer 43:2207–2214.
16. Miller WR. 1990. Endocrine treatment for breast cancers: biological rationale and current progress. J Steroid Biochem Mol Biol 37:467–480.
17. Sutherland DJ, Mobbs BG. 1992. Hormones and cancer. In Tannock IF, Hill RP, eds. The Basic Science of Oncology, 2nd ed. New York: McGraw-Hill, Health Professions Division, pp. 207–232.
18. Lippman ME. 1988. Steroid hormone receptors and mechanisms of growth regulation of human breast cancer. In Lippman ME, Lichtner AS, Danforth DN, eds. Diagnosis and Management of Breast Cancer. Philadelphia: W.B. Saunders, pp. 327–347.
19. Editorial. 1960. Androgens and estrogens in the treatment of disseminated mammary carcinoma. Retrospective study of nine hundred forty-four patients. Report of the Council on Drugs. JAMA 172:135–147.
20. Carter AC, Sedransk N, Kelley RM, Ansfield FJ, Ravdin RG, Talley RW, Potter NR. 1977. Diethylstilbestrol: recommended dosages for different categories of breast cancer patients. Report of the Cooperative Breast Cancer Group. JAMA 237:2079–2080.
21. Pritchard KI, Sutherland DJA. 1989. Diagnosis and therapy of breast cancer: the use of endocrine therapy. Hematol Oncol Clin North Am 3:765–805.

22. Minton MJ, Knight RK, Rubens RD, Hayward JL. 1981. Corticosteroids for elderly patients with breast cancer. Cancer 48:883–887.
23. Bruera E, Roca E, Cedaro L, Carraro S, Chacon R. 1985. Action of oral methylprednisolone in terminal cancer patients: a prospective randomized double-blind study. Cancer Treat Rep 69:751–754.
24. Lippman M, Bolan G, Huff K. 1976. The effects of estrogens and antiestrogens on hormone-responsive human breast cancer in long-term tissue culture. Cancer Res 36:4595–4601.
25. Wakeling AE. 1993. The future of new pure antiestrogens in clinical breast cancer (review). Breast Cancer Res Treat 25:1–9.
26. Litherland S, Jackson IM. 1988. Antioestrogens in the management of hormone-dependent cancer. Cancer Treat Rev 15:183–194.
27. Manni A. 1987. Tamoxifen therapy of metastatic breast cancer. J Lab Clin Med 109:290–299.
28. Henderson IC. 1991. Endocrine therapy of metastatic breast cancer. In Harris JR, Hellman S, Henderson IC, Kinne DW, eds. Breast Diseases, 2nd ed. New York: Lippincott, pp. 559–603.
29. Canney PA, Griffiths T, Latief TN, Priestman TJ. 1987. Clinical significance of tamoxifen withdrawal response (letter). Lancet 1:36.
30. Buckley MM, Goa KL. 1989. Tamoxifen. A reappraisal of its pharmacodynamic and pharmacokinetic properties, and therapeutic use (review). Drugs 37:451–490.
31. Malet C, Gompel A, Spritzer P, Bricout N, Yaneva H, Mowszowicz I, Mauvais-Jarvis P. 1988. Tamoxifen and hydroxytamoxifen isomers versus estradiol effects on normal human breast cells in culture. Cancer Res 48:7193–7199.
32. Karnik PS, Kulkarni S, Liu XP, Budd GT, Bukowski RM. 1994. Estrogen receptor mutations in tamoxifen-resistant breast cancer. Cancer Res 54:349–353.
33. Katzenellenbogen BS. 1991. Antiestrogen resistance: mechanisms by which breast cancer cells undermine the effectiveness of endocrine therapy (editorial; comment). J Natl Cancer Inst 83:1434–1435.
34. Paik S, Hartmann DP, Dickson RB, Lippman ME. 1994. Antiestrogen resistance in ER positive breast cancer cells (review). Breast Cancer Res Treat 31:301–307.
35. Mauvais-Javis P, Baudot N, Castaigne D, Banzet P, Kuttenn F. 1986. Trans-4-Hydroxytamoxifen concentration and metabolism after local percutaneous administration to human breast. Cancer Res 46:1521–1525.
36. Murphy C, Fotsis T, Pantzar P, Adlercreutz H, Martin F. 1987. Analysis of tamoxifen, N-desmethyltamoxifen and 4-hydroxytamoxifen levels in cytosol and KCl-nuclear extracts of breast tumours from tamoxifen treated patients by gas chromatography-mass spectrometry (GC-MS) using selected ion monitoring (SIM). J Steroid Biochem 28:609–618.
37. Osborne CK, Wiebe VJ, McGuire WL, Ciocca DR, DeGregorio MW. 1992. Tamoxifen and the isomers of 4-hydroxytamoxifen in tamoxifen-resistant tumors from breast cancer patients. J Clin Oncol 10:304–310.
38. Wiebe VJ, Osborne CK, McGuire WL, DeGregorio MW. 1992. Identification of estrogenic tamoxifen metabolite(s) in tamoxifen-resistant human breast tumors. J Clin Oncol 10:990–994.
39. Wolf DM, Langan-Fahey SM, Parker CJ, McCague R, Jordan VC. 1993. Investigation of the mechanism of tamoxifen-stimulated breast tumor growth with nonisomerizable analogues of tamoxifen and metabolites. J Natl cancer Inst 85:806–812.
40. Clarysse A. 1985. Hormone-induced tumor flare (editorial). Eur J Cancer Clin Oncol 21:545–547.
41. Plotkin D, Lechner JJ, Jung WE, Rosen PJ. 1978. Tamoxifen flare in advanced breast cancer. JAMA 240:2644–2646.
42. Rose DP, Fischer AH, Jordan VC, 1981. Activity of the antioestrogen trioxifene against N-Nitrosomethylurea-induced rat mammry carcinomas. Eur J Cancer Clin Oncol 17:893–898.
43. Witte RS, Pruitt B, Tormey DC, Moss S, Rose DP, Falkson G, Carbone PP, Ramirez G, Falkson H, Pretorius FJ. 1986. A phase I/II investigation of trioxifene mesylate in advanced breast cancer. Clinical and endocrinologic effects. Cancer 57:34–39.

44. Lee RW, Buzdar AU, Blumenschein GR, Hortobagyi GN. 1986. Trioxifene mesylate in the treatment of advanced breast cancer. Cancer 57:40–43.
45. Anttila M, Valavaara R, Kivinen S, Maenpaa J. 1990. Pharmacokinetics of toremifene. J Steroid Biochem 36:249–252.
46. Kangas L. 1990. Introduction to toremifene (review). Breast Cancer Res Treat 16 (Suppl):S3–S7.
47. Valavaara R. 1990. Phase II trials with toremifene in advanced breast cancer: a review. Breast Cancer Res Treat 16 (Suppl):S31–S35.
48. Stenbygaard LE, Herrstedt J, Thomsen JF, Svendsen KR, Engelholm SA. 1993. Toremifene and tamoxifen in advanced breast cancer — a double-blind cross-over trial. Breast Cancer Res Treat 25:57–63.
49. Vogel CL, Shemano I, Schoenfelder J, Gams RA, Green MR. 1993. Multicenter phase II efficacy trial of toremifene in tamoxifen-refractory patients with advanced breast cancer. J Clin Oncol 11:345–350.
50. Kawamura I, Mizota T, Lacey E, Tanaka Y, Manda T, Shimomura K, Kohsaka M. 1993. The estrogenic and antiestrogenic activities of droloxifene in human breast cancers. Jpn J Pharmacol 63:27–34.
51. Buzdar AU, Kau S, Hortobagyi GN, Theriault RL, Booser D, Holmes FA, Walters R, Krakoff IH. 1994. Phase I trial of droloxifene in patients with metastatic breast cancer. Cancer Chemother Pharmacol 33:313–316.
52. Bruning PF. 1992. Droloxifene, a new anti-oestrogen in postmenopausal advanced breast cancer: preliminary results of a double-blind dose-finding phase II trial. Eur J Cancer 28A:1404–1407.
53. Deschenes L. 1991. Droloxifene, a new antiestrogen, in advanced breast cancer. A double-blind dose-finding study. The Droloxifene 002 International Study Group. Am J Clin Oncol 14 (Suppl 2):S52–S55.
54. Bellmunt J, Sole L. 1991. European early phase II dose-finding study of droloxifene in advanced breast cancer. Am J Clin Oncol 14 (Suppl 2):S36–S39.
55. Haarstad H, Gundersen S, Wist E, Raabe N, Mella O, Kvinnsland S. 1992. Droloxifene — a new anti-estrogen. A phase II study in advanced breast cancer. Acta Oncol 31:425–428.
56. Stein RC, Dowsett M, Cunningham DC, Davenport J, Ford HT, Gazet JC, Coombes RC. 1990. Phase I/II study of the anti-oestrogen zindoxifene (D16726) in the treatment of advanced breast cancer. A Cancer Research Campaign Phase I/II Clinical Trials Committee study. Br J Cancer 61:451–453.
57. Coombes RC, Jarman M, Dowsett M. 1993. New endocrine agents for the treatment of breast cancer. Recent Results in Cancer Res 127:267.
58. Wakeling AE. 1990. Therapeutic potential of pure antioestrogens in the treatment of breast cancer (review). J Steroid Biochem Mol Biol 37:771–775.
59. Wakeling AE. 1990. Novel pure antiestrogens. Mode of action and therapeutic prospects. Ann NY Acad Sci 595:348–356.
60. Poulin R, Merand Y, Poirier D, Levesque C, Dufour JM, Labrie F. 1989. Antiestrogenic properties of keoxifene, trans-4-hydroxytamoxifen, and ICI 164,384, a new steroidal antiestrogen, in ZR-75-1 human breast cancer cells. Breast Cancer Res Treat 14:65–76.
61. Thompson EW, Katz D, Shima TB, Wakeling AE, Lippman ME, Dickson RB. 1989. ICI 164,384, a pure antagonist of estrogen-stimulated MCF-7 cell proliferation and invasiveness. Cancer Res 49:6929–6934.
62. Bronzert DA, Davidson N, Lippman M. 1986. Estrogen and antiestrogen resistance in human breast cancer cell lines (review). Adv Exp Med Biol 196:329–345.
63. Gottardis MM, Jiang SY, Jeng MH, Jordan VC. 1989. Inhibition of tamoxifen-stimulated growth of an MCF-7 tumor variant in athymic mice by novel steroidal antiestrogens. Cancer Res 49:4090–4093.
64. Wakeling AE, Bowler J. 1992. ICI 182,780, a new antioestrogen with clinical potential (review). J Steroid Biochem Mol Biol 43:173–177.

65. Wakeling AE, Dukes M, Bowler J. 1991. A potent specific pure antiestrogen with clinical potential. Cancer Res 51:3867–3873.
66. DeFriend DJ, Howell A, Nicholson RI, et al. 1994. Investigation of a new pure antiestrogen (ICI 182,780) in women with primary breast cancer. Cancer Res 54:408–414.
67. Howell A, DeFriend D, Robertson J, Blamey R, Walton P. 1995. Response to a specific antioestrogen (ICI 182,780) in tamoxifen-resistant breast cancer (see comments). Lancet 345:29–30.
68. Bakker GH, Setyono-Han B, Portengen H, De Jong FH, Foekens JA, Klijn JG. 1990. Treatment of breast cancer with different antiprogestins: preclinical and clinical studies. J Steroid Biochem Mol Biol 37:789–794.
69. Schneider MR, Michna H, Nishino Y, Neef G, el Etreby MF. 1990. Tumor-inhibiting potential of ZK 112.993, a new progesterone antagonist, in hormone-sensitive, experimental rodent and human mammary tumors. Anticancer Res 10:683–687.
70. Cunningham D, Gazet J, Ford HT, Coombes RC. 1987. Oral gestrinone: a novel antiprogestin with no antitumor activity in endocrine-sensitive breast cancer. Cancer Treat Rep 71:1091–1092.
71. Perrault DJ, Logan DM, Stewart DJ, Bramwell VH, Paterson AH, Eisenhauer EA. 1988. Phase II study of flutamide in patients with metastatic breast cancer. A National Cancer Institute of Canada Clinical Trials Group study. Invest New Drugs 6:207–210.
72. Manni A, Santen RJ. 1988. Clinical use of aromatase inhibitors in the treatment of breast cancer (review). Cancer Treat Res 39:67–81.
73. Santen RJ, Worgul TJ, Lipton A, Harvey H, Boucher A, Samojlik E, Wells SA. 1982. Aminoglutethimide as treatment of postmenopausal women with advanced breast carcinoma. Ann Intern Med 96:94–101.
74. Stuart-Harris RC, Smith IE. 1984. Aminoglutethimide in the treatment of advanced breast cancer. Cancer Treat Rev 11:189–204.
75. Goss PE, Gwyn KM. 1994. Current perspectives on aromatase inhibitors in breast cancer (review). J Clin Oncol 12:2460–2470.
76. Bolufer P, Ricart E, Lluch A, Vazquez C, Rodriguez A, Ruiz A, Llopis F, Garcia-Conde J, Romero R. 1992. Aromatase activity and estradiol in human breast cancer: its relationship to estradiol and epidermal growth factor receptors and to tumor-node-metastasis staging. J Clin Oncol 10:438–446.
77. Lawrence BV, Lipton A, Harvey HA, Santen RJ, Wells SA Jr, Cox CE, Smart EK. 1980. Influence of estrogen receptor status on response of metastatic breast cancer to aminoglutethimide therapy. Cancer 45:786–791.
78. Wander HE, Blossey HC, Nagel GA. 1986. Aminoglutethimide in the treatment of premenopausal patients with metastatic breast cancer. Eur J Cancer Clin Oncol 22:1371–1374.
79. Brufman G, Biran S. 1990. Second line hormonal therapy with aminoglutethimide in metastatic breast cancer. Acta Oncol 29:717–720.
80. Messeih AA, Lipton A, Santen RJ, Harvey HA, Boucher AE, Murray R, Ragaz J, Buzdar AU, Nagel GA, Henderson IC. 1985. Aminoglutethimide-induced hematologic toxicity: worldwide experience. Cancer Treat Rep 69:1003–1004.
81. Foster AB, Jarman M, Leung CS, Rowlands MG, Taylor GN, Plevey RG. 1985. Analogues of aminoglutethimide: selective inhibition of aromatase. J Med Chem 28:200–204.
82. Haynes BP, Jarman M, Dowsett M, Mehta A, Lonning PE, Griggs LJ, Powles T, Stein R, Coombes RC. 1991. Pharmacokinetics and pharmacodynamics of the aromatase inhibitor 3-ethyl-3-(4-pyridyl)piperidine-2,6-dione in patients with postmenopausal breast cancer. Cancer Chemother Pharmacol 27:367–372.
83. Plourde PV, Dyroff M, Dowsett M, Demers L, Yates R, Webster A. 1995. ARIMIDEX: a new oral, once-a-day aromatase inhibitor (review). J Steroid Biochem Mol Biol 53:175–179.
84. Jonat W, Howell A, Blomqvist C, Eiermann W, Winblad G, Tyrrell C, Mauriac L, Roche H, Lundgren S, Hellmund R, Azab M. 1996. A randomised trial comparing two doses of the new selective aromatase inhibitor anastrozole (Armidex) with megestrol acetate in postmenopausal patients with advanced breast cancer. Eur J Cancer 32A:404–412.

85. Dowsett M. 1991. Inhibitors of steroidogenic enzymes for the treatment of breast cancer (review). J Steroid Biochem Mol Biol 39:805–809.
86. Williams CJ, Barley VL, Blackledge GR, Rowland CG, Tyrrell CJ. 1993. Multicentre cross over study of aminoglutethimide and trilostane in advanced postmenopausal breast cancer. Br J Cancer 68:1210–1215.
87. Brodie AM, Wing LY, Goss P, Dowsett M, Coombes RC. 1986. Aromatase inhibitors and the treatment of breast cancer. J Steroid Biochem 24:91–97.
88. Pickles T, Perry L, Murray P, Plowman P. 1990. 4-hydroxyandrostenedione — further clinical and extended endocrine observations. Br J Cancer 62:309–313.
89. Stein RC, Dowsett M, Hedley A, Davenport J, Gazet JC, Ford HT. 1990. Treatment of advanced breast cancer in postmenopausal women with 4-hydroxyandrostenedione. Cancer Chemother Pharmacol 26:75–78.
90. Hoffken K, Jonat W, Possinger K, et al. 1990. Aromatase inhibition with 4-hydroxyandrostenedione in the treatment of postmenopausal patients with advanced breast cancer: a phase II study. J Clin Oncol 8:875–880.
91. Possinger K, Jonat W, Hoffken K. 1994. Formestane in the treatment of advanced postmenopausal breast cancer. Ann Oncol 5 (Suppl 7):S7–S10.
92. Zilembo N, Bajetta E, Noberasco C, Buzzoni R, Vicario G, Bono A, Laffranchi A, Biasi G, Dolci S, Bichisao E. 1995. Formestane: an effective first-line endocrine treatment for advanced breast cancer. J Cancer Res Clin Oncol 121:378–382.
93. Perez Carrion R, Alberola Candel V, Calabresi F, et al. 1994. Comparison of the selective aromatase inhibitor formestane with tamoxifen as first-line hormonal therapy in postmenopausal women with advanced breast cancer. Ann Oncol 5 (Suppl 7):S19–S24.
94. Coombes RC, Goss PE, Dowsett M, Hutchinson G, Cunningham D, Jarman M. 1987. 4-Hydroxyandrostenedione treatment for postmenopausal patients with advanced breast cancer. Steroids 50:245–252.
95. Zilembo N, Noberasco C, Bajetta E, et al. 1995. Endocrinological and clinical evaluation of exemestane, a new steroidal aromatase inhibitor. Br J Cancer 72:1007–1012.
96. Lipton A, Harvey HA, Demers LM, Hanagan JR, Mulagha MT, Kochak GM, Sanders SI, Santen RJ. 1990. A phase I trial of CGS 16949A. A new aromatase inhibitor. Cancer 65:1279–1285.
97. Demers LM, Lipton A, Harvey HA, Hanagan J, Mulagha M, Santen RJ. 1993. The effects of long term fadrozole hydrochloride treatment in patients with advanced stage breast cancer. J Steroid Biochem Mol Biol 44:683–685.
98. Santen RJ, Demers LM, Lynch J, et al. 1991. Specificity of low dose fadrozole hydrochloride (CGS 16949A) as an aromatase inhibitor. J Clin Endocrinol Metab 73:99–106.
99. Raats JI, Falkson G, Falkson HC. 1992. A study of fadrozole, a new aromatase inhibitor, in postmenopausal women with advanced metastatic breast cancer. J Clin Oncol 10:111–116.
100. Bhatnagar AS, Hausler A, Schieweck K, Lang M, Bowman R. 1990. Highly selective inhibition of estrogen biosynthesis by CGS 20267, a new non-steroidal aromatase inhibitor (review). J Steroid Biochem Mol Biol 37:1021–1027.
101. Perez N, Borja J. 1992. Aromatase inhibitors: clinical pharmacology and therapeutic implications in breast cancer. J Int Med Res 20:303–312.
102. Lipton A, Demers LM, Harvey HA, Kambic KB, Grossberg H, Brady C, Adlercruetz H, Trunet PF, Santen RJ. 1995. Letrozole (CGS 20267). A phase I study of a new potent oral aromatase inhibitor of breast cancer. Cancer 75:2132–2138.
103. Iveson TJ, Smith IE, Ahern J, Smithers DA, Trunet PF, Dowsett M. 1993. Phase I study of the oral nonsteroidal aromatase inhibitor CGS 20267 in postmenopausal patients with advanced breast cancer. Cancer Res 53:266–270.
104. Dowsett M, Johnston SRD, Doody D, et al. 1994. The clinical and endocrine effects of the oral aromatase inhibitor vorozole in human breast cancer (abstract). Proc ASCO 13:71.
105. Goss PE, Clark R, Ambus U, et al. 1994. Phase II study of vorozole (R 83842) a new aromatase inhibitor in postmenopausal women with advanced breast cancer (abstract). Proc ASCO 13:88.

106. Vinholes J, Paridains R, Piccart MJ, et al. 1994. An EORTC breast group phase II study of vorozole (R 83842), a new aromatase inhibitor in advanced breast cancer (abstract). Proc ASCO 13:105.
107. Goldenberg IS, Waters N, Ravdin RS, Ansfield FJ, Segaloff A. 1973. Androgenic therapy for advanced breast cancer in women. A report of the Cooperative Breast Cancer Group. JAMA 223:1267–1268.
108. Manni A, Arafah BM, Pearson Oh. 1981. Androgen-induced remissions after antiestrogen and hypophysectomy in stage IV breast cancer. Cancer 48:2507–2509.
109. Peters TG, Lewis JD, Wilkinson EJ, Fuhrman TM. 1977. Danazol therapy in hormone-sensitive mammary carcinoma. Cancer 40:2797–2800.
110. Coombes RC, Dearnaley D, Humphreys J, Gazet JC, Ford HT, Nash AG, Mashiter K, Powles TJ. 1980. Danazol treatment of advanced breast cancer. Cancer Treat Rep 64:1073–1076.
111. Coombes RC, Perez D, Gazet JC, Ford HT, Powles TJ. 1983. Danazol treatment for advanced breast cancer. Cancer Chemother Pharmacol 10:194–195.
112. Brodovsky HS, Holroyde CP, Laucius JF, Dugery C, Serbin J. 1987. Danazol in the treatment of women with metastatic breast cancer. Cancer Treat Rep 71:875–876.
113. Pronzato P, Amoroso D, Ardizzoni A, Bertelli G, Conte PF, Michelotti A, Rosso R. 1987. A phase II study of danazol in metastatic breast cancer. Am J Clin Oncol 10:407–409.
114. Huggins C, Yang NC. 1962. Induction and extinction of mammary cancer. Science 137:257–262.
115. Petru E, Schmahl D. 1987. On the role of additive hormone monotherapy with tamoxifen, medroxyprogesterone acetate and aminoglutethimide. in advanced breast cancer. Klin Wochen 65:959–966.
116. Liber J, Rose C, Salimtschik M, Mouridsen HT. 1981. Treatment of advanced breast cancer with progestins. Acta Obstet Gynecol Scand — Suppl 101:39–46.
117. Haller DG, Glick JH. 1986. Progestational agents in advanced breast cancer: an overview. Semin Oncol 13:2–8.
118. Pannuti F, Martoni A, Piana E, et al. Progestins in breast cancer. In Pannuti F, ed. Hormonotherapy: Results and Perspectives. Pavia (Italy): Edizioni, pp. 207–222.
119. Parazzini F, Colli E, Scatigna M, Tozzi L. 1993. Treatment with tamoxifen and progestins for metastatic breast cancer in postmenopausal women: a quantitative review of published randomized clinical trials (review). Oncology 50:483–489.
120. Sedlacek SM, Horwitz KB. 1991. The role of progestins and progesterone receptors in the treatment of breast cancer. Steroids 44:467–483.
121. Pannuti F, Martoni A, Di Marco AR, et al. 1979. Prospective, randomized clinical trial of two different high dosages of medroxyprogesterone acetate (MAP) in the treatment of metastatic breast cancer. Eur J Cancer 15:593–601.
122. Della Cuna GR, Calciati A, Strada MRB, Bumma C, Campio L. 1978. High dose medroxyprogesterone acetate (MPA) treatment in metastatic carcinoma of the breast: a dose–response evaluation. Tumori 64:143–149.
123. Cortes Funes H, Madrigal PL, Perez Mangas G, et al. 1983. Medroxyprogesterone acetate at two different doses for the treatment of advanced breast cancer. In Campio L, Robustelli Della Cuna G, Taylor RW, eds. Role of Medroxyprogesterone in Endocrine Related Tumors, 2nd ed. New York: Raven Press, pp. 77–83.
124. Cavalli F, Goldhirsch A, Jungi F, Martz G, Mermillod B, Alberto P. 1984. Randomized trial of low-versus high-dose medroxyprogesterone acetate in the induction treatment of postmenopausal patients with advanced breast cancer. J Clin Oncol 2:414–419.
125. Gallagher CJ, Cairnduff F, Smith IE. 1987. High dose versus low dose medroxyprogesterone acetate: a randomized trial in advanced breast cancer. Eur J Cancer Clin Oncol 23:1895–1900.
126. Sedlacek SM. 1988. An overview of megestrol acetate for the treatment of advanced breast cancer. Semin Oncol 15:3–13.

127. Brufman G, Isacson R, Haim N, Gez E, Sulkes A. 1994. Megestrol acetate in advanced breast carcinoma after failure to tamoxifen and/or aminoglutethimide. Oncology 51:258–261.
128. Muss HB, Case LD, Capizzi RL, et al. 1990. High-versus standard-dose megestrol acetate in women with advanced breast cancer: a phase III trial of the Piedmont Oncology Association. J Clin Oncol 8:1797–1805.
129. Muss HB, Case LD, Atkins JN, et al. 1994. Tamoxifen versus high-dose oral medroxyprogesterone acetate as initial endocrine therapy for patients with metastatic breast cancer: a Piedmont Oncology Association study (see comments). J Clin Oncol 12:1630–1638.
130. DeSombre ER, Johnson ES, White WF. 1976. Regression of rat mammary tumors effected by a gonadoliberin analog. Cancer Res 36:3830–3833.
131. Klijn JG. 1992. LH-RH agonists in the treatment of metastatic breast cancer: ten years' experience (review). Recent Results Cancer Res 124:75–90.
132. Belchetz PE, Plant TM, Nakai Y, Keogh EJ, Knobil E. 1978. Hypophysial responses to continuous and intermittent delivery of hypopthalamic gonadotropin-releasing hormone. Science 202:631–633.
133. Conn PM, Crowley WF Jr. 1991. Gonadotropin-releasing hormone and its analogues (see comments) (review). N Engl J Med 324:93–103.
134. Harris AL, Carmichael J, Cantwell BM, Dowsett M. 1989. Zolodex: endocrine and therapeutic effects in post-menopausal breast cancer. Br J Cancer 59:97–99.
135. Eidne KA, Flanagan CA, Millar RP. 1985. Gonadotropin-releasing hormone binding sites in human breast carcinoma. Science 229:989–991.
136. Miller WR, Scott WN, Morris R, Fraser HM, Sharpe RM. 1985. Growth of human breast cancer cells inhibited by a luteinizing hormone-releasing hormone agonist. Nature 313:231–233.
137. Bajetta E, Zilembo N, Buzzoni R, Celio L, Zampino MG, Colleoni M, Oriana S, Attili A, Sacchini V, Martinetti A. 1994. Goserelin in premenopausal advanced breast cancer: clinical and endocrine evaluation of responsive patients. Oncology 51:262–269.
138. Kaufmann M, Jonat W, Kleeberg U, et al. 1989. Goserelin, a depot gonadotrophin-releasing hormone agonist in the treatment of premenopausal patients with metastatic breast cancer. German Zoladex Trial Group. J Clin Oncol 7:1113–1119.
139. Hardy JR, Powles TJ, Judson IR, Sinnett HD, Ashley SE, Coombes RC, Ellin CL. 1990. Combination of tamoxifen, aminoglutethimide, danazol and medroxyprogesterone acetate in advanced breast cancer. Eur J Cancer 26:824–827.
140. Mouridsen HT, Salimtschik M, Dombernowsky P, Gelshoj K, Palshof T, Daehnfeldt JL, Rose C. 1980. Therapeutic effect of tamoxifen versus combined tamoxifen and diethylstilboestrol in advanced breast cancer in postmenopausal women. Eur J Cancer Suppl 1:107–110.
141. Ingle JN, Twito DI, Schaid DJ, et al. 1988. Randomized clinical trial of tamoxifen alone or combined with fluoxymesterone in postmenopausal women with metastatic breast cancer. J Clin Oncol 6:825–831.
142. Ingle JN, Green SJ, Ahmann DL, Long HJ, Edmonson JH, Rubin J, Chang MN, Creagan ET. 1986. Randomized trial of tamoxifen alone or combined with aminoglutethimide and hydrocortisone in women with metastatic breast cancer. J Clin Oncol 4:958–964.
143. Bezwoda WR, Meyer K. 1990. Effect of alpha-interferon, 17 beta-estradiol, and tamoxifen on estrogen receptor concentration and cell cycle kinetics of MCF 7 cells. Cancer Res 50:5387–5391.
144. Seymour L, Bezwoda WR. 1993. Interferon plus tamoxifen treatment for advanced breast cancer: in vivo biologic effects of two growth modulators. Br J Cancer 68:352–356.
145. Cobleigh MA, Dowlatshahi K, Deutsch TA, et al. 1993. Phase I/II trial of tamoxifen with or without fenretinide, an analog of vitamin A, in women with metastatic breast cancer. J Clin Oncol 11:474–477.
146. Vink-van Wijngaarden T, Pols HA, Buurman CJ, van den Bemd GJ, Dorssers LC,

Birkenhager JC, van Leeuwen JP. 1994. Inhibition of breast cancer cell growth by combined treatment with vitamin D3 analogues and tamoxifen. Cancer Res 54:5711–5717.
147. Candi E, Melino G, De Laurenzi V, Piacentini M, Guerrieri P, Spinedi A, Knight RA. 1995. Tamoxifen and somatostatin affect tumours by inducing apoptosis. Cancer Lett 96:141–145.
148. Lissoni P, Barni S, Meregalli S, Fossati V, Cazzaniga M, Esposti D, Tancini G. 1995. Modulation of cancer endocrine therapy by melatonin: a phase II study of tamoxifen plus melatonin in metastatic breast cancer patients progressing under tamoxifen alone. Br J Cancer 71:854–856.
149. Binder SC, Flynn WJ, Pass LM. 1977. Endocrine ablative therapy of metastatic breast cancer. CA 27:1–9.

14. The regulation of estrogen receptor expression and function in human breast cancer

Anne T. Ferguson, Rena G. Lapidus, and Nancy E. Davidson

1. Introduction

Estrogen and estrogen receptor (ER) play an important role in the development and function of the mammary gland. During mammary gland development, the hypothalamus and pituitary gland signal changes in the level of plasma estrogen, which is associated with proliferation of the mammary epithelial cells, leading to branching of ducts and formation of alveolar structures called lobules. Normal mammary epithelial cells express low basal levels (0–37 fmol/mg cytosol protein) of ER, and immunohistochemical studies show that about 7% of normal breast epithelial cells stain positively for ER [1,2]. These levels fluctuate during the menstrual cycle in conjunction with the cyclic changes in estrogen [3]. Definitive evidence that ER plays a pivotal role in normal mammary development was demonstrated using transgenic mice that were homozygously deleted for the gene. Adult female ER knockout mice develop mammary glands with only vestigial ducts present at the nipples [4].

Estrogen and ER also play a significant role in the development and progression of breast cancer as well as in the treatment and outcome of breast cancer patients [5]. A majority of breast cancers express the ER gene and synthesize ER protein. Immunohistochemical staining of ER-positive tumors demonstrates that ER expression is heterogeneous, and approximately 70% of the tumor cells stain positively for ER [6]. These tumors tend to be more differentiated and less aggressive. Because they are dependent on estrogen for growth, they are often responsive to hormonal therapies. In contrast, approximately 30% of mammary carcinomas lack ER as defined by immunohistochemical analysis or ligand binding assay. Tumors lacking ER are generally associated with a more aggressive disease course and poorer clinical outcome [7]. Most importantly, since these cancers can grow in the absence of estrogen, they rarely respond to hormonal therapies.

The ER belongs to a superfamily of nuclear hormone receptors that includes the progesterone, retinoic acid, vitamin D, glucocorticoid, androgen, and thyroid hormone receptors. The structure of these proteins can be divided into six conserved, functional domains, A–F ([8]; figure 1). The A/B region in the amino-terminal end of the protein shows the greatest variability in

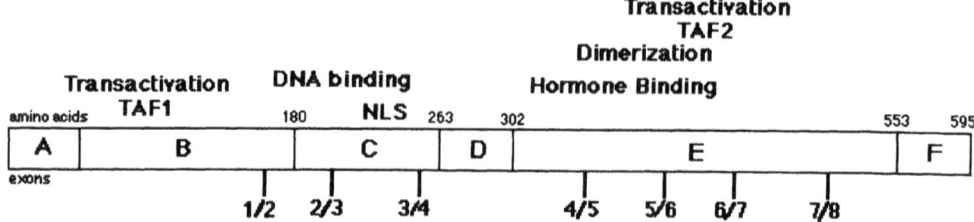

Figure 1. Structure of the ER gene and protein. Exons 1–8 and functional domains, A–F, encompassing the 595 amino acids of the 67-kDa protein, are shown. A/B: constitutive transcriptional activation function (TAF1); C: DNA binding domain containing two zinc-finger motifs and a nuclear localization signal (NLS); D: hinge domain; E: estrogen-inducible transactivation function (TAF2); F: unknown function [8,22].

sequence and size, whereas regions C and E are the most conserved, suggesting that these regions have functions common to all the steroid receptors.

The A/B domain of the ER protein contains a constitutive, estrogen-independent transcriptional activation function, TAF1 [9]. Domain C possesses two zinc-finger DNA binding motifs responsible for protein recognition of *cis*-acting estrogen response elements (EREs) [10]. The nuclear localization signal is located at the carboxy terminus of the DNA binding domain. This sequence is important for the nuclear localization of the receptor in the absence of ligand. The D or hinge region may be involved in estrogen-mediated transcriptional repression [11], while the E domain contains the hormone binding site, the region required for stable dimerization of the receptor, and a second estrogen-inducible transcriptional activation function, TAF2 [9]. The function of the F domain is presently unclear, but it may interact with cell type-specific factors that regulate ER function [12].

A scheme of estradiol and ER-mediated gene expression is outlined in figure 2. Normally, the heat shock proteins hsp 27, hsp 70, and hsp 90 associate with inactive ER in the absence of estradiol [13]. Estradiol binding to ER displaces the heat shock proteins and causes phosphorylation of the receptor at serine residues within the TAF1 domain. This estrogen binding also causes a conformational change in the protein that allows for a productive interaction and transcriptional synergism between TAF1 an TAF2 [14]. These changes allow for receptor homodimerization and subsequent binding to *cis*-acting elements within enhancers of target genes. Association with various accessory factors permits interaction of the steroid receptor with the basal transcriptional machinery leading to activation of estrogen-responsive genes such as progesterone receptor (PR; [15]), pS2 [16], c-*myc* [17], and TGF-α [18]. These receptor-mediated effects ultimately lead to the proliferation of ER-positive tumor cells. Antiestrogens, such as the pure antagonistic ICI compounds, ICI 182,680 and ICI 164,384, block ER homodimerization, whereas the mixed agonist–antagonist tamoxifen prevents the interaction of ER with its accessory factors [19].

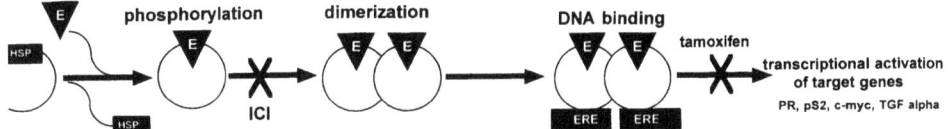

Figure 2. Estrogen-induced gene expression. Estrogen (E) binding to ER causes release of heat shock proteins (HSP) and phosphorylation within the TAF1 domain of ER, receptor homodimerization, binding to estrogen response elements (EREs) within the enhancers of estrogen-responsive genes, and finally transcriptional activation of target genes such as progesterone receptor (PR), pS2, the proto-oncogene c-*myc*, and transforming growth factor-α (TGFα). The pure antiestrogens ICI 182,680 and ICI 164,384 block transcription by preventing receptor dimerization and the antagonist/partial agonist tamoxifen blocks interaction of the active receptor with its cofactors [10,19].

Table 1. Frequency of hormone receptor expression in breast cancer and initial response to endocrine therapy

Tumor phenotype	Frequency of phenotype	Response rate to hormonal therapy
ER+/PR+	41%	75–80%
ER+/PR−	30%	20–30%
ER−/PR+	2%	40–45%
ER−/PR−	27%	<10%

The ER and PR status of breast cancer specimens is closely linked to patient response to endocrine therapy. As shown in table 1, approximately 40% of primary breast carcinomas express PR. Since PR gene expression is an estrogen-mediated event, the presence of PR suggests that the ER is functional. Such ER-positive/PR-positive or ER-negative/PR-positive tumors are generally responsive to hormonal therapies such as ovarian ablation or antiestrogen treatment. However, about 60% of tumors lack PR and have diminished responses. Half these tumors lack both ER and PR and rarely respond to endocrine therapy. The remainder of tumors contain ER that is apparently not fully functional, since PR is absent; these tumors are only moderately responsive to endocrine interventions.

Since estrogens and ER play a pivotal role in the development and progression of breast cancer as well as the treatment and outcome of breast cancer patients, mechanisms underlying regulation of ER gene expression and function are key areas of study. This chapter will review our current understanding of this complex field in normal and malignant breast cells, with a focus on alterations to the ER DNA coding sequence; regulation of ER gene expression at the transcriptional, posttranscriptional, and posttranslational levels; and ER interactions with proteins that modulate its activity.

2. Alterations in ER gene structure

2.1. ER gene amplification

The ER gene was initially cloned from the ER-positive human breast cancer cell line, MCF-7, in 1986 [20,21]. Located on chromosome 6q25.1, the human ER gene is made up of eight exons spanning more than 140 kb [22].

One possible explanation for overexpression of the ER gene in ER-positive tumors may be amplification of the ER gene. Nevertheless, few instances of ER gene amplification within human breast cancer cell lines or primary breast cancers have been reported. Using Southern analysis, Watts et al. found two- to threefold amplification of the ER gene in 1 of 29 ER-positive tumors and found no amplification in nine cell lines [23]. Nembrot et al. did not detect gene amplification in eight ER-negative tumors but found that 6 of 14 ER-positive tumors displayed amplification ranging from 1.6- to 3-fold [24]. Unexpectedly, there was no correlation between the level of ER gene amplification and the level of ER expression. Hence, ER gene amplification does not account for the increase in ER gene expression found in ER-positive breast carcinomas.

2.2. Deletions/insertions and rearrangements

A number of mechanisms could account for loss of ER in breast cancers, including deletions, insertions, rearrangements, or point mutations of the ER gene. Homozygous deletion of the region of chromosome 6 carrying the ER gene has not been reported. Although loss of heterozygosity (LOH) of this region is noted in 80%–90% of breast cancers, there is no significant difference in frequency of LOH between ER-positive and ER-negative breast cancers [25]. Moreover, studies fail to show major alterations of the remaining ER allele in ER-negative human breast cancers [23,26,27]. A more detailed analysis using polymerase chain reaction (PCR) demonstrated that DNAs from 12 of 12 ER-negative and 14 of 14 ER-positive breast tumors had a complete set of eight exons of normal size, which eliminates the possibility that the remaining allele contains deletions/insertions or rearrangements greater than 20 nucleotides in length [28].

Point mutations that cause functional alterations of the ER protein are also rare. Roodi et al. sequenced the majority of the ER coding region of DNAs from 118 ER-positive tumors and 70 ER-negative tumors [29]. Previously undescribed neutral polymorphisms were noted in codons 10, 87, 243, 325, and 594 in both ER-positive and ER-negative breast tumors. Two missense mutations were identified in 1 of 70 ER-negative breast tumors, one at codon 69 in the N-terminal region of the protein and the other at codon 396, within the hormone binding domain [29]. In another study, DNAs from 8 of 66 ER-positive breast cancers contained a mutation in codon 86 that causes reduced binding to estradiol [30]. These mutations as well as others that have been

Table 2. Some estrogen receptor mutants in human breast cancer biopsies and cell lines

Domain	RNA change	Protein change	Effect on ER function	References
A/B	C to G	Asn to Lys at 69	Unknown	29
	C to T	Ala to Val at 86	Decreased estradiol binding	30
C	In-frame deletion	259–412 deleted	No estradiol binding; no nuclear localization	91
D	T to C	Leu to Pro at 296	Unknown	63
E/F	A to ?	Glu to Val at 352	Unknown	31
	A to G	Met to Val at 396	Unknown	29
	G deleted	ER truncated at 419	No estradiol binding	91
	Replacement	ER truncated at 455	No estradiol binding	31
	T deleted	ER truncated at 438	Tamoxifen resistant	31
	Insertion of bases	80-kDa protein	Unknown	92
	G to T	Asp to Tyr at 351	Stimulated by tamoxifen	32

reported are listed in table 2. It is important to note that these analyses were carried out on DNAs from primary breast cancers. The status of the ER gene in metastatic lesions has not been examined.

2.3. ER gene mutations associated with antiestrogen resistance

In order to determine whether ER gene mutations are associated with tamoxifen resistance, several laboratories looked for mutations in DNAs from tamoxifen-resistant tumors using single-stranded conformation polymorphism and DNA sequencing. For example, Karnik et al. [31] examined DNAs from 15 tamoxifen-responsive and 15 tamoxifen-resistant primary breast cancers and five tumor/metastasis pairs from patients who developed metatstatic disease while receiving adjuvant tamoxifen. One point mutation and one 42 base pair insertion were found in two separate tamoxifen-resistant tumors from a total of 20 tumors. Also, a single missense mutation in 1 of the 20 tamoxifen-sensitive tumors was observed. Therefore, ER gene mutations in tamoxifen-resistant tumors are infrequent and do not appear to account for tamoxifen resistance in the majority of tumors.

Still work has continued using in vivo model systems to identify new ER gene mutations in tamoxifen-resistant tumors. For example, a point mutation (T $\rightarrow$ A at codon 351) in the ligand binding domain of the ER gene was found in an MCF-7 tumor grown in an athymic nude mouse treated with tamoxifen [32]. Since tumor was growth-stimulated by tamoxifen, this cell line is a good model to examine tamoxifen resistance in vitro. Stable transfection of this mutant into the ER-negative cell line, MDA-MB-231, showed that the protein altered the pharmacology of 4-OH tamoxifen from an estrogen antagonist to an estrogen agonist, while pure antiestrogens remained antagonistic [33].

Using a similar tamoxifen-stimulated MCF-7 tumor mouse model system, no mutations were found in the A/B or E regions of the ER gene [34]. These results suggest that the ER gene is normal in these tumors and another mechanism may be responsible for altered response to tamoxifen.

In conclusion, there are currently no significant polymorphisms, deletions, rearrangements, or point mutations of the ER gene that can explain its loss of expression or altered function in the majority of hormone-resistant breast cancers. However, it is important to note that breast tumors are a heterogeneous population of normal and malignant cells, and current techniques may not be sufficiently sensitive to identify ER mutations that are in low abundance. In addition, most studies have focused on primary rather than metastatic lesions. It is possible that single-cell PCR-based sequencing methods and/or studies of metastatic deposits may reveal more changes in the ER gene than are currently documented.

3. Regulation of the ER gene expression

3.1. Differential promoter usage

The ER gene has two major promoters that yield two unique transcripts encoding the same-size gene product (figure 3). The P1 transcription initiation site is located 233 base pairs upstream of the translational start site, while the second initiation site, P2, is located approximately 1500 base pairs further upstream [35,36]. Results from quantitative reverse transcriptase PCR (RT PCR) studies demonstrate that transcripts from normal mammary epithelial cells are initiated equally at these two sites, whereas transcripts from ER-positive breast cancer cell lines are initiated predominantly at P1 with minor start sites at P2 and P0 [37–39]. Interestingly, the P2 start site is primarily

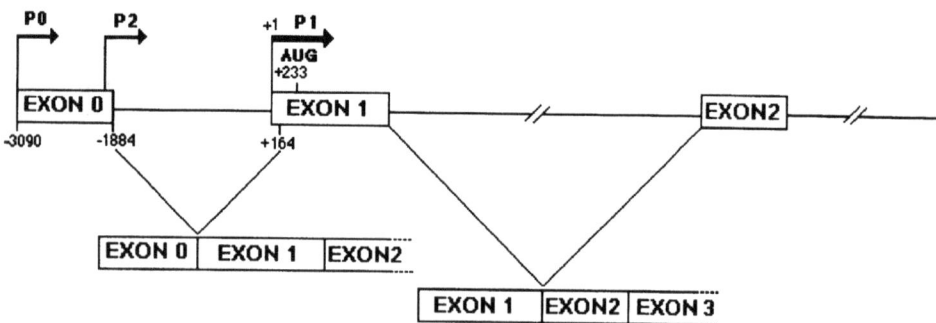

Figure 3. The initiation sites used for ER transcription. The three promoters are labeled P0, P1, and P2. Transcripts from normal mammary epithelial cells are initiated equally from P1 and P2, whereas transcripts from breast tumor cells are initiated primarily at P1 with minor start sites at P0 and P2 [35–39].

utilized in other estrogen target tissues, normal uterine cells, and primary osteoblasts, as well as osteosarcomas [37]. These results suggest that one mechanism of ER gene regulation may be through differential, tissue-specific promoter utilization. ER transcripts with unique 5' untranslated regions could exhibit variable stability due to different 5' secondary structure or altered transcriptional and translational efficiencies. For instance, it is possible that the ER mRNA transcript originating form P1 is more stable in some primary breast cancers, allowing accumulation of ER protein as seen in the ER-positive tumor cell phenotype.

3.2. Methylation of the ER-gene CpG island

One possible mechanism for lack of ER gene expression is loss of ER transcription. The ER-negative breast cancer cell lines, MDA-MB-231, MDA-MB-468, and Hs578t, lack ER mRNA as shown by Northern analysis [40]. Weigel and deConinck [41] confirmed the loss of ER transcription using nuclear run-on assays in MDA-MB-231 cells. Although immunohistochemistry indicates that ER-negative primary human breast cancers lack detectable levels of ER protein, a large survey using in situ hybridization to study ER transcripts in these cancers has not yet been reported.

One epigenetic mechanism that may block the transcription of the ER gene in ER-negative breast cancer cells is methylation of cytosine-rich areas, termed *CpG islands*, located in the 5' regulatory regions of genes [42]. DNA methyltransferase (DMT) is the enzyme that methylates cytosines that are 5' to guanosines. In normal somatic cells, CpG islands are unmethylated, with the exception of transcriptionally silent genes on the inactive X chromosome and some imprinted genes [43,44]. Methylation of these islands has been shown to inhibit transcription directly or to stabilize chromatin in a conformation that prevents transcription [45]. In contrast, in cancer cells, there tends to be a global hypomethylation in the bulk genome with a corresponding hypermethylation of CpG islands, resulting in loss of gene expression (figure 4). Hypermethylation of the CpG islands of the von-Hippel–Lindau, p16, and p15 tumor suppressor genes and the correlation of hypermethylation to lack of transcription has been well documented [46–48].

The ER gene has also been studied as a target for silencing via methylation. Initial studies that focused on the methylation status of the body of the ER gene failed to show any correlation between methylation and ER expression [23,49,50]. However, more recent studies directed at the CpG island in the 5' transcriptional regulatory region and first exon of the gene have established a clear correlation between ER CpG island methylation and lack of ER gene expression in breast cancer cell lines and primary breast tumors. Using established human breast cancer cell lines, Ottaviano et al. showed that absence of ER gene expression in ER-negative cells is associated with increased DMT mRNA and activity as well as extensive methylation of the ER CpG island (figure 5; [40]). A functional role for methylation is supported by studies in

DNA Methylation Changes in Cancer

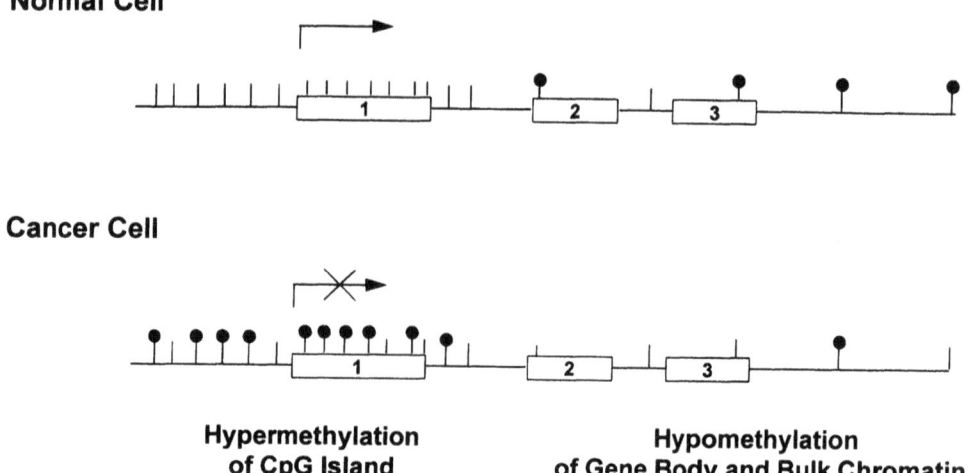

Figure 4. DNA methylation changes in cancer. Arrow indicates transcription initiation. Lines depict CpG dinucleotides; the solid circles denote methylated cytosines that are 5' to guanosines. Exons 1, 2, and 3 of a hypothetical gene are shown.

which two human ER-negative breast cancer cell lines were treated with the demethylating agents 5-aza-2'-deoxycytidine (deoxyC) or 5-azacytidine, resulting in the demethylation of the ER gene CpG island, reexpression of the ER gene, and production of protein [51]. Two assays confirmed that the newly produced ER was functional. First, stable clones of ER-negative MDA-MB-231 cells, transfected with a construct containing two estrogen response elements from the vitellogenin gene 5' to luciferase as a reporter gene, were treated with deoxyC in the presence of estrogen. Increasing luciferase activity at 3, 5, and 7 days posttreatment verified ER action. Second, the reexpression of the ER-regulated PR gene was demonstrated after deoxyC treatment of both MDA-MB-231 and Hs578t ER-negative cells.

In order to confirm that methylation of the ER-gene CpG island was not a cell culture artifact, the methylation status of the ER-gene CpG island in primary breast cancers was also studied. No methylation of the ER-gene CpG island was observed in DNAs from any normal tissue examined, including breast, thyroid, lung, kidney, bone marrow, epithelium, cervix, endometrium, or circulating mononuclear cells [40,52]. Also, 53 tumors that were defined as ER positive by ligand binding assay and immunohistochemistry were unmethylated at multiple sites in the ER-gene CpG island. In contrast, hypermethylation was observed in 9 of 39 ER-negative tumor DNAs at the Not I restriction enzyme recognition site in the ER-gene CpG island (table 3).

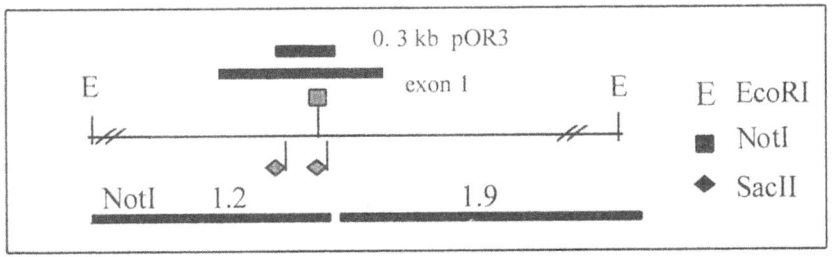

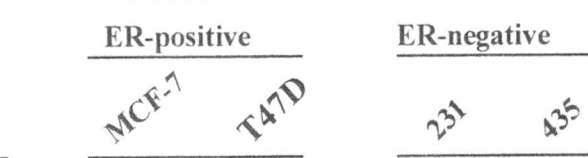

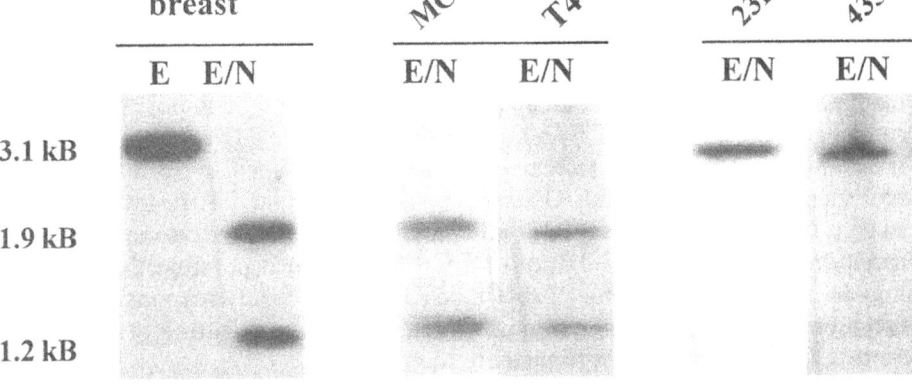

Figure 5. Southern blot analysis demonstrating different methylation patterns in the ER gene CpG island in ER-positive and ER-negative human breast cancer cell lines. Lane 1: EcoRI (E) digested normal breast DNA (3.1 kb DNA fragment); Lane 2: EcoRI/NotI (E/N) digested DNA from normal breast (1.9- and 1.2-kb DNA fragments); Lanes 3 and 4: EcoRI/NotI digested DNA from two ER-positive cell lines, MCF-7 and T47D (1.9- and 1.2-kb DNA fragments); Lanes 5 and 6: EcoRI/NotI digested DNA from two ER-negative cell lines, MDA-MD-231(231) and MDA-MB-435(435) (3.1-kb DNA fragment). Methylation of CpG dinucleotides within the NotI recognition site prevents digestion with this enzyme. Consequently, methylation is identified by presence of 3.1-kb DNA fragment.

Table 3. Methylation of the Not I site in the ER-gene CpG island in human breast tissues [52]

Tissue type	Gene phenotype	Methylation
Primary breast cancers	ER+/PR+	0/29 methylated
	ER+/PR−	0/24 methylated
	ER−/PR−	9/39 methylated
Metastases	ER−/PR−	2/2 methylated
Normal breast	ER+/PR−	0/9 methylated

These data suggest that ER-gene CpG island methylation may play a role in gene silencing in a subset of ER-negative human breast cancers.

3.3. Transcription factors

Altered expression of transacting factors that are responsible for ER transcription may also play a role in loss of ER gene expression. Weigel et al. identified an important *cis*-acting regulatory element that binds a protein that is present in ER-positive but not in ER-negative breast cancer cells [53]. Using a transient expression assay, they showed that DNA sequences from +132 to +201 of the 5' untranslated region enhance ER transcription. Results from mutational analysis within this region and competitive gel shift assays allowed the definition of a distal, high-affinity binding site (+182 to +201) and a proximal, low-affinity binding site (+132 to +171) (refer to figure 3).

A 30-kDa protein, called ERF-1 (estrogen receptor factor-1), was identified that binds to these two sites. ERF-1 is expressed at low levels in normal human mammary epithelial cells and at higher levels in three ER-positive breast cancer cell lines (MCF-7, T47D, and BT-20) and in two ER-positive endometrial carcinoma cell lines (RL95-2 and ECC-1) as shown by Southwestern blotting and gel shifts. The ERF-1 protein is absent in the ER-negative breast cancer cell line, MDA-MB-231, and in the two ER-negative endometrial carcinoma cell lines, HEC 1B and HEC 1A. Thus, it is possible that ERF-1 may be a common regulatory protein of ER in hormonally responsive breast carcinomas in vitro. Isolation, identification, and characterization of the ERF-1 protein in primary breast tissues are in progress.

3.4. Other transcriptional regulators of ER

Human breast cancer cell lines growing in tissue culture provide an excellent model system for the study of ER gene regulation by a variety of factors. Estrogen, antihormones, peptide growth factors, cadmium, and sodium butyrate all downregulate ER at either the transcriptional and/or posttranscriptional levels.

ER is transcriptionally and posttranscriptionally autoregulated, and this activity is dependent on the growth history of the cells and their ER content [54–56]. When ER is present at high levels, the addition of estradiol downregulates ER mRNA as determined by using MCF-7 clones that have higher levels of ER expression. In contrast, when ER is less abundant, as in the T47D cell line, the addition of estradiol results in a 2.5-fold increase in ER mRNA [55]. Nuclear run-on assays performed with MCF-7 cells treated with 1 nM estradiol showed a 90% decrease in transcription within one hour of treatment followed by a 4- to 5-fold increase within three hours. However, steady-state levels of ER mRNA and protein remained low for up to 48 hours. These data indicate that estradiol initially downregulates ER transcription but that the low steady state levels of ER are maintained by an unknown posttranscriptional mechanism [56].

Although the antiestrogens, 4-OH tamoxifen (4-OHT) and LY117018, do not affect ER mRNA levels in the MCF-7 cell line, tamoxifen treatment may decrease the level of ER protein in primary tumor cells [55–59]. Results from one study using serial biopsies taken prior to and eight weeks after tamoxifen treatment demonstrated a significant decrease in the level of ER within tamoxifen-treated tumors [58]. A second study that monitored the changes in ER content of tumors during their progression to tamoxifen resistance found that de novo resistance directly correlates with loss of ER [59]. The underlying molecular mechanism responsible for the tamoxifen-associated decrease in ER remains unknown.

Another steroid compound, the progestin R5020, downregulates ER mRNA and protein in the ER-positive cell line T47D. However, the combination of the antiprogestin RU486 and R5020 did not inhibit this downregulation [54,55], which suggests that control of ER by progestin is not mediated directly through PR.

While epidermal growth factor (EGF) and insulin-like growth factor I (IGF-1) do not significantly alter the level of ER in MCF-7 cells, exposure of these cells to transforming growth factor β causes a 20% decrease in the level of ER RNA, which is coincident with inhibition of cell growth [55].

Another inhibitory effect on ER gene expression is observed with the heavy metal cadmium. Nuclear run-on analysis using MCF-7 cells demonstrates that cadmium represses ER gene expression by 60% within 24 hours of exposure [60]. Other heavy metals did not affect ER transcription, which suggests that this outcome is not a general effect of heavy metals.

Finally, the differentiating agent sodium butyrate also has an inhibitory effect on ER transcription [61]. A three-hour exposure of MCF-7 cells to 3 mM sodium butyrate led to an 80% decrease in ER mRNA and protein. This decrease is coincident with a decrease in the rate of transcriptional initiation, which was not affected by cycloheximide, demonstrating that the effect of butyrate is not dependent on protein synthesis. The epigenetic and molecular effects of this compound are unknown.

In summary, findings from tissue culture studies have led to the identification of many agents that may be involved in the control of ER transcription. One or more of those just discussed, as well as new, unrecognized compounds, may inhibit hormone responsiveness in breast cancer.

4. Posttranscriptional regulation of ER

In addition to the many factors that influence ER RNA synthesis, ER expression and function is posttranscriptionally regulated by three different mechanisms, namely, differential RNA stability, alternative RNA splicing, and posttranslational modification. Agents like 12-O-tetradecanolphorbol-13-acetate or TPA affect the stability of the ER transcript. Once ER transcripts are synthesized, differential use of splice donor and acceptor sites can produce variant ER RNAs, some of which translate into nonfunctional as well as alternative-function proteins. Lastly, different extracellular and intracellular signaling pathways may regulate ER function by stimulating ER phosphorylation, leading to activation of ER and estrogen-responsive gene expression. The significance of each of these three regulatory mechanisms with respect to altered expression and function of ER in human breast cancer is reviewed below.

4.1. RNA stability

The possibility that stabilization of ER mRNA might play a role in ER regulation has been demonstrated by studies using the tumor-promoting agent, TPA, that activates the AP-1 transcription factor signal transduction pathway and also downregulates ER [62]. After treatment of the MCF-7 cell line with 100 nM TPA, the concentration of ER decreases by 80% as measured by enzyme immunoassay and ligand binding assays. RNase protection studies showed a parallel decrease in ER mRNA, but nuclear run-on assays failed to show a decrease in the rate of transcription initiation. An RNA half-life study indicated that regulation occurs by a posttranscriptional mechanism that causes destabilization of ER mRNA.

4.2. ER RNA splice variants

The role of ER mRNA splice variants in determining hormone response or resistance is a major area of investigation. It has been suggested that these variants may be responsible for several breast tumor phenotypes, including ER-positive/PR-negative, ER-negative/PR-positive, and hormone-resistant ER-positive tumors. One hypothesis to explain the biological significance of variants is that ER mRNA is alternatively spliced at a low frequency in normal cells. During tumor progression, the resultant variant proteins give the cells a growth advantage, so cells that express the variants at a higher level predominate in the population. A major flaw of the proposal is that variant ER proteins corresponding to the ER RNA splice variants have only been identified in a single cell line and have not yet been detected in primary human tumors. Furthermore, the RNA variants are always found in conjunction with wild-type (WT) ER RNA, and they are frequently detected in normal as well as malignant tissues. Therefore, the true functional significance of the variants remains to be established.

To date, three classes of ER variant RNAs have been identified in established breast cancer cell lines and/or clinical samples. These RNAs encode proteins with different function as determined by in vitro expression analysis. The first is the constitutively active ERΔE5 variant receptor that is active in

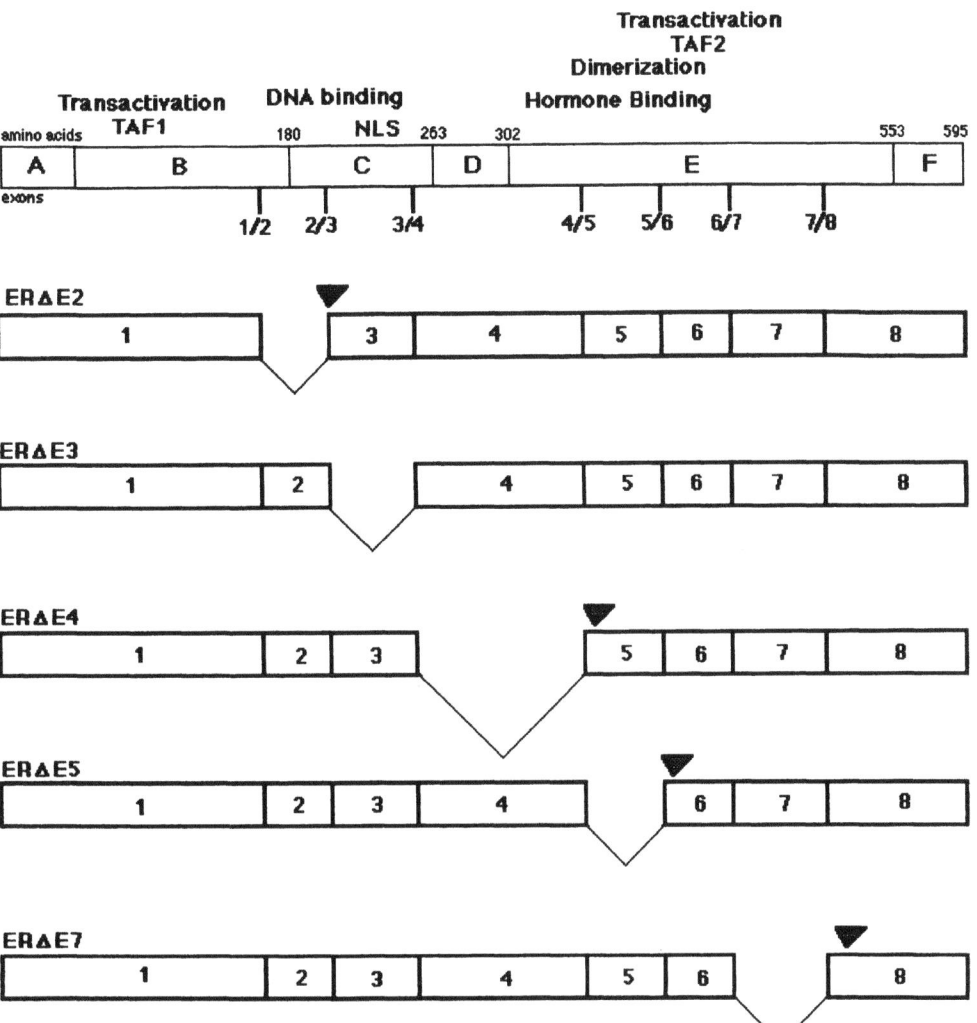

Figure 6. Structure of ER RNA splice variants. Exons 1–8 and corresponding functional domains A–F are shown. Exons that are deleted by alternative splicing are not shown, and premature termination of translation is indicated by arrowhead [65,71,72,77].

the absence of ligand. The second class includes variant receptors that are themselves inactive but prevent the function of normal ER, consequently behaving as dominant-negative variants. These proteins lack the DNA binding domain and/or part of the *trans*-activation domain and include the ERΔE3 and ERΔE7 variants [13,63]. A third class, or which ERΔE2 is representative, is completely inactive alone or in conjunction with WT ER (figures 6, 7). The three types of variants are described in greater detailed below.

VARIANT	MW	tumor type	binds hormone	binds ERE	dimerization	transcriptional activation	references
ERΔE2	17kD	ER+/PR+	no	no	no	inactive	71
ERΔE3	61kD	ER+/PR+ ER+/PR-	ND	no	no	dominant negative	13,71,72
ERΔE4	54kD	ER+/PR+	ND	ND	ND	inactive	76,77,78
ERΔE5	42kD	ER+/PR+ ER+/PR- ER-/PR+	no	yes	yes	constitutively active	63,64,65,66,67
ERΔE7	52kD	ER+/PR+ ER+/PR-	ND	yes	yes?	dominant negative	71,73,74,75

Figure 7. Structure and function of the ER RNA variants found in human breast cancers. RNA splice variants are described in relation to predicted molecular weight (MW), tumor types in which the RNAs have been detected, and functional characteristics of the resultant proteins as determined by in vitro analysis. ND: not determined.

4.2.1. The constitutively active variant: ERΔE5. The ERΔE5 variant lacks exons 5–8 and has a predicted molecular weight of approximately 40 kDa. When ERΔE5 and WT ER are overexpressed in tissue culture cells, the two proteins can be coimmunoprecipitated using an amino terminal-specific antibody, which indicates that this variant forms heterodimers with WT ER [65]. Consequently, this variant is thought to act by forming either homodimers or heterodimers with WT ER to activate transcription, even in the presence of antiestrogen, because it lacks the interactive hormone binding domain.

When expressed in yeast, the constitutively active variant can activate transcription of an estrogen-responsive reporter gene in the absence of estradiol, but at a twofold lower level than WT ER [64,65]. Since the protein lacks the hormone binding domain, it cannot be detected by conventional ligand binding assays or by immunocytochemistry using antibodies targetted to this domain of the protein. Therefore, this variant protein may be functional in tumors that are assayed as ER positive but are unresponsive to endocrine therapies.

One study showed that stable overexpression of ERΔE5 in an ER-positive cell line leads to an antiestrogen-resistant, estrogen-responsive phenotype ([13]; unpublished results). These data suggest than ERΔE5 may predominate in ER-positive tumors that are either initially or subsequently unresponsive to antiestrogen treatments. However, conflicting results were found using an inducible ERΔE5 system. The results of this study suggested that expression of the variant was not sufficient to induce estrogen-independent transcription or cell growth or antiestrogen resistance [66].

In order to determine the biological relevance of this variant, primary tumor tissue was examined by RNase protection and RT PCR analysis for the presence of ERΔE5-variant RNA [63,67]. ERΔE5 RNA was detectable in ER-positive/PR-positive, ER-positive/PR-negative, and ER-negative/PR-positive tumors and was always found in excess of WT ER RNA, but was not detected in ER-negative/PR-negative tumors. There was a higher ratio of ERΔE5 to WT ER RNA in ER-negative tumors that expressed PR and pS2 [68]. Nonetheless, the ratio of ERΔE5 to WT ER was no different in tamoxifen-resistant mammary cancer specimens than in control tumor tissue, suggesting that ERΔE5 is unlikely to be responsible for tamoxifen resistance in most breast cancers.

4.2.2. The dominant-negative variants: ERΔE3 and ERΔE7. Fifty percent of all hormone-resistant breast carcinomas are ER positive, and the presence of dominant-negative ER variants may be one explanation for this seemingly enigmatic observation. These variants both are transcriptionally inactive proteins and are thought to interfere with wild-type protein function by one or more of three possible mechanisms [69,70]. First, if the variant receptor has an intact dimerization domain, it can form transcriptionally inactive heterodimers with WT ER. Secondly, if the variant protein has an intact DNA binding domain, it can compete with WT ER for its DNA binding site. Lastly, if the variant protein has intact TAF1 and/or TAF2 domains, it can compete for coactivators that physically interact with these domains of the protein and cause squelching of transcription.

One group described an ER variant lacking exon 3, ERΔE3, with a predicted molecular weight of 61 kDa, that would lack a significant portion of the DNA binding domain [71,72]. In vitro characterization demonstrated that the protein is unable to bind to an ERE and also prevents WT ER from binding. Transient transfection of HeLa cells with equimolar amounts of ERΔE3 and WT ER along with an estrogen-responsive reporter gene plasmid led to significant inhibition of normal estrogen-stimulated transcription. The mechanism of ERΔE3-mediated inhibition is either by direct interaction with WT ER and formation of heterodimers incapable of binding to EREs or by squelching of a coactivator that interacts with the intact TAF1 and TAF2 domains of ERΔE3. ERΔE3 and WT ER RNAs were found to be expressed at equal levels in ER-positive/PR-positive and ER-positive/PR-negative tumors [13].

A second ER variant, the 51-kDa ERΔE7 protein, lacks all of exons 7 and 8, so the protein is predicted to lack a significant part of the hormone binding, transactivation, and dimerization domains. It is unclear whether ERΔE7 is actually a dominant-negative variant or simply an inactive variant. This truncated protein does not bind to EREs in vitro, presumably due to lack of the dimerization domain required for paired protein binding to two ERE half-sites [71,73]. However, one report suggests that the protein is able to reduce the binding of WT ER to ERE in vitro [73]. When ERΔE7 and WT ER are cotransfected into mammalian cells with an estrogen-responsive reporter construct, ERΔE7 has no effect on the level of transactivation by WT ER [71]. In contrast, when these two proteins are coexpressed in yeast, ERΔE7 caused a 60% decrease in transactivation by WT ER [73]. A 50-kDa protein found in human breast tumor tissue, which has the molecular weight expected of the

ERΔE7 variant and does not bind to ERE in vitro, was also shown to form both homodimers and heterodimers with WT ER [74]. This finding suggests that the non-DNA binding ERΔE7 variant may act by forming a heterodimer with WT ER, thus preventing WT ER interaction with an ERE and subsequent transcriptional activation. This variant has been detected in both ER-positive/PR-positive and ER-positive/PR-negative human breast tumors and the ER-positive/PR-positive cell lines T47D and MCF-7 [71,73,75,76].

4.2.3. The inactive variant: ERΔE2. In the ER-positive cell line T47D, Wang and Miksicek [71] identified a splice variant, ERΔE2, that is prematurely terminated after exon 1. The predicted molecular weight of the protein is 17kDa, and it would comprise only the amino terminal transactivation domain. Cotransfection of a high molar excess of ERΔE2 with WT ER and an estrogen-responsive reporter gene construct into HeLa cells led to only modest inhibition of WT ER function, presumably due to inefficient titration of coactivators that interact with the TAF1 domain of the variant protein.

4.2.4. Variant of uncertain significance: ERΔE4 variant. Yet another RNA splice variant, ERΔE4, lacks exon 4, which includes part of the hinge and hormone binding domains. It was detected along with WT ER in MCF-7 and ZR-75-1 cells and in one tumor specimen, but was not found in MDA-MB-231 cells [76–78]. The biological function of ERΔE4 remains to be determined.

4.3. Phosphorylation

Phosphorylation of steroid receptors influences their hormone and DNA binding activities as well as receptor recycling. Therefore, regulation of phosphorylation may be another mechanism to control both the level and function of ER [79]. In the presence of estrogen and antiestrogens, ER phosphorylation increases by 3- to 8-fold [80,81]. Phosphoaminoacid and two-dimensional tryptic phosphopeptide analysis revealed that the sites of phosphorylation enhanced by estrogen and antiestrogens are within the amino terminal A/B domain or TAF1 at serines 104, 106, and 118 [81]. Mutation of serine 118 to an alanine prevents this residue from being phosphorylated and leads to a decrease in the transcriptional activity of ER without affecting DNA binding or the nuclear localization of ER, whereas mutation of the serine to the negatively charged residue glutamic acid creates a receptor that is transcriptionally active in the absence of estrogen [80]. Simultaneous mutation of all three serines to alanine leads to a 40% reduction in transcription as assayed by using transient transfections [81]. Therefore, phosphorylation of these sites is important for the normal transcriptional activity of ER.

Recently, it was demonstrated that both estradiol and phorbol ester cause phosphorylation of serine 118 and that greater than 30% of cellular estrogen receptor is phosphorylated at this residue [82]. Also, the TAF1 region of ER was shown to be phosphorylated at serine 118 in vitro and in vivo by mitogen-activated protein kinase (MAPK) [83]. Furthermore, the transcriptional activity and phosphorylation of ER can be induced by the growth factors, EGF and IGF, which act via the receptor tyrosine kinase-Ras-Raf-MAPK signaling pathway [83].

5. Proteins that interact with ER to regulate its function

Recently, several ER-associated proteins have been identified. These proteins are thought to be required for productive interaction of ER with the basal transcriptional machinery. Consequently, their absence or modification may result in aberrant ER function. For example, although a tumor cell possesses ER, it may lack a coactivator required for ER stimulatory activity or may possess a corepressor that inhibits ER function. This cell would be characterized as ER positive by standard biochemical or immunohistochemical assays but would actually lack ER function, rendering it unresponsive to endocrine therapies.

It has been proposed that hormone-induced conformational changes in the ER protein expose the hormone binding domain to permit interaction with these accessory proteins. Estrogen antagonists may induce a distinct conformational change in the receptor that impairs its ability to interact with coactivators to transactivate gene expression. This may be the mechanism whereby antiestrogens inhibit estrogen-induced transcription.

Techniques such as immuno-, steroid- and site-specific DNA affinity chromatography as well as screening of expression libraries with radiolabeled receptor protein have been used to identify proteins that associate with ER in vitro and are required for ER activity. A number of ER-associated proteins interact with the TAF2 domain of ER. The utilization of an ^{35}S-labeled GST-TAF2 fusion protein as a probe for Far Western blot analysis of ZR75-1, HeLa, and COS-1 cell proteins led to the identification of 160-kDa, 140-kDa, and 80-kDa proteins called RIP160, RIP140, and RIP80, respectively [84,85]. An association between ER and RIP160 is required for ER activity, is dependent on estrogen, and is blocked by antiestrogens [84]. Using similar methodologies, Halachmi et al. identified a 160-kDa protein, ERAP160, in the human breast cancer cell line MCF-7. ERAP160 also exhibits estrogen-dependent and antiestrogen-blocked interactions with ER [86]. In addition, a new TATA binding protein-associated factor, human $TAF_{II}30$, was found to interact with the TAF2 region of ER and is required for ER-stimulated transcription [87]. However, its interaction with ER is unaffected by estrogen or antiestrogens, so its relative importance in estrogen-induced transcription is unclear.

Using a yeast two-hybrid system, a novel 125-kDa protein, termed *steroid receptor coactivator-1* (SRC-1), that also binds to the TAF2 domain of ER was identified [88]. The amino terminal domain of SRC-1 specifically interacts with ligand-bound steroid receptors, and its carboxy domain is presumed to interact with the basal transcriptional machinery. SRC-1 is required for a 14-fold increase in receptor-mediated transcriptional activation in the presence of ligand. However, the presence of antagonists inhibits SRC-1-activated gene expression. In another study, which attempted to identify proteins required for ER to bind to its *cis*-acting estrogen-responsive element, proteins of 55 kDa (a protein disulfide isomerase family member), 48 kDa, and 45 kDa, as well as hsp70, were identified [89].

Recently, a new protein was found that interacts with the amino-terminal region of the receptor, possibly TAF1. This protein, RAP46, is a highly hydrophilic receptor-associated protein that binds with high affinity to ER in the presence of antiestrogens, does not require the presence of estrogen, and does not interact with ER in the presence of heat shock proteins [90]. This ubiquitously expressed 46-kDa protein also interacts with other steroid receptors such as glucocorticoid and thyroid receptors. Interestingly, approximately 200 amino acids at the amino terminal region of RAP46 have 80% amino acid sequence identity to the Bcl-2-associated protein, BAG-1.

In summary, most studies have focused on identification of proteins that interact with the hormone-inducible *trans*-activation domain or TAF2 of ER. Those proteins, whose interaction with ER is dependent on estrogen and blocked by antiestrogens, are thought to act as coactivators of estrogen-responsive transcription. The identification of multiple factors that interact with the TAF2 domain of ER to regulate its function suggests that the mechanisms of steroid receptor activation and inactivation are extremely complex. It is possible that in the future, new proteins that interact with the A/B, D, and F domains may also be identified.

6. Conclusion

Hormonal responsiveness is a critical determinant of breast cancer progression and management. Response to endocrine therapy is highly correlated with ER status of tumor cells, so identification of the mechanisms that regulate ER expression in normal and malignant breast tissues is of high priority. Increased ER expression is associated with a more indolent clinical course and improved response to hormonal approaches. This finding could potentially result from amplification of the ER gene, stabilization of the transcript, and/or increased efficiency of translation. Gene amplification is not a common finding in cell lines or breast cancers, so it is unlikely to be a major factor in this phenotype. However, several studies have indicated that differential promoter usage, which can produce transcripts with increased half-life and translation efficiency, may lead to higher basal levels of ER protein. This area is worth further exploration.

Conversely, de novo or acquired hormonal resistance is a common feature of many breast cancers. Approximately one third of breast cancers lack ER gene expression and are seldom hormone responsive. Studies on both cell lines and primary breast cancer specimens have shown that mutations in the ER coding region are rare and do not account for the majority of breast cancers that lack ER gene expression. Alternatively, this loss of ER expression may be a consequence of transcriptional inactivation through *cis*-acting mechanisms like aberrant methylation of the ER CpG island in the regulatory region of the ER gene, loss of important transacting factors, or a combination of the two. Indeed, most ER-negative human breast cancer cell lines and about 25% of ER-negative primary breast tumors exhibit evidence of ER-gene CpG island hypermethylation that may alter the binding of critical transcriptional activators in the ER promoter region. Alternatively, loss of expression or function of transcription factors such as ERF-1 that are required for basal or enhanced ER gene expression may play a significant role in loss of ER transcription.

A more common clinical scenario is the ER-positive cancer that is hormone independent. In this situation, posttranscriptional and posttranslational events may play a role in loss of ER function. The possibility that ER RNA splice variants may be involved is intriguing. For example, the ERΛE5 may allow cells to grow in the absence of estrogen, while ERΛE3 and ERΛE7 may inhibit normal ER protein function. The functional significance of these types of variants in human breast cancer is uncertain because they are always expressed in conjunction with WT ER and are also frequently expressed in normal tissues. Finally, since putative proteins that correspond to these splice variants have not been detected with any frequency in human breast cancer specimens, the contribution of the variants to progression to estrogen independence and hormone resistance is not yet established.

Posttranslational modification of ER via phosphorylation of serines, particularly serine 118, is required for full ER activity. Since mutations were not found in these residues, the possibility that alterations in cell signaling pathways, such as the tyrosine kinase receptor–ras–raf–MAPK pathway that leads to ER phosphorylation, are associated with loss of ER function should be addressed in experimental studies.

On the other hand, cells with WT ER may have altered expression of accessory proteins that are required for the interaction of ER with the basal transcriptional machinery. Several recent studies have identified cofactors that physically interact with ER either to activate or to inhibit its function. Once these proteins are further characterized, it should be possible to screen for their presence in tumor samples. The loss of a coactivator or gain of a corepressor may be a novel mechanism whereby normal ER function is lost in apparently ER-positive tumor cells.

In conclusion, normal ER gene expression and function may be altered by a variety of mechanisms. Some pathways lead to enhanced expression of ER in cancer cells, rendering them sensitive to the mitogenic effects of estrogen. These cancers may be effectively managed with interventions like ovarian ablation, aromatase inhibitors or antiestrogens. In contrast, the majority of breast tumors arise or evolve to a hormone-unresponsive state and are poorly responsive to endocrine maneuvers. Improved understanding of the pathways that lead to loss of ER protein and/or function should allow the development of better predictive indicators and novel therapeutic approaches to target these estrogen-independent cancers.

Acknowledgments

We would like to thank Dr. Paula M. Vertino for her design of figure 4. This work was supported by American Cancer Society Grants PF4231 (A.T.F.) and BE237 (N.E.D.) and by the Susan G. Komen Foundation (R.G.L.).

References

1. Peterson OW, Hoyer PE, Van Deurs B. 1987. Frequency and distribution of estrogen positive cells in normal, non-lactating human breast tissue. Cancer Res 47:5748-5751.
2. Ricketts D, Turnbull L, Ryall G, Bakshi R, Raswon NSB, Gazet J-C, Nolan C, Coombes RC. 1991. Estrogen and progesterone receptor in the normal female breast. Cancer Res 51:1817-1822.
3. Markopoulus C, Berger U, Wilson P, Gazet J, Coombes RC. 1988. Oestrogen receptor content of normal breast cells and breast carcinoma throughout the menstrual cycles. Br Med J 296:1349-1351.
4. Korach KS. 1994. Insights from the study of animals lacking functional estrogen receptor. Science 266:1524-1527.
5. Murdoch FE, Fritsch M, Gorski J. 1988. The estrogen receptor: mechanism of action and relationship to human breast cancer. ISI Atlas of Science: Pharmacology, pp. 267-275.
6. Osborne CK. 1985. Heterogeneity in hormone receptor status in primary and metastatic breast cancer. Semin Oncol 12:317-326.
7. McGuire WL. 1978. Hormone receptors: their role in predicting prognosis and response to endocrine therapy. Semin Oncol 5:428-433.
8. Kumar V, Green S, Stack G, Berry M, Jin JR, Chambon P. 1987. Functional domains of the human estrogen receptor. Cell 51:941-951.
9. Tora L, White J, Brou C, Tasset D, Webster N, Scheer E, Chambon P. 1989. The human estrogen receptor has two independent nonacidic transcriptional activation functions. Cell 59:477-487.
10. Klein-Hitpass L, Tsai SY, Greene GL, Clark JH, Tsai MJ, O'Malley BW. 1989. Specific binding of estrogen receptor to the estrogen response element. Mol Cell Biol 9:43-49.
11. Adler S, Waterman ML, Rosenfeld MG. 1988. Steroid receptor-mediated inhibition of rat prolactin gene expression does not require the receptor DNA-binding domain. Cell 52:685-695.
12. Montano MM, Muller V, Trobaugh A, Katzenellenbogen BS. 1995. The carboxy-terminal F domain of the human estrogen receptor: role in the transcriptional activity of the receptor and the effectiveness of antiestrogens as estrogen antagonists. Mol Endocrinol 9:814-825.
13. Fuqua SAW, Chamness GC, McGuire WL. 1993. Estrogen receptor mutations in breast cancer. J Cell Biochem 51:135-139.
14. Kraus WL, McInerney EM, Katzenellenbogen BS. 1995. Ligand-dependent, transcriptionally productive association of the amino- and carboxyl-terminal regions of a steroid hormone nuclear receptor. Proc Natl Acad Sci USA 92:12314-12318.
15. Read LD, Snider CE, Miller JS, Greene GL, Katzenellenbogen BS. 1988. Ligand-modulated regulation of progesterone receptor messenger ribonucleic acid and protein in human breast cancer cell lines. Mol Endocrinol 2:263-271.
16. Jakowlev SB, Breathnach R, Teltsa JM, Masaikowski P, Chambon P. 1984. Sequence of pS2

mRNA induced by estrogen in the human breast cancer cell line, MCF-7. Nucleic Acids Res 12:2861–2878.
17. Dubik D, Shiu RPC. 1988. Transcriptional regulation of c-*myc* oncogene expression by estrogen in hormone-responsive human breast cancer cells. J Biol Chem 263:12705–12708.
18. Bates SE, Davidson NE, Valverius EM, Freter CE, Dickson RB, Tam JP, Kudlow JE, Lippman ME, Salomon DS. 1988. Expression of transforming growth factor α and its messenger ribonucleic acid in human breast cancer: its regulation by estrogen and its possible functional significance. Mol Endocrinol 2:543–555.
19. Katzenellenbogen BS, Fang H, Ince BA, Pakdel F, Reese JC, Wooge CH, Wrenn CK. 1993. Extrogen receptors: ligand discrimination and antiestrogen action. Breast Cancer Res Treat 27:17–26.
20. Greene GL, Hilna P, Waterfield M, Baker A, Hort Y, Shine J. 1986. Sequence and expression of human estrogen receptor complementary DNA. Science 231:1150–1154.
21. Green S, Walter P, Kumar V, Krust A, Bornet J-M, Argos P, Chambon P. 1986. Human oestrogen receptor cDNA: sequence, expression and homology to v-erb- A. Nature 320:134–139.
22. Ponglikitmonkol M, Green S, Chambon P. 1988. Genomic organization of the human oestrogen receptor gene. EMBO J 7:3385–3388.
23. Watts CK, Handel ML, King RJB, Sutherland RL. 1992. Oestrogen receptor gene structure and function in breast cancer. J Steroid Biochem Mol Biol 41(3):3–9.
24. Nembrot M, Quintana B, Mordoh J. 1990. Estrogen receptor gene amplification is found in some estrogen receptor-positive human breast tumors. Biochem Biophys Res Commun 166:601–607.
25. Fujii H, Marsh C, Cairns P, Sidransky D, Gabrielson E. 1996. Genetic divergence in the clonal evolution of breast cancer. Cancer Res 56:1493–1497.
26. Hill SM, Fuqua SAW, Chamness GC, Greene GL, McGuire WL. 1989. Estrogen receptor expression in human breast cancer associated with an estrogen receptor gene restriction fragment length polymorphism. Cancer Res 49:145–148.
27. Parl FF, Cavener DR, Dupont WD. 1989. Genomic DNA analysis of the estrogen receptor gene in breast cancer. Breast Cancer Res Treat 14:57–64.
28. Yaich L, Dupont WD, Cavener DR, Parl FF. 1992. Analysis of the PvuII restriction fragment polymorphism and exon structure of the estrogen receptor gene in breast cancer and peripheral blood. Cancer Res 52:77083.
29. Roodi N, Bailey LR, Kao W-Y, Verrier CS, Yee CJ, Dupont WD, Parl FF. 1995. Estrogen receptor gene analysis in estrogen receptor-positive and receptor-negative primary breast cancer. J Natl Cancer Inst 87:446–451.
30. Garcia T, Sanchez M, Cox JL, Shaw PA, Ross JB, Lehre S, Schachter B. 1989. Identification of a variant form of the human estrogen receptor with an amino acid replacement. Nucleic Acid Res 17:8364.
31. Karnik PS, Kulkarni S, Liu X-P, Budd GT, Bukowski RM. 1994. Estrogen receptor mutation in tamoxifen-resistant cancer. Cancer Res 54:349–353.
32. Wolf DM, Jordan VC. 1994. The estrogen receptor from a tamoxifen stimulated MCF-7 tumor variant contains a point mutation in the ligand binding domain. Br Cancer Res Treat 31:129–138.
33. Catherino W, Wolf DM, Jordan VC. 1995. A naturally occurring estrogen receptor mutation results in increased estrogenicity of a tamoxifen analog. Mol Endocrinol 9:1053–1062.
34. Osborne CK, Fuqua SAW. 1994. Mechanisms of tamoxifen resistance. Breast Cancer Res Treat 32:49–55.
35. Grandien KFH, Berkenstam A, Nilsson S, Gustafson JA. 1993. Localization of DNase I hypersensitive sites in the human estrogen receptor gene correlates with the transcriptional activity of the two differentially used promoters. J Mol Endocrinol 10:269–277.
36. Keaveney M, Klug J, Dawson MT, Nestor PV, Nielan JG, Forde RC, Gannon F. 1991. Evidence for a previously unidentified upstream exon in the human oestrogen receptor gene. J Mol Endocrinol 6:111–115.

37. Grandien K, Bacikdahl M, Ljunggren O, Gustafsson JA, Berkenstam A. 1995. Estrogen target tissue determines alternative promoter utilization of the human estrogen receptor gene in osteoblasts and tumor cell lines. Endocrinology 136:2223–2229.
38. Piva R, Bianchi N, Aguiari GL, Gambari R, del Senno L. 1993. Sequencing of an RNA transcript of the human estrogen receptor gene: evidence for a new transcriptional event. J Steroid Biochem Mol Biol 46:531–538.
39. Weigel RJ, Crooks DL, Iglehart JD, deConinck EC. 1995. Quantitative analysis of the transcriptional start sites of estrogen receptor in breast carcinoma. Cell Growth Differ 6:707–711.
40. Ottaviano YL, Issa J-P, Parl FF, Smith HS, Baylin SB, Davidson NE. 1994. Methylation of the estrogen receptor gene CpG island marks loss of estrogen receptor expression in human breast cancer cells. Cancer Res 54:2552–2555.
41. Weigel RJ, deConinck EC. 1993. Transcriptional control of estrogen receptor in estrogen receptor negative breast carcinoma. Cancer Res 53:3472–3474.
42. Bird AP. 1986. CpG-rich islands and the function of DNA methylation. Nature 321:209–213.
43. Li E, Beard and Jaenisch R. 1993. Role of DNA methylation in genomic imprinting. Nature 366:362–365.
44. Mohandas T, Sparkes RS, Shapiro LJ. 1981. Reactivation of an inactive human X chromosome: evidence for X inactivation by DNA methylation. Science 211:393–396.
45. Antequera F, Boyes J, Bird A. 1990. High levels of *de novo* methylation and altered chromatin structure at CpG islands in cell lines. Cell 62:503–514.
46. Herman JG, Latif F, Weng Y, Lerman MI, Zbar B, Liu S, Samid D, Duan DS, Gnarra JR, Linehan WM, Baylin SB. 1994. Silencing of the VHL-tumor suppressor gene by DNA methylation in renal carcinoma. Proc Natl Acad Sci USA 91:9700–9704.
47. Herman JG, Merlo A, Mao L, Lapidus RG, Issa J-P, Davidson NE, Sidransky D, Baylin SB. 1995. Inactivation of the CDKN2/p16/MST1 gene is frequently associated with aberrant DNA methylation in all common human cancers. Cancer Res 55:4525–4530.
48. Herman JG, Jen J, Merlo A, Baylin SB. 1996. Hypermethylation-associated inactivation indicates a tumor suppressor role for p15^{INK4B1}. Cancer Res 56:722–727.
49. Piva R, Rimondi AP, Hanau S, Maestri I, Alvisi A, Kumar VL, del Senno L. 1990. Different methylation of oestrogen receptor DNA in human breast carcinomas with and without oestrogen receptor. Br J Cancer 61:270–275.
50. Falette NS, Fuqua SAW, Chamness GC, Cheah MS, Greene GL, McGuire WL. 1990. Estrogen receptor gene methylation in human breast tumors. Cancer Res 50:3974–3978.
51. Ferguson AT, Lapidus RG, Baylin SB, Davidson NE. 1995. Demethylation of the estrogen receptor gene in estrogen receptor-negative breast cancer cells can reactivate estrogen receptor gene expression. Cancer Res 55:2279–2283.
52. Lapidus RG, Ferguson AT, Ottaviano YL, Parl FF, Smith HS, Weitzman SA, Baylin SB, Issa J-PJ, Davidson NE. 1996. Methylation of estrogen and progesterone receptor genes 5' CpG islands correlates with lack of ER and PR gene expression in breast tumors. Clin Cancer Res 2:805–810.
53. deConinck EC, McPherson LA, Weigel RJ. 1995. Transcriptional regulation of estrogen receptor in breast carcinomas. Mol Cell Biol 15: 2191–2196.
54. Berkenstam A, Glaumann H, Martin M, Gustafsson J, Norstedt G. 1989. Hormonal regulation of estrogen receptor messenger ribonucleic acid in T47D$_{co}$ and MCF-7 breast cancer cells. Mol Endocrinol 3:22–28.
55. Read LD, Greene GL, Katzenellenbogen BS. 1989. Regulation of estrogen receptor messenger ribonucleic acid and protein levels in human breast cancer cell lines by sex steroid hormones, their antagonists and growth factors. Mol Endocrinol 3:295–304.
56. Saceda M, Lippman ME, Chambon P, Lindsey RL, Ponglkitmongkol M, Puente M, Martin MB. 1988. Regulation of the estrogen receptor in MCF-7 cells by estradiol. Mol Endocrinol 2:1157–1162.
57. Saceda M, Lippman ME, Lindsey RK, Puerte M, Martin MB. 1989. Role of estrogen receptor-

dependent mechanism in the regulation of estrogen receptor mRNA in MCF-7 cells. Mol Endocrinol 3:1782–1787.
58. Lundren S, Soreide JA, Lea DA. 1994. Influence of tamoxifen on the tumor content of steroid hormone receptors (ER, PgR and AR) in patients with primary breast cancers. Anticancer Res 14:1313–1316.
59. Johnston SRD, Seccani-Jotti G, Smith IE, Salter J, Newby M, Coppen M, Ebbs SR, Dowsett M. 1995. Changes in estrogen receptor, progesterone receptor and pS2 expression in tamoxifen resistant human breast cancers. Cancer Res 55:3331–3338.
60. Garcia-Morales P, Saceda M, Kenney N, Kim N, Salomon DS, Gottardis MM, Solomon HB, Shollier PE, Jordan VC, Martin MB. 1994. Effect of cadmium on estrogen receptor levels and estrogen-induced responses in human breast cancer cells. J Biol Chem 269:1–6.
61. deFazio A, Chiew Y, Donoghue C, Lee CSL, Sutherland RL. 1992. Effect of sodium butyrate on estrogen receptor and epidermal growth factor receptor gene expression in human breast cancer cell lines. J Biol Chem 267:18008–18012.
62. Saceda M, Knabbe C, Dickson RB, Lippman ME, Bronzer D, Lindsey RK, Gottardis MM, Martin MB. 1991. Post-transcriptional destabilization of estrogen receptor mRNA in MCF-7 cells by 12-O-Tetradecanoylphorbol-13-acetate. J Biol Chem 266:17809–17814.
63. McGuire WL, Chamness GC, Fuqua SAW. 1992. Estrogen receptor varians in clinical breast cancer. Mol Endocrinol 5:1571–1577.
64. Fuqua SAW, Fitzgerald SD, Chamness GC, Tandon AK, McDonnell DP, Nawaz Z, O'Malley BW, McGuire WL. 1991. Variant human breast tumor estrogen receptor with constitutive transcriptional activity. Cancer Res 51:105–109.
65. Castles CG, Fuqua SAW, Klotz DM, Hill SM. 1993. Expression of a constitutively active estrogen receptor variant in the estrogen receptor-negative BT-20 human breast cancer cell line. Cancer Res 53:5934–5939.
66. Rhea D, Parker MG. 1996. Effects of an exon 5 variant of the estrogen receptor in MCF-7 breast cancer cells. Cancer Res 56:1556–1563.
67. Zang Q, Borg A, Fuqua SAW. 1993. An exon 5 deletion variant of the estrogen receptor frequently coexpressed with wild-type estrogen receptor in human breast cancer. Cancer Res 53:5882–5884.
68. Daffada AAI, Johnston SRD, Smith IE, Detre S, King N, Dowsett M. 1995. Exon 5 deletion variant estrogen receptor messenger RNA expression in relation to tamoxifen resistance and progesterone receptor/pS2 status in human breast cancer. Cancer Res 55:288–293.
69. Schodin DJ, Zhuang Y, Shapiro DJ, Katzenellenbogen BS. 1995. Analysis of mechanisms that determine dominant negative estrogen receptor effectiveness J Biol Chem 270:31163–31171.
70. Yen PM, Chin WW. 1994. Molecular mechanisms of dominant negative activity by nuclear hormone receptors. Mol Endocrinol 8:1450–1454.
71. Wang Y, Miksicek RJ. 1991. Identification of a dominant negative form of the human estrogen receptor. Mol Endocrinol 8:1707–1715.
72. Miksicek RJ, Lei Y, Wang Y. 1993. Exon Skipping gives rise to alternatively spliced forms of the ER in breast tumor cells. Breast Cancer Res Treat 26:163–174.
73. Fuqua SAW, Fitzgerald SD, Allred DC, Elledge RM, Nawaz Z, McDonnell DP, O'Malley W, Greene GL, McGuire WL. 1992. Inhibition of estrogen receptor action by a naturally occurring variant in human breast tumors. Cancer Res 52:483–486.
74. Scott GK, Kushner P, Vigne JL, Benz CC. 1991. Truncated forms of DNA-binding estrogen receptors in human breast cancer. J Clin Invest 88:700–706.
75. Murphy LC, Dotzlaw H. 1989. Variant ER mRNA species detected in human breast cancer biopsy samples. Mol Endocrinol 3:687–693.
76. Koehorst SGA, Jacobs HM, Thijssen JHH, Blankenstein MA. 1993. Wild type and alternatively spliced estrogen receptor messenger RNA in human meningioma tissue and MCF-7 breast cancer cells. J Steroid Biochem Mol Biol 45:227–233.
77. Pfeffer U, Fecarotta E, Castagnetta L, Vidali G. 1993. Estrogen receptor variant messenger RNA lacking exon 4 in estrogen-responsive human breast cancer cell lines. Cancer Res 53:741–743.

78. Murphy LC, Dotzlaw H, Hamerton J, Schwarz J. 1993. Investigation of the origin of variant, truncated estrogen receptor-like mRNAs identified in some human breast cancer biopsy samples. Breast Cancer Res Treat 26:149–161.
79. Kuiper GG, Brinkmann AO. 1994. Steroid hormone receptor phosphorylation: is there a physiological role? Mol Cell Endocrinol 100:103–107.
80. Ali S, Metzger D, Bonet JM, Chambon P. 1993. Modulation of transcriptional activation by ligand-dependent phosphorylation of the human oestrogen receptor A/B region. EMBO J 12:1153–1160.
81. LeGoff P, Montano MM, Schodin DJ, Katzenellenbogen BS. 1994. Phosphorylation of the human estrogen receptor. J Biol Chem 269:4458–4466.
82. Joel PB, Traish AM, Lannigan DA. 1995. Estradiol and phorbol ester cause phosphorylation of serine 118 in the human estrogen receptor. Mol Endocrinol 9:1041–1052.
83. Kato S, Endoh H, Masuhiro Y, et al. 1995. Activation of the estrogen receptor through phosphorylation by mitogen-activated protein kinase. Science 270:1491–1494.
84. Cavailles V, Dauvois S, Danielian PS, Parker MG. 1994. Interaction of proteins with transcriptionally active estrogen receptors. Proc Natl Acad Sci USA 91:10009–10013.
85. Cavailles V, Dauvois S, L'Horset F, Lopez G, Hoare S, Kushner PJ, Parker MG. 1995. Nuclear factor RIP140 modulates transcriptional activation by the estrogen receptor. EMBO J 14:3741–3751.
86. Halachmi S, Marden E, Martin G, MacKay H, Abbondanza C, Brown M. 1994. Estrogen receptor-associated proteins: possible mediators of hormone-induced transcription. Science 264:1455–1458.
87. Jacq X, Brou C, Lutz Y, Davidson I, Chambon P, Tora L. 1994. Human $TAF_{II}30$ is present in a distinct TFIID complex and is required for transcriptional activity by the estrogen receptor. Cell 79:107–117.
88. Ornate SA, Tsai SY, Tsai MJ, O'Malley BW. 1995. Sequence and characterization of a coactivator for the steroid hormone receptor superfamily. Science 270:1354–1357.
89. Landel CC, Kushner PJ, Greene GL. 1994. The interaction of human estrogen receptor with DNA is modulated by receptor-associated proteins. Mol Endocrinol 8:1407–1419.
90. Zeiner M, Gehring U. 1995. A protein that interacts with members of the nuclear hormone receptor family: identification and cDNA cloning. Proc Natl Acad Sci USA 92:11465–11469.
91. Graham ML, Kreet NL, Miller LA, Leslie KK, Gordon DF, Wood WM, Wei LL, Horwitz KB. 1990. T47Dco cells, genetically unstable and containing estrogen receptor mutations are a model for the progression of breast cancers hormone resistance. Cancer Res 50:6208–6217.
92. Pink JJ, Jiang SY, Fritsch M, Jordan VC. A unique MCF-7 human breast cancer cell line expressing an 80 kD estrogen receptor 1994 (abstract 1651). Proc Am Assoc Cancer Res 35:276.

Index

A

Alkaline phosphatase, in prostate cancer prognosis, 76
Allium compounds. See also *Phytochemicals*.
  anticancer effects of, 109
5-Alpha-reductase inhibitors, in prostate cancer, 79
Aminoglutethimide
  in breast cancer, 150, 238–240
  in endometrial cancer, 99
  in prostate cancer, 75
Amyloidosis, in multiple myeloma, 13
Anastrozole, in breast cancer, 240
Androgens
  in breast cancer, 242
  in endometrial cancer, 99
Angiogenesis, phytochemical inhibition of, 119
Antiandrogens
  in breast cancer, 238
  in prostate cancer, 74–75, 78–79
Antibody, anti-Id, 52
Antiestrogens. See also *Tamoxifen*.
  in breast cancer, 143–149, 233–237
Antigens, tumor, 35–36
Antigen supplementation, in vaccine therapy, 37–38
Anti-idiotype antibody vaccine therapy, 51–66. See also *Cellular vaccine therapy*.
  animal model of, 54–55
  in B-cell lymphoma, 56–57
  in breast cancer, 65–66
  cellular response to, 59, 63–64
  clinical response to, 59–61, 64
  in colorectal cancer, 55, 56, 61–65
  humoral responses to, 62
  immune network hypothesis in, 51–54
  in melanoma, 56, 66
  in T-cell lymphoma, 57–61
  T-cell-dependent antigens in, 53–54
  toxicity of, 59, 64
Antioxidants. See also *Phytochemicals*.
  anticancer effects of, 108, 116
Antiprogestins, in breast cancer, 149, 237–238
Apoptosis, phytochemical induction of, 117
Arachidonic acid, phytochemical inhibition of, 117
Arimidex, in breast cancer, 150
Aromatase inhibitors, in breast cancer, 150–151, 238–242

B

B-cell lymphoma, anti-idiotype antibody vaccine therapy in, 56–57
Beta-carotene
  in cancer prevention, 111
  structure of, 112
Biopsy, for endometrial carcinoma, 203–204
Bone
  hormone replacement effects on, 217
  ovarian ablation effects on, 176
  tamoxifen effect on, 217
Bone marrow transplantation, in chronic myelogenous leukemia, 4
Bowman-Birk inhibitor. See also *Phytochemicals*.
  anticancer effects of, 119, 123
Breast
  endogenous regulators of, 115
  epithelial differentiation of, 141–142
  hormone replacement effects on, 218–221
Breast cancer
  aminoglutethimide in, 238–240
  anastrozole in, 240
  androgens in, 242
  antiandrogens in, 238
  antiestrogens in, 143–149, 233–237
  anti-idiotype antibody vaccine therapy in, 65–66
  antiprogestins in, 149, 237–238

279

Breast cancer *(Continued)*
  aromatase inhibitors in, 150–151, 238–242
  in Asian populations, 107, 108
  atamestane in, 241
  caffeine and, 126
  calusterone in, 242
  combination endocrine therapy in, 244–245
  combination oral contraceptive in, 151–152
  contralateral, 218–219
  cyproterone acetate in, 238
  DMBA-induced rat model of, 137–138
  droloxifene in, 236–237
  epidermal growth factor in, 232
  estrogen receptors in, 255–274. See also *Estrogen receptors.*
  exemestane in, 241
  fadrozole in, 241
  fenretinide in, 142–143, 245
  fluoxymesterone in, 242
  flutamide in, 238
  gestrinone in, 238
  gonadotropin releasing factor agonists in, 243–244
  goserelin prevention in, 150
  growth factors in, 232, 233
  after hormone replacement therapy, 220–221
  hormone replacement therapy stimulation of, 221–222
  hormone-exposure model of, 139–141
  4-hydroandrostenedione in, 240–241
  ICI 164,384 in, 237
  ICI 182,780 in, 237
  idoxifene in, 237
  imidazoles in, 241
  incidence of, 108
  letrozole in, 241
  luteinizing hormone-releasing hormone analogues in, 150, 243–244
  medroxyprogesterone acetate in, 242–243
  megestrol acetate in, 242–243
  melatonin in, 245
  metastatic, 231–246. See also *Metastatic breast cancer.*
  1-methyl-1,4-androstadiene-3,7-dione in, 241
  mifepristone in, 237
  onaprostone in, 237–238
  ovarian ablation treatment of, 159–177. See also *Ovarian ablation.*
  pathogenesis of, 136–141
  phytochemical prevention of, 107–127. See also *Phytochemicals.*
  phytoestrogens and, 118–119
  post-treatment hormone replacement therapy and, 209–224. See also *Hormone replacement therapy.*
  prednisolone in, 233
  pregnancy-related protection in, 137, 141–142
  progestins in, 242–243
  progression of, 140–141
  pyridoglutethimide in, 240
  retinoids in, 142–143
  risk factors for, 136–141, 219
  RU486 prevention of, 149
  somatostatin in, 245
  tamoxifen in, 143–149, 146–147, 181–206, 211–214, 233–237. See also *Tamoxifen.*
  tamoxifen resistance of, 259–260
  tamoxifen-associated endometrial carcinoma and, 199–203
  terioxifene mesylate in, 235
  testololactone in, 241, 242
  testosterone in, 242
  toremifene in, 236
  transforming growth factors in, 232
  trilostane in, 240
  vitamin D in, 245
  vorozole in, 241
  zindoxifene in, 237
Breast cancer patients
  fracture in, 217
  hormone replacement therapy in, 209–224. See also *Hormone replacement therapy.*
  hot flashes in, 214–215
  vaginal symptoms in, 215–216
Busulfan, in chronic myelogenous leukemia, 3

C

Caffeine. See also *Phytochemicals.*
  anticancer effects of, 126
Calusterone, in breast cancer, 242
Carcinoembryonic antigen (CEA), in colorectal cancer, 61, 64–65
Carcinogenesis, 136–141
Carotenoids. See also *Phytochemicals.*
  anticancer effects of, 108, 116, 117, 120
Casodex, in prostate cancer, 74
Cellular vaccine therapy, 35–47. See also *Anti-idiotype antibody vaccine therapy.*
  antigen supplementation in, 37–38
  in colorectal cancer, 41–44
  cyclophosphamide-induced immunopotentiation in, 36–37
  cytokine gene—enhanced, 44–45
  in melanoma, 36–44
  in metastatic melanoma, 39–41

microbial adjuvants in, 36
in non-small cell lung cancer, 41–44
remissions with, 45–46
in renal cell cancer, 41–44
in residual melanoma, 36–39
Chemotherapy
amenorrhea with, 174–175, 210
in chronic myelogenous leukemia, 3, 4, 5–6
in colorectal cancer, 23–28
in endometrial cancer, 99–100
in multiple myeloma, 13–14
in non-small cell lung cancer, 30
oophorectomy with, 163–165
vs. ovarian ablation, 174–175
Chlormadinone acetate, in prostate cancer, 78
2-Chlorodeoxyadenosine (cladribine), in hairy cell leukemia, 12
Cholesterol, hormone replacement effects on, 217
Chronic myelogenous leukemia, 1–7
acute phase of, 2–3
chemotherapy in, 3, 4, 5–6
chronic phase of, 2
clinical features of, 1–3
interferon-alpha in, 4–7
interferon-gamma in, 6
Ph¹ chromosome in, 1, 6
treatment of, 3–6
Cladribine (2-chlorodeoxyadenosine), in hairy cell leukemia, 12
Clomiphene citrate, in endometrial cancer, 99
Clonidine, for hot flashes, 214
Coagulation, tamoxifen effect on, 217
Colorectal cancer
anti-idiotype antibody vaccine therapy in, 55, 56, 61–65
cellular vaccine therapy in, 41–44
fluorouracil and interferon-alpha and leucovorin in, 25–26
fluorouracil and interferon-alpha in, 23–28
interferon-alpha in, 23–28
Corticosteroid therapy, in breast cancer, 233
Coumarins. See also *Phytochemicals.*
anticancer effects of, 109, 122
CpG island methylation, in estrogen receptor gene expression, 261–264
Cucurmin, anticancer effects of, 125–126
Cyclophosphamide, in vaccine therapy, 36–37
Cyproterone acetate
in breast cancer, 238
in prostate cancer, 73
Cytarabine, in chronic myelogenous leukemia, 4
Cytokines, in vaccine therapy, 44–45

Cytokine therapy
in melanoma, 44, 45
in renal cell cancer, 44–45

D
Danazol, in breast cancer, 242
2-Deoxycoformycin (pentostatin), in hairy cell leukemia, 12
Diallyl sulfide, structure of, 112
Diethylstilbestrol, in prostate cancer, 72–73
Dithiolthiones. See also *Phytochemicals.*
anticancer effects of, 108
Droloxifene, in breast cancer, 234, 236–237

E
Ellagic acid
anticancer effects of, 125–126
structure of, 113
Endometrial cancer, 89–103
adjuvant progestin therapy in, 92–93
advanced, 93–99
aminoglutethimide in, 99
biopsy screening for, 203–204
in breast cancer patients, 201–203
clomiphene citrate in, 99
combination therapy in, 99–100
gonadotropin-releasing hormone agonists in, 98–99
histological grade of, 95
hormone replacement therapy in, 100–101
incidence of, 108
methyltrienolone in, 99
phytochemical prevention of, 107–127. See also *Phytochemicals.*
progesterone receptors in, 95–96
progestin therapy in, 91–96
radiation therapy in, 100
RU-486 (mifepristone) in, 99
screening for, 203–205
stage I and II, 91–93
tamoxifen therapy in, 96–98
tamoxifen-associated, 186, 195–196, 199–203
transvaginal sonography screening for, 204–205
Endometrial polyps, tamoxifen-associated, 197–199
Endometrium
endogenous regulators of, 115
hormonal effects on, 89–90, 91
hormone replacement effects on, 217–218
tamoxifen effects on, 195–206. See also *Endometrial cancer.*
Enzymes, phytochemical induction of, 116

281

Epidermal growth factor, in breast cancer, 232
ERAP160 protein, 271
Esophageal cancer, interferon-alpha in, 28
Estrogen, in breast cancer development, 139–141
Estrogen cream, for vaginal atrophy, 216
Estrogen receptors, 255–274. See also *Estrogen receptor gene.*
  constitutively active variant of, 268–269
  dominant-negative variants of, 269–270
  inactive variant of, 270
  mRNA splice variants of, 266–271
  phosphorylation of, 270–271
  RNA stability of, 266
  tamoxifen administration and, 145–146
Estrogen receptor factor-1, 264
Estrogen receptor gene, 255–257
  amplification of, 258
  autoregulation of, 264–265
  CpG island methylation in, 261–264
  deletions of, 258
  growth factor effects on, 265
  point mutations in, 258–260
  posttranscriptional regulation of, 265–271
  promoters of, 260–261
  R5020 effects on, 265
  regulation of, 260–265
  sodium butyrate effects on, 265
  tamoxifen effects on, 265
  transcription of, 260–265
  tumor tamoxifen resistance and, 259–260
Estrogen receptor-associated proteins, 272–272
Estrogen replacement therapy. See *Hormone replacement therapy.*
Exemestane, in breast cancer, 241

F

Fadrozole, in breast cancer, 241
Fenretinide, in breast cancer, 142–143, 245
Fiber. See also *Phytochemicals.*
  anticancer effects of, 108, 114, 122
Finasteride, in prostate cancer, 79
Flavonoids. See also *Phytochemicals.*
  anticancer effects of, 109, 116, 117, 123
Fluorouracil, in colorectal cancer, 23–28
Flutamide
  in breast cancer, 238
  in prostate cancer, 74, 76–77, 79
Fluoxymestrone, in breast cancer, 242
Folic acid. See also *Phytochemicals.*
  anticancer effects of, 108, 117, 122
  structure of, 113
Fruits, anticancer effects of, 110, 111, 114, 120

G

Gastric cancer, interferon-alpha in, 28
Genes, phytochemical effects on, 117
Gene therapy, in melanoma, 44, 45
Genistein
  anticancer effects of, 117, 118, 119
  structure of, 113
Gestrinone, in breast cancer, 238
Glucosinolates. See also *Phytochemicals.*
  anticancer effects of, 109
Glycyrrhetinic acid
  anticancer effects of, 117
  structure of, 113
Gonadotropin-releasing hormone agonists
  in breast cancer, 243–244
  in endometrial cancer, 98–99
Goserelin (Zoladex)
  in breast cancer, 150
  ovarian ablation with, 175–176
  in prostate cancer, 73–74
gp37 antigen, in T-cell lymphoma, 60
Green tea. See also *Phytochemicals.*
  anticancer effects of, 125–126
Growth factors
  in breast cancer, 232, 233
  estrogen receptor gene effects of, 265

H

Hairy cell leukemia, 8–12
  cladribine (2-chlorodeoxyadenosine) in, 12
  clinical features of, 8–9
  interferon-alpha in, 9–12
  laboratory features of, 9
  pentostatin (2-deoxycoformycin) in, 12
Heart disease
  estrogen replacement therapy effect on, 210
  hormone replacement effects on, 217
  ovarian ablation effects on, 176
  tamoxifen effect on, 188
Hepatoma, interferon-alpha in, 29
HLA-B7 antigen, in melanoma gene therapy, 45
HLA-DR antigen, in hairy cell leukemia, 9–10
Hormone replacement therapy, 140, 209–224
  bone effects of, 217
  breast cancer prognosis after, 220–221
  as breast cancer risk factor, 219
  breast cancer stimulation by, 221–222
  in breast cancer survivors, 222–223
  breast effects of, 218–221
  cardiovascular effects of, 217
  coagulation effects of, 217
  contralateral breast cancer and, 218–219
  in endometrial cancer, 100–101

endometrial effects of, 217–218
standard of care for, 211
tamoxifen and, 212–214
Hot flashes, in breast cancer patients, 214–215
Human chorionic gonadotropin, in breast cancer prevention, 142
4-Hydroandrostenedione, in breast cancer, 240–241
Hydroxyprogesterone caproate, in endometrial cancer, 91–96
Hypercalcemia, in multiple myeloma, 13
Hypothalamic-pituitary-gonadal-prostatic axis, in prostate cancer, 69–71

I

ICI 164,384, in breast cancer, 234, 237
ICI 182,780, in breast cancer, 234, 237
Idiotypes
  of immunoglobulins, 51–53
  regulatory, 52–53
Idoxifene, in breast cancer, 234, 237
Imidazoles, in breast cancer, 241
Immune network hypothesis, 51–54
Immunoglobulin(s)
  idiotypes of, 51–52
  in multiple myeloma, 13
Immunoglobulin genes, in hairy cell leukemia, 9
Immunopotentiation, cyclophosphamide-induced, 36–37
Immunotherapy, 51. See also *Anti-idiotype antibody vaccine therapy; Cellular vaccine therapy.*
  immune network hypothesis in, 51–54
Indole-3-carbinol, structure of, 112
Indoles. See also *Phytochemicals.*
  anticancer effects of, 109, 116
Infection, in hairy cell leukemia, 9
Inositol hexaphosphate (phytic acid). See also *Phytochemicals.*
  anticancer effects of, 109
Insulin-like growth factors, in breast cancer, 213–214
Interferon-alpha
  in agnogenic myeloid metaplasia, 7
  antibodies to, 11
  in chronic myelogenous leukemia, 4–7
  in colorectal cancer, 23–28
  in esophageal cancer, 28
  in gastric cancer, 28
  in hairy cell leukemia, 9–12
  in hepatoma, 29
  in lymphoma, 14–15
  in multiple myeloma, 14
  in non-small cell lung cancer, 30
  in pancreas cancer, 29
  in polycythemia vera, 7
  in primary thrombocythemia, 7
  side effects of, 5, 11
Interferon-alpha 2a, in hairy cell leukemia, 11
Interferon-alpha 2b, in hairy cell leukemia, 11
Interferon-gamma, in chronic myelogenous leukemia, 6
Interleukin-10, in melanoma, 46
Isoflavones. See also *Phytochemicals.*
  anticancer effects of, 109, 116, 117, 118, 124
Isothiocyanates. See also *Phytochemicals.*
  anticancer effects of, 109

K

Ketoconazole, in prostate cancer, 75

L

Letrozole, in breast cancer, 241
Leucovorin, in colorectal cancer, 25–26
Leukapheresis, in chronic myelogenous leukemia, 3
Leukemia
  hairy cell, 8–12. See also *Hairy cell leukemia.*
  myelogenous, 1–7. See also *Chronic myelogenous leukemia.*
Lignans. See also *Phytochemicals.*
  anticancer effects of, 109, 118
d-Limonene. See also *Phytochemicals.*
  anticancer effects of, 125
  structure of, 113
Lung cancer
  interferon-alpha in, 30
  vaccine therapy in, 41–44
Lupron (Leuprolide), in prostate cancer, 73–74
Luteinizing hormone-releasing hormone (LHRH) agonists
  in breast cancer, 150, 243–244
  ovarian ablation with, 175–176
  in prostate cancer, 73–74
Lymphoma
  anti-idiotype antibody vaccine therapy in, 56–61
  interferon-alpha in, 14–15

M

Mammography, hormone replacement therapy effect on, 218
Medroxyprogesterone acetate
  in breast cancer, 242–243
  in endometrial cancer, 91–96
  for hot flashes, 214

Megestrol acetate
  in breast cancer, 242–243
  in endometrial cancer, 91–96
  for hot flashes, 214
  in prostate cancer, 73
Melanoma
  anti-idiotype antibody vaccine therapy in, 56, 66
  cytokine injections in, 45
  cytokine-secreting vaccine therapy in, 44
  gene therapy in, 44, 45
  interleukin-10 in, 46
  transforming growth factor beta in, 46
  vaccine therapy in, 36–44
  vaccine-related remission of, 45–46
Melanoma cells
  antigen supplementation of, 37–38
  cytokine gene transduction of, 44–45
  vaccine production from, 37
Melatonin, in breast cancer, 245
Melphalan, in multiple myeloma, 13–14
Metastatic breast cancer, 231–246. See also *Breast cancer.*
  androgens in, 242, 246
  antiandrogens in, 238, 246
  antiestrogens in, 233–237, 246
  antiprogestins in, 237–238, 246
  aromatase inhibitors in, 238–242, 246
  combination endocrine therapy in, 244–245, 246
  gonadotropin releasing hormone agonists in, 243–244, 246
  progestins in, 242–243, 246
1-Methyl-1,4-androstadiene-3,7-dione, in breast cancer, 241
Methyldopa, for hot flashes, 214
Methyltrienolone, in endometrial cancer, 99
Mifepristone (RU-486)
  in breast cancer, 149, 237
  in endometrial cancer, 99
Multiple myeloma, 12–14
  chemotherapy in, 13–14
  clinical features of, 13
  interferon-alpha in, 14
  laboratory features of, 13
  treatment of, 13–14
Myelogenous leukemia, chronic, 1–7. See also *Chronic myelogenous leukemia.*

N

Natural killer cells, in hairy cell leukemia, 9
Nephropathy, in multiple myeloma, 13
Nilutamide, in prostate cancer, 74
Nolvadex. See *Tamoxifen.*

Non-small cell lung cancer
  interferon-alpha in, 30
  vaccine therapy in, 41–44

O

Onaprostone, in breast cancer, 237–238
Oophorectomy, 135, 150, 159–165. See also *Ovarian ablation.*
  chemotherapy with, 163–165
  estrogen receptors and, 160
Oral contraceptive, in breast cancer prevention, 151–152
Orchiectomy, in prostate cancer, 72
Organosulfur compounds. See also *Phytochemicals.*
  anticancer effects of, 108, 122–123
Ovarian ablation, 159–177, 231–232
  adjuvant, 160–163
  in breast cancer prevention, 149–151
  chemotherapy-induced, 174–175, 210
  contralateral breast cancer after, 172
  late effects of, 167, 169, 171, 176
  medical, 165–166, 174–176
  radiation-induced, 175–176
  in women over 50, 167
  in women under 50, 166–167, 168–173
  Zoladex-induced, 175–176

P

Pancreas cancer, interferon-alpha in, 29
Pentostatin (2-deoxycoformycin), in hairy cell leukemia, 12
Ph[1] chromosome, in chronic myelogenous leukemia, 1
Phytic acid (inositol hexaphosphate). See also *Phytochemicals.*
  anticancer effects of, 109
Phytochemicals, 107–127
  angiogenesis inhibition by, 119
  anticancer mechanisms of, 111, 114–120
  antioxidant effects of, 116
  antiproliferative effects of, 117
  apoptosis induction by, 117
  arachidonic acid inhibition by, 117
  clinical trials of, 127
  enzyme induction by, 116
  epidemiology of, 113–114
  hormone activity modulation by, 118–119
  structures of, 112
  tissue differentiation effects of, 118
  tumor gene modulation by, 117
  tumor initiation prevention by, 116–117
  tumor invasion inhibition by, 119

tumor promotion blockade by, 117–119
   types of, 107–113
Phytoestrogens, anticancer effects of, 118–119
Polycythemia vera, interferon-alpha in, 7
Polyphenols. See also *Phytochemicals.*
   anticancer effects of, 109, 116, 125–126
Prednisolone, in breast cancer, 233
Prednisone, in multiple myeloma, 13–14
Pregnancy, in breast cancer prevention, 137, 141–142
Premarin, for vaginal atrophy, 216
Progesterone receptors. See also *Estrogen receptors.*
   in breast cancer, 257
   in endometrial cancer, 95–96, 97–98
Progestins
   in advanced endometrial cancer, 93–96
   antiestrogenic effect of, 140
   in breast cancer development, 139–141
   in breast cancer treatment, 242–243
   in early endometrial cancer, 91–93
Prostate cancer, 69–81
   adrenalectomy for, 76
   5-alpha reductase inhibitors in, 79
   antiandrogen withdrawal in, 78–79
   antiandrogens in, 74–75, 79
   combination hormone therapy for, 76–77
   detection of, 69
   early versus delayed therapy in, 78
   hypothalamic-pituitary-gonadal-prostatic axis in, 69–71
   medical castration for, 72–74
   orchiectomy for, 72
   preprostatectomy hormonal therapy in, 79–80
   pre—radiation hormonal therapy in, 80–81
   prognosis for, 75–76
   steroidogenesis inhibitors for, 75
Prostatectomy, neoadjuvant hormonal therapy with, 79–80
Prostate-specific antigen, in prostate cancer prognosis, 76
Protease inhibitors. See also *Phytochemicals.*
   anticancer effects of, 109, 119, 123
Pseudopregnancy, in breast cancer prevention, 141–142
Pyridoglutethimide, in breast cancer, 240

Q

Quercetin, structure of, 112

R

R5020, estrogen receptor gene effects of, 265

Radiation therapy
   in endometrial cancer, 100
   for ovarian ablation, 175–176
   in prostate cancer, 80–81
RAP46 protein, 272
Renal cell cancer
   cytokine-secreting vaccine therapy in, 44–45
   vaccine therapy in, 41–44
Replens, for vaginal atrophy, 216
Retinoids. See also *Phytochemicals.*
   anticancer effects of, 117, 119, 120
   in breast cancer prevention, 142–143
RIP80 protein, 271
RIP160 protein, 271
RU–486 (mifepristone)
   in breast cancer, 149, 237
   in endometrial cancer, 99

S

Saponins. See also *Phytochemicals.*
   anticancer effects of, 109, 124
Seaweed polysaccharides. See also *Phytochemicals.*
   anticancer effects of, 126
Secoisolariciresinol, structure of, 113
Selenium. See also *Phytochemicals.*
   anticancer effects of, 108, 116, 121–122
β-Sitosterol, structure of, 113
Sobrerol, anticancer effects of, 125
Sodium butyrate, estrogen receptor gene effects of, 265
Somatostatin, in breast cancer, 245
Soy, anticancer effects of, 118
Spironolactone, in prostate cancer, 75
Splenectomy
   in chronic myelogenous leukemia, 3–4
   in hairy cell leukemia, 9
Steroid receptor coactivator–1, 271–272
Sterols. See also *Phytochemicals.*
   anticancer effects of, 109, 124

T

Tamoxifen
   ATLAS trial of, 189–190
   ATTOM trial of, 190
   in breast cancer prevention, 143–149, 212
   in breast cancer treatment, 146–147, 181–206, 211–214
   cardiovascular benefit of, 188
   coagulation effects of, 217
   ECOG trial of, 189
   in endometrial cancer treatment, 96–98
   endometrial cancer with, 186, 195–196, 199–203. See also *Endometrial cancer.*

285

Tamoxifen *(Continued)*
  endometrial effects of, 195–206
  endometrial hyperplasia with, 198–199
  endometrial polyps with, 197–199
  estrogen receptor gene effects of, 265
  fenretinide with, 143
  hormone replacement therapy and, 212–214
  isomers of, 235
  metabolite E of, 196
  NSABP B14 trial of, 184–187, 189, 200–201, 213
  overview analysis of, 181–183
  postmenopausal bone density and, 147–148
  resistance to, 183–184
  Scottish trial of, 187–188, 189
  side effects of, 148
  tumor cell effects of, 144–146, 213
  tumor flare with, 235
  tumor growth with, 183
  tumor resistance to, 259–260
  vaginal epithelial effects of, 196–197
T-cell lymphoma, anti-idiotype antibody vaccine therapy in, 57–61
Terioxifene mesylate, in breast cancer, 235
Terpenes. See also *Phytochemicals.*
  anticancer effects of, 109, 125
Testololactone, in breast cancer, 241, 242
Testosterone
  in breast cancer, 242
  in prostate cancer prognosis, 76
Thiocyanates. See also *Phytochemicals.*
  anticancer effects of, 109
Thrombocythemia, interferon-alpha in, 7
α-Tocopherol, structure of, 112
Toremifene, in breast cancer, 234, 236
Transcription factors, in estrogen receptor gene expression, 264

Transforming growth factors
  in breast cancer, 232
  in melanoma, 46
Transvaginal sonography, in endometrial carcinoma, 204–205
Trioxifene mesylate, in breast cancer, 234

U

Ultrasonography, in endometrial carcinoma, 204–205

V

Vaccine therapy
  anti-idiotype antibody, 51–66. See also *Anti-idiotype antibody vaccine therapy.*
  cellular, 35–47. See also *Cellular vaccine therapy.*
Vaccinia virus, in melanoma gene therapy, 45
Vagina, tamoxifen effects on, 196–197
Vaginal atrophy, in breast cancer patients, 215–216
Vegetables. See also *Phytochemicals.*
  anticancer effects of, 110, 111, 114, 116, 120, 126–127
Vitamin C. See also *Phytochemicals.*
  anticancer effects of, 108, 110, 111, 120
  structure of, 112
Vitamin D, in breast cancer, 245
Vitamin E. See also *Phytochemicals.*
  anticancer effects of, 108, 111, 116, 120–121
Vorozole, in breast cancer, 241

Z

Zindoxifene, in breast cancer, 234, 237
Zoladex (goserelin)
  in breast cancer, 150
  ovarian ablation with, 175–176
  in prostate cancer, 73–74

CPSIA information can be obtained
at www.ICGtesting.com
Printed in the USA
LVHW051406150523
747041LV00003B/246